# The Autonomous Cruiser: The Complete Guide to Cruising For and With Disabled Travellers

*by Michele Monro*

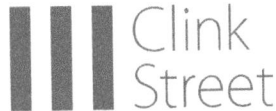

*Published by Clink Street Publishing 2021*

*Copyright © 2021*

*First edition.*

*The author asserts the moral right under the Copyright, Designs and Patents Act 1988 to be identified as the author of this work.*

*All rights reserved. No part of this publication may be reproduced, stored in a retrieval system or transmitted, in any form or by any means without the prior consent of the author, nor be otherwise circulated in any form of binding or cover other than that with which it is published and without a similar condition being imposed on the subsequent purchaser.*

*ISBN:*
*978-1-913962-49-4 - paperback*
*978-1-913962-50-0 - ebook*

*The spelling throughout the book may vary between English and American. It is not necessarily a spelling error but something I have had to honour otherwise certain details, like American company names, website addresses and quotes would be incorrect.*

***Caveat:*** *Every care has been taken to ensure that all details in this book are current and up-to-date at the time of going to press, but because of the constant changes in the travel sector I cannot make any guarantees that it is error-free and apologise if something is now inaccurate or outdated.*

*Information included has been given in good faith on the basis of the information provided to me by the cruise lines and services listed and taken from official government websites, public sector information licensed under the Open Government License v3.0. and recognised charities. It has been produced to provide help and assistance to disabled passengers and their support companion but don't use the information contained within this book as your only source of reference, it is only offered as a selection of the marketplace and in all cases, you need to clarify with a professional body the information is current and accurate before travelling.*

*Inclusion of any company, whether cruise, plane, ferry, train, taxi, coach or hotel is not an endorsement of that provider, they are merely suggestions. I am not affiliated, associated, authorised, endorsed by or in any way officially connected with any cruise company or any of its subsidiaries. I have no direct or indirect business relationship with any private operator listed and inclusion of any company must not be taken as an endorsement of that company. Exclusion of any company or private operator must not be taken in any way on the quality or probity of such company*

*I do not accept any responsibility or liability for any/all inaccuracies or omissions held within the information or any such consequence that might occur as a result of any/all inaccuracies or omissions. and accept no responsibility for any error or misrepresentation. All liability, disappointment, negligence or other damage caused by the reliance on the information contained in this guide, or in any company or individual mentioned, or in the event of any company or individual ceasing to trade, is hereby excluded. Any decisions based on information contained in the information is your sole responsibility.*

*All rights reserved. No part of this publication may be reproduced, stored in a retrieval system, or transmitted, in any form or by any means, electronic, mechanical, photocopying, recording or otherwise, without the prior written permission of the copyright owner.*

*This book is sold subject to the condition that it shall not, by way of trade or otherwise, be lent, resold, hired out or otherwise circulated without the copyright holder's prior written consent in any form of binding or cover other than that in which it is published and without a similar condition being imposed on the subsequent purchaser.*

© Michele Monro

*To my son Maxwell who always inspires me to be the best I can be and for loving me just the way I am. I thank you for your patience, understanding and commitment in helping me complete something very dear to my heart. I couldn't have done it without you. xx*

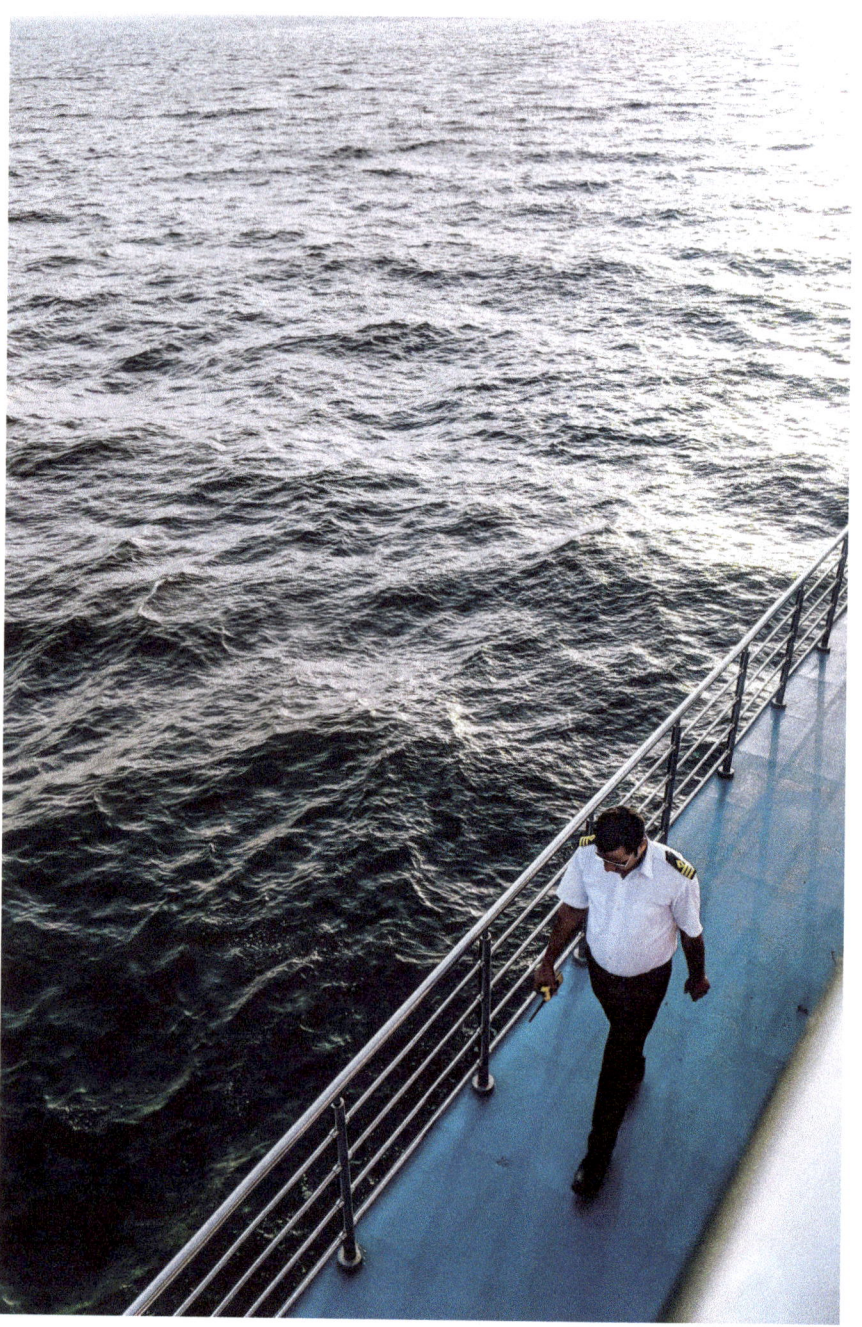

Credit: Billeasy, Unsplash

# Contents

**Foreword** ............................................................. 15

## Where to Start? ............................................. 19

**Armed to Cruise** ...................................................... 19
**Passenger Restrictions** ............................................. 20
**Special Needs** .......................................................... 23
Travelling with Pre-existing Illness .................................. 23
Travelling with Special Dietary Considerations ................. 23
Travelling with Prescriptions & Medication ...................... 25
Travelling with Epilepsy ................................................ 25
Travelling with Diabetes ............................................... 26
Travelling with Heart Disease ........................................ 27
Travelling with Dementia .............................................. 27
Travelling with Cognitive, Intellectual & Developmental Disabilities ... 28
Travelling with a Breathing Disorder ............................... 29
Travelling with Kidney Disease ...................................... 29
Travelling with a Visual Impairment ................................ 31
Travelling with a Hearing Impairment .............................. 32

**Travelling Companions** ............................................. 34
Caregivers & Chaperones .............................................. 34
Service Dogs ............................................................... 35

**Accessibility: Your cruising questions answered** ........... 46

**Disability Apps** ........................................................ 61

**Cruise Choices** ........................................................ 67

**European River Cruising** .......................................... 70

**Old vs New** ............................................................. 73

**Dress Codes** ........................................................... 77

**Where to Go?** ......................................................... 78

| | |
|---|---|
| Tendering at Sea | 87 |
| **Where to Go From?** | 90 |
| **UK Cruise Ports** | 90 |
| **Armed to Fly** | 91 |
| Fly-cruises | 91 |
| Wheelchair Advice | 94 |
| Travelling to the Airport | 97 |
| Airport Guides | 100 |
| Car Park Assistance | 100 |
| Delayed or Missed Flight | 101 |
| Checked Luggage/Carry-on Bags | 101 |
| Security & Customs | 102 |
| **Special Needs** | 103 |
| Flying with Pre-existing Illness | 103 |
| Flying with Prescriptions and Medication | 103 |
| Flying with Epilepsy | 103 |
| Flying with Diabetes | 104 |
| Flying with Heart Disease | 105 |
| Flying with Dementia | 107 |
| Flying with Cognitive, Intellectual & Developmental Disabilities | 108 |
| Flying with a Breathing Disorder | 109 |
| Flying with Kidney Disease | 110 |
| Flying with a Visual Impairment | 110 |
| Flying with a Hearing Impairment | 112 |
| Pre-flight Checklist | 114 |
| Return Journey | 115 |
| Lost/Delayed Luggage | 115 |
| Transfers | 116 |
| In-flight Tips | 117 |
| Pre- or Post-cruise Accommodation | 117 |
| **Armed to Fly Apps** | 119 |
| **Who to Go With?** | 120 |
| Best for Romantics | 122 |
| Best for Weddings | 123 |
| Best for Luxury Offerings | 125 |
| Best for Spas | 127 |
| Best for Disability | 128 |
| Best for Seniors | 138 |
| Best for Families with Children | 139 |

Best for Expedition & Adventure ... 145
Best for Budget Cruises ... 146
Best for Food & Wine Lovers ... 148
Best for Enrichment: ... 151
Best for After Dark ... 153
Best for Solo Travellers: ... 155
Best Foreign Brands ... 156
Best European River Cruises ... 158

## Smoking Onboard ... 161

## Religious Services ... 162

## Where to Sleep? ... 165
Accessible Cabins ... 165
Cabin Grade ... 167
Cabin Size ... 169
Balconies ... 169
Suites ... 173
Family Cabins ... 173
Single Cabins ... 174
Spa Cabins ... 174
Cabin Location ... 175
Upgrades ... 177

## When to Book? ... 179

## How to Book? ... 181
Cruise Line Agents ... 181
Independent Cruise Specialists & Accessible Travel Agents ... 182
The Fine Print ... 183
Hidden Costs ... 184

## Booking Confirmation ... 188

# Before You Go ... 191

## Holiday Admin/The Bureaucratic Stuff ... 191

## Passports & Visas ... 191

## Vaccinations ... 193

## Prescriptions & Medication ... 194

## Travel Money ... 196

## Staying in Touch ... 199

| | |
|---|---|
| Cruise Booking Confirmation | 199 |
| Flight Booking Confirmation | 200 |
| Tickets & Boarding Passes | 200 |
| Online Check-In | 200 |
| Boarding Documents | 202 |
| Baggage Allowance | 202 |
| Travel Insurance | 203 |
| **Special Needs** | **207** |
| Travelling with Compromised Immune Systems | 207 |
| Travelling with Epilepsy | 209 |
| Travelling with Diabetes | 209 |
| Travelling with Heart Disease | 211 |
| Travelling with Dementia | 212 |
| Travelling with Cognitive, Intellectual & Developmental Disabilities | 213 |
| Travelling with a Breathing Disorder | 214 |
| Travelling with Kidney Disease | 216 |
| Travelling with a Visual Impairment | 217 |
| Travelling with a Hearing Impairment | 217 |
| **Rental Equipment** | **218** |
| **Equipment Insurance** | **219** |
| **Pregnancy** | **220** |
| **Pre-planning** | **220** |
| Children's Clubs | 220 |
| Gifts | 221 |
| Dining | 221 |
| Specialty Dining | 221 |
| Drinks Packages | 222 |
| Swimming Pools | 223 |
| Spa Treatments | 223 |
| **Ports and Shore Excursions** | **225** |
| Cruise Line Bookings | 226 |
| Independent Tour Operators | 228 |
| Private Tour Guides | 230 |
| Going It Alone | 231 |
| Local Customs | 236 |
| Local Events | 237 |

| | |
|---|---|
| Getting to the Cruise Terminal | 238 |
| UK Cruise Ports | 238 |
| Pier Transfers | 238 |
| Luggage Services | 239 |
| Door-to-Door Cruise Transfers | 242 |
| Coach Transfers | 245 |
| Airport Lounges | 245 |
| Must Have Buys | 246 |
| Cruise Apps | 250 |
| Dress Codes | 251 |
| The Ultimate Cruise Packing List | 253 |
| Leaving Home Checklist | 268 |

## Life Onboard — 273

| | |
|---|---|
| Embarkation | 273 |
| Cruise Ship Etiquette | 283 |
| Bon Appétit - Cruise Ship Dining | 291 |
| That's Entertainment | 296 |
| Meetings | 304 |
| Bridge Visits | 304 |
| Children's Clubs | 305 |
| Swimming Pools | 306 |
| Spa Centres | 307 |
| Shopping | 314 |
| Duty-free | 315 |
| Photo Gallery | 318 |
| Onboard Savings | 318 |
| Onboard Apps | 326 |
| Ship Visits | 329 |

Port Calls ........................................................................................... 329
Tendering Protocol ......................................................................... 333
Don't Miss the Ship ........................................................................ 334
Port Apps .......................................................................................... 336
Travel Scams .................................................................................... 340
Technology at Sea ........................................................................... 348
Phone Apps ...................................................................................... 352
Safety & Security ............................................................................. 354
Disembarkation ............................................................................... 360

# Directory — 367

## UK Cruise Ports — 367

### Cruising from Southampton — 395
Cruise Terminals .............................................................................. 396
Domestic Flights .............................................................................. 398
Driving ................................................................................................ 400
Southampton Car Park Services .................................................. 401
Rail Travel ......................................................................................... 403
Coach Travel .................................................................................... 405
Ferry Services .................................................................................. 407
Transfer Services ............................................................................ 407

### Disabled Facilities on Your Favourite Cruise Lines — 409

### Smoking Facilities — 431

### Travel Planning Disability Resources — 438
Accessible Shore Excursions ........................................................ 439
Accessible Travel News, Reviews & Practical Advice ............. 440
Blind/Impaired Sight ...................................................................... 443
Breathing Disorders & Oxygen .................................................... 443
Car Services ..................................................................................... 444
Cognitive, Intellectual and Developmental Disabilities ....... 445
Companion/Carer Service ............................................................ 446
Deaf/Impaired Hearing ................................................................. 448
Diabetes ............................................................................................ 448
Dialysis .............................................................................................. 449
Epilepsy ............................................................................................. 450
Equipment Rental .......................................................................... 451

Travel Equipment Insurance ... 452
Travel Health Protection Comparison Site ... 453
Travel Health Protection ... 454
Wheelchair Accessibility Resources ... 456

## Accessible Travel Agents ... 457

## Independent Cruise Specialists ... 462

## Travel Planning Website Directory ... 465
Cruising ... 469
Travel Money ... 470
Communication ... 471
Foreign Language ... 472
Government Services ... 472

## Cruise Line Directory ... 473
Ocean Cruise Lines ... 473
Expedition & Adventure Cruise Lines ... 480
River Cruises ... 485
Cargo, Container & Freighter Ship Voyages ... 489

## Cruise Lingo Glossary ... 492

## Ship's Codes ... 496

## Tender Ports ... 498

# About the Author ... 509

# Contributions ... 511

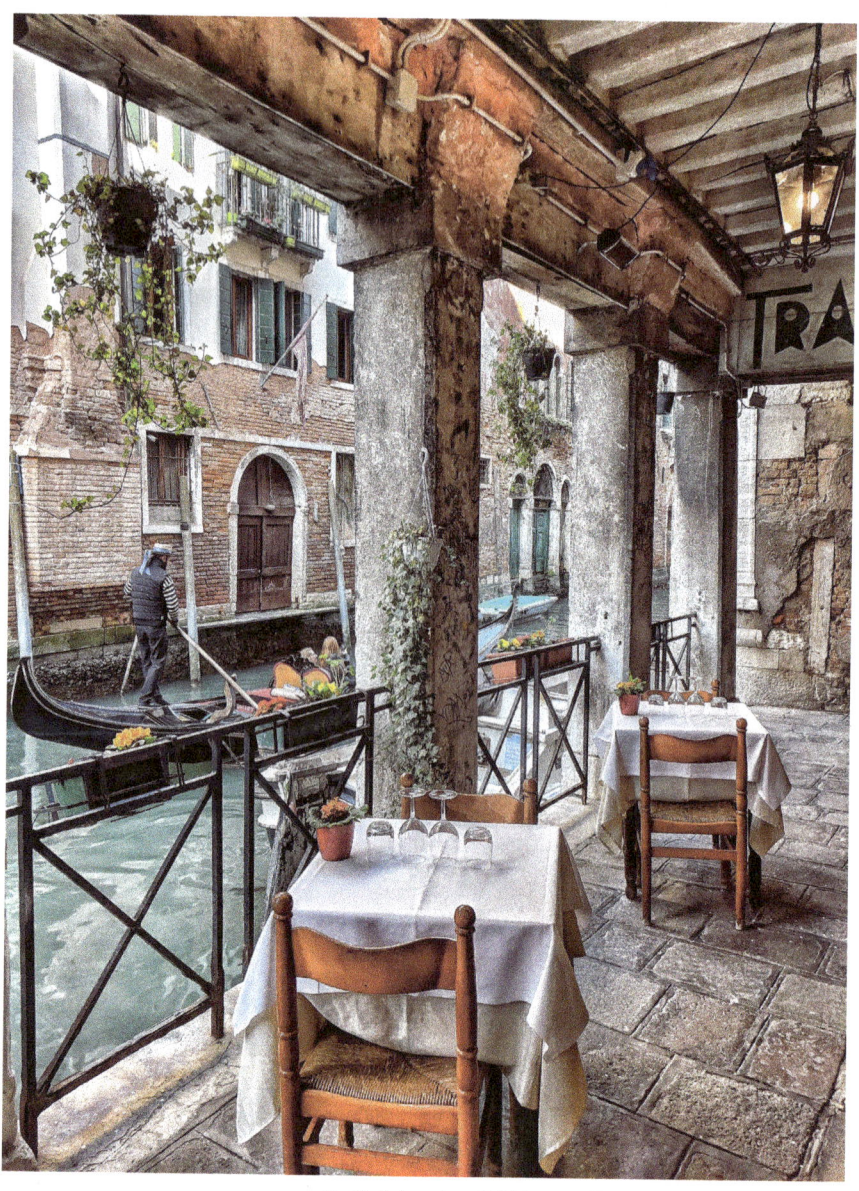

Credit: Sotoportego Del Magazen, Venice - Igor Oliyarnik, Unsplash

# Foreword

I have been cruising for more than forty years, the last eleven working as a guest speaker on Celebrity, P&O, Princess Cruises, Cunard, Cruise and Maritime, Fred Olsen and Royal Caribbean. Twenty-five years ago I was diagnosed with multiple sclerosis, after which I began to notice the lack of information available for people with limited mobility; places I had visited previously presented obstacles that I hadn't encountered before.

Information on accessibility is hard to find and the internet is filled with dead sites - with no one policing the web pages, you can source information only to find it is out-of-date and has been for some time. For example, one woman planned a dream trip to Venice as a surprise for her husband who is a permanent wheelchair user. She set off, husband in tow, thinking she had planned the perfect trip. Sadly, when they arrived, she found several bridge lifts had been disabled two years earlier, leaving the couple unable to access the city's key areas.

As much as I love travelling across the sea, a lack of destination information has been a constant annoyance, with ships never telling you exactly where in the city you will be docking until the night before or whether the port is accessible; P&O don't even advertise the docking times, making it impossible to pre-plan a day ashore.

With the evolution of the cruising industry one thing hasn't changed: the travel industry's inability to provide a disabled traveller with what they need to plan and enjoy a stress-free adventure.

I emailed Princess Cruises' special services with questions relating to the accessibility of their island, Princess Cay, as the only information on the internet was that it had "ramps for easy access." An automated email promised me a reply within ten business days, but when I finally received a response, it was sketchy at best. Their main concern was that I knew their rules governing tender use for disabled passengers and they attached a medical questionnaire. The bottom of the email informed me "we can supply the information requested; however, we are unable to advise if you will be able to ride the water shuttle." I asked a simple question and never got the information requested.

One of the dozens of challenging but common ports is Copenhagen's Langelinie quay, one of three cruise terminals servicing the city. It is fabulously placed for tourists, with many key sights reachable by foot, including The Little Mermaid statue. A hop-on-hop-off bus stops across the road from the port exit, as do the cruise lines' shuttle buses, tour excursion coaches and taxis, but it is an incredibly busy street, running more than half a mile. Upon exiting the cruise berth's wire-fenced compound you are forced to cross the street as only one side has a pavement; the problem is that there isn't one dropped kerb along the entire stretch of road, despite cruise companies complaining to the port authorities for the past few years. If you are travelling in a manual chair, it isn't too difficult if you are being pushed, as the chair can simply be tilted to mount the pavement, but electric wheelchairs and scooters don't have that option. The result is often defiant tourists braving the two-way traffic and dodging the port delivery trucks, fuel tankers and tour buses that use the road - it is incredibly dangerous and an accident waiting to happen.

Halfway down the pier's street, beneath the stone arches of Langelinie's old harbour-front warehouses, lies a great outlet shopping arcade accessible via eight steel-framed steps. The wheelchair lifts broke several years ago and remain broken. Ignorance isn't bliss, it is unacceptable.

I have searched high and low for a website that could offer up this kind of information but to no avail; instead, the average tourist is left none the wiser. I believe information is power: the power to be able to control our choices and know what we are going to come up against when we drop anchor in a desirable location.

Everyone experiences different degrees of mobility. For those that can manage a few steps, there is a good and varied choice of accessible tour options, but for those that are permanent wheelchair users, choices can be more limited. Having trawled through thousands of websites and articles and interviewed countless company representatives within the travel sector, I've found there are those that are willing to go that extra mile to make cruising more accessible, you just have to know where to look.

I decided to address all of these issues with a series of cruise books dedicated to disabled people who want to cruise on their own terms. This general how-to on cruising is the first, aimed at giving you the power to take control, make your own choices and organise the perfect seafaring holiday, getting the best out of both the ship and its destinations. The books that will follow are dedicated port guides and will offer an in-depth look at what each location offers in terms of accessibility, addressing issues like whether the port is easy to disembark at, what facilities are at the terminal and what the destination offers its disabled guests. It will give you the ability to get the most out of each destination and not waste precious time in working out what to do or how to do it.

Living with a disability presents a lot of obstacles, but a cruise holiday doesn't have to be one of them. Bon voyage.

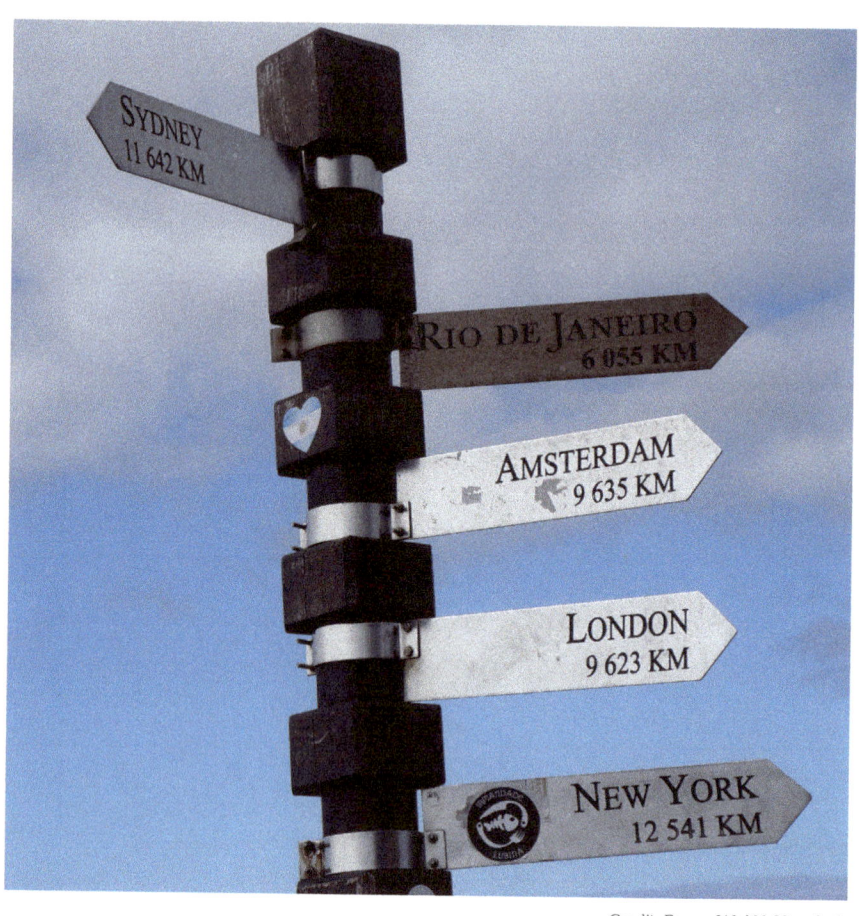

Credit: Bruno Wolff, Unsplash

# Where to Start?

Planning the perfect cruise holiday is no easy task, especially if you have some form of disability - it requires careful consideration to ensure you pick the right destination, the right time of year and the right ship for your disability. Are you looking for sunshine, snow, culture, scenery, beaches, history, cosmopolitan cities, tropical islands, food, a themed trip or a shopping spree? Finding a cruise that ticks all of your boxes used to be difficult as options were limited, but nowadays you'll be spoilt for choice - all it takes is a little forethought and some light reading.

## Armed to Cruise

You might not realise you have certain rights when it comes to travel, but knowing what you're entitled to should give you the confidence to make your first booking.

Any cruise ship passenger departing from the United Kingdom or anywhere in the European Union is governed by an EU Regulation that empowers you with rights if you are "any person whose mobility when using transport is reduced as a result of any physical disability (sensory or locomotor, permanent or temporary), intellectual disability or impairment, or any other cause of disability, or as a result of age, and whose situation needs appropriate attention and adaptation to his (or her) particular needs of the service made available to all passengers."

Your rights as a disabled passenger apply throughout your dealings with a ferry or cruise operator, whether before, during or after travel. Generally speaking, your booking has to be treated exactly the same as it would with any other traveller, at the same cost but with any added assistance needed to travel. However, there are some exceptions - your cruise line can refuse a booking or deny boarding if:

- Your disability would prevent you from evacuating the vessel within 30 minutes in an emergency.
- If the ship, its terminal or the infrastructure of the port could impact on your safety.
- If the cruise line's allocation of adapted cabins has been reached.
- If you attempt to bring any restricted medical equipment on board - it is your responsibility to check what restrictions your preferred cruise line has in place.

If you use a specially adapted electric wheelchair that is considered too heavy or large for certain areas of the ship you may be provided with an alternative to use onboard. However, if your medical equipment satisfies the guidelines set in place by the carrier, you can take it onboard with you at no additional cost.

If a passenger cannot take care of their own feeding, dressing or toiletry needs unassisted, the cruise company can insist they are accompanied by a physically able companion who can provide the necessary assistance.

You are within your rights to request embarkation disability assistance at the cruise terminal but you need to inform your chosen cruise company at least 48 hours before travel. An attendant will help you at check-in, escort you through security, and take you onto the ship. The procedure will be reversed on disembarkation at your home port. The attendant can accompany you to the public bathroom within the terminal but you must be able to take care of yourself once inside the cubicle.

## Passenger Restrictions

Expectant mothers are not allowed to travel after a certain point in their pregnancy, typically during their third trimester or if they will be more than 24 weeks on the day of disembarkation. A doctor's letter or medical certificate is required stating that mother and baby are both in good physical health, fit to travel, that the pregnancy is not high-risk and the estimated due date. If you discover you are pregnant after making a booking, and you will be more than 24 weeks by the final date of your cruise, you should receive a refund but a doctor's letter will be needed and must be supplied on stamped, practice-headed paper.

Avoid destinations with the threat of malaria as certain antimalarial medications are not safe to take when pregnant. Remote areas might lack land-based hospitals and the standards of healthcare you might expect. The Caribbean in particular has experienced the Zika virus and this is particularly dangerous to you and your unborn foetus. Make sure you research your destination thoroughly for any health risks and speak to your doctor before booking a cruise.

***Insurance Tip:*** *You must disclose your pregnancy to your travel insurance company and make sure the cover protects your unborn baby. Make sure you always travel with your maternity notes.*

Although there are a few exceptions such as MSC, babies must be 6 months old at the time of embarkation to sail to most cruise destinations, and 12 months old for trans-ocean crossings, exotic fly-cruises or world cruises.

In order to travel unaccompanied, passengers will need to be at least 18 or 21 years old, depending on the cruise line.

Like duty-free sales, the casino is only open once the ship is outside of UK territorial waters, typically 12 miles from shore and if the itinerary includes visiting an overseas port. The gaming area will not open at all on British Isles cruises as the ship never leaves UK territorial waters. British cruise lines have a minimum age limit of 18 to gamble while the American lines impose a minimum age of 21 and this applies to all casino table play, slot machines and bingo. If you are embarking in an overseas port, the same 12-mile offshore rules will apply.

Most cruise lines adopt the age requirement of the territory in which they're sailing for purchasing and drinking alcohol onboard ships - 21 when in US waters, but only 18 in most of Europe, South America, Asia, Australia and New Zealand. That being said, there are several cruise companies, such as Carnival, Seabourn, and Regent Seven Sea Cruises, that apply a minimum drinking age of 21 to all destinations. Bartenders, security and duty-free shop staff will ask for ID or your cruise card, which is encoded with your age, and will refuse service if a passenger is underage, rowdy or over-intoxicated.

For those cruise lines who have their own private islands included on an itinerary, the same age will apply that is enforced on board their ship, even if the country's legal drinking age is younger. Check with the individual cruise lines for their policy if this is important to you.

***Alcohol Warning:*** *Don't get caught buying a drink for an underage passenger, or trying to sneak alcohol on the ship; the risks of getting caught are high and the punishment severe.*

Aside from the United States that enforces a 21 years old age limit on alcohol, most other ports of call have a legal age limit of 18 years old. If a destination's legal age limit is younger than onboard the ship, the cruise line has no jurisdiction over you drinking alcohol in that port. If you get caught drinking underage in a port of call, you are subject to the laws of that country.

Trying to sneak alcohol on the ship is a popular pastime among passengers but security is wise to most tricks. The days when you could sneak alcohol through in an Evian bottle have long gone as everything seen on the security scanners that are deemed suspicious will be inspected. The same videos that you watch on YouTube of the best smuggling methods are also watched by the cruise line's staff and most hidden contraband will be confiscated from your suitcase and withheld at the end of your cruise.

Cruise lines' strict drinking policy when it comes to consumption or trying to sneak alcohol on the ship is not taken lightly. Royal Caribbean state, *"Alcoholic beverages seized on embarkation day will not be returned. Security may inspect containers (water bottles, soda bottles, mouthwash, luggage etc.) and will dispose of containers holding alcohol. Guests who violate any alcohol policies, (over consume, provide alcohol to people under age 21, demonstrate irresponsible behaviour, or attempt to conceal alcoholic items at security and or luggage check points or any other time), may be disembarked or not allowed to board, at their own expense, in accordance with our Guest Conduct Policy."*

In this security-conscious age, bridge visits have generally been stopped for safety reasons, though some cruise lines include it as part of a 'Behind-the-Scenes' tour. A hefty fee will be applied to your onboard account for the privilege of visiting some back of house areas that are considered the heartbeat of cruise operations, including the engine room, main galley, laundry room and the theatre's backstage area, typically finishing with a glass of champagne with the captain in his command centre.

That being said, some cruise lines do it differently. Windstar Cruises, whose yacht-like ships show that they pride themselves on being anything but ordinary, invite their clientele to visit the bridge whenever they want. This 'Open Bridge' policy is also present on Star Clippers, Sea Cloud Cruises, Quark Expeditions and UnCruise Adventures. Windstar have even gone one step further, having recently unveiled a new suite onboard its Wind Surf yacht; at first, this might not seem strange, but it's actually an officer's suite within a crew-only area just behind the ship's bridge - it has to be the ultimate behind-the-scenes cruising experience.

## Special Needs

### Travelling with Pre-existing Illness

The sheer number of UK ports being used as embarkation points for cruises means the need to fly or travel long distances to get on a ship is a thing of the past, making cruising much more accessible to travellers with pre-existing conditions or disabilities. Most cruise ships have seen deck space given over to modern medical centres with a full complement of professional doctors and nurses added to the cruise line's payroll.

Thousands of people with pre-existing medical conditions are now able to travel safely, provided that the necessary precautions are considered in advance. The World Health Organisation suggests "those who have underlying health problems such as cancer, heart or lung disease, anaemia and diabetes, who are on any form of regular medication or treatment, who have recently had surgery or been in hospital, or who are concerned about their fitness to travel for any other reason should consult their doctor or a travel medicine clinic before deciding to travel."

*Transfusion Precaution:* *Make and carry a record of your blood type.*

### Travelling with Special Dietary Considerations

When considering a trip away from home, it is important to make sure your dining preferences can be catered to if you need a special diet. Food intolerances and allergies are easily managed if you know the foods to avoid. Cruise lines will do their best to make your holiday as perfect and stress-free as possible, and will be happy to provide special menus if you request them at the time of booking. Also, advise your cruise agent when making the booking if you need your food blended because of a medical condition and speak to the maître d' once on board.

A number of health conditions, including impaired kidney function, Crohn's disease and diabetes, need a meal plan in place that controls the intake of certain foods and nutrients. Characterised by elevated sugar levels, diabetes doesn't as much need a special diet as a regular dining regime. Eating patterns are essential for diabetics taking medication to control their condition, and skipping meals can lead to dangerously low blood glucose levels. Choosing the right cruise ship may prove very important as not only do they vary in size but in the amount of eating venues onboard and most importantly, the times they are open.

**Dietary Essential:** *Guests with food allergies should discuss any special diets or food sensitivities at the time of booking as some cruise lines require a 90-day notice period to implement special requests.*

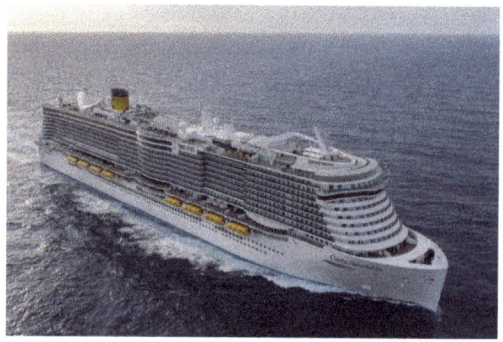
Credit: Costa Smeralda – Costa Cruises

All the mainstream cruise ships have excellent food options, especially Carnival, who cover all special dietary requests including vegetarian, vegan, low cholesterol, food intolerances and gluten-free. Norwegian Cruise Lines go one step further by providing a special services coordinator who will work with you to determine precisely the sort of diet you would like to adopt. You will need to notify them of your particular needs 30 days before your departure date.

AIDA also caters to guests with food allergies or intolerances. Buffet restaurants always provide gluten and lactose-free meals. Furthermore, any guests suffering from specific food intolerances will need to register these at the time of booking. On the day of embarkation, an appointment is arranged with the kitchen chef, who will explain the various restaurants available onboard and provide valuable insight into the meals that will not conflict with your intolerances. A 'special diets bar' is available on nine of the twelve AIDA ships.

Several of the big cruise brands have been granted halal certification and serve halal meals in the main dining room to meet the needs of their guests. Meals need to be pre-ordered at least two months in advance and are typically prepared off the ship, prepacked and frozen for use during the cruise.

No ship offers 100% kosher facilities, but certain lines will send out a menu before your sailing date, and the meals will be sent pre-packaged to the cruise ship by a specialised supplier. Costa and Windstar do not offer kosher meals, but allow guests to bring their own pre-packaged meals onboard which are subsequently heated up and served in the main dining room. Some cruise lines need as much as 90 days' notice prior to sailing to accommodate a dietary requirement, so advise the cruise line as soon as you make your booking.

***Cruise Tip:*** *It's unlikely that your kosher or halal meals will be loaded onto the ship until late afternoon, so you need to make alternative arrangements for embarkation day.*

***Cruise Essential:*** *Choose your cruise dates carefully as getting off a docked ship is a problem on Shabbos because you cannot carry your key card. Naked flames are prohibited in staterooms, so you need to get battery-operated candles.*

If you don't want to worry about your next kosher dining option, then why not book a dedicated cruise? Kosherica is the leader in Glatt Kosher (Cholov Yisroel, Pas Yisroel) cruises and tours and offers year-round sailings (*kosherica.com*), while Kosher-Cruise provides competitive prices on several cruise lines throughout the year (*kosher-cruise.com*). Kosher Riverboat Cruises offer all-inclusive 5* luxury sailings which include gourmet cuisine, an open bar, fabulous entertainment, all tours, lecture programs and airport transfers (*kosherrivercruise.com*).

## Travelling with Prescriptions & Medication
Please refer to the relevant section in 'Before You Go'.

## Travelling with Epilepsy
Patients with controlled epilepsy can generally enjoy cruise travel safely, but they should be aware of the potential seizure threshold-lowering effects of dehydration, delayed meals, hypoxia and disturbed circadian rhythm that, without proper care, can all happen quite easily whilst at sea. Some people's seizures are also triggered because of excitement, anxiety or fatigue, all of which can happen as the result of a long day, but are easily avoided with sufficient down time. Certain seizure medicines need to be stored in a cool place - if yours do, make sure to book a cabin that has a fridge, or contact

your preferred cruise line about providing one. Finally, consider the best time of year to travel as extreme humidity and heat can trigger complications. It's tempting to drink a lot to stay hydrated but too much liquid can also cause a seizure.

The International Bureau of Epilepsy offers a free downloadable booklet which is excellent for anyone undertaking a trip, with general travel advice that covers insurance, medication reminders and first-aid instructions (*https://www.ibe-epilepsy.org/publications/ibe-travellers-handbook*).

## Travelling with Diabetes

The climate of your destination is an important consideration when booking a trip as a diabetic - hot weather increases the risk of hypos as your insulin will be absorbed more quickly, whereas cold weather works in the opposite way and insulin will be absorbed more slowly. Sun damage is one of the biggest health risks for most diabetics, another reason it might be best not to opt for an extremely hot itinerary.

***Hypo Needs:*** *Treat a hypo immediately by eating or drinking a fast-acting carbohydrate, such as a tube of glucose gel, glucose tablets, a small juice carton, a sugary drink or a handful of jelly babies. Also, it's always wise to carry a glucagon pen in case of a severe attack.*

Some diabetics worry that the test of avoiding all the treats, cakes and desserts onboard may be too much, but most cruise lines offer plenty of healthier, low calorie and low-fat meals. The buffets are often laden with fresh fruit and salad bars, low-fat dressings, sugar-free desserts and even the ice cream cabinets have low calorie options. Disney is excellent at catering for children and adults with type 1 diabetes, with low carbohydrate options and fresh foods.

***Medical Need:*** *Most cruise lines provide refrigerators in certain staterooms suitable for storing insulin.*

When it comes to managing diabetes whilst away, some form of exercise each day is just as important as your diet - make sure to book a cruise with facilities which take your fancy, like a well-equipped gym or a running track.

## Travelling with Heart Disease

While the medical staff certainly have the best qualifications and significant experience in emergency treatment, they are still limited in what they can offer if you do suffer a heart attack. The medical centres on ships are not hospitals, they are more akin to small clinics and if an emergency does occur, the doctor will focus on stabilising the patient and evacuating them to a land-based unit for further treatment.

Newer vessels carry a well-stocked medical centre with standard diagnostic tools, x-ray and airway equipment, EKG machines, cardiac monitors, defibrillators, pulse oximeters and oxygen. Each ship has an onboard pharmacy that carries basic supplies, but they are unlikely to stock your particular prescription, so it is essential that you carry more than you need in case of travel delays.

All things considered, with careful planning there is no reason why someone with a heart condition can't travel safely. If you have either angina or heart failure, extreme weather can put an added strain on your heart - it may be best to avoid climates where temperatures will be extremely hot or very cold. Also, talk to your medical care team about your plans to travel and make sure to discuss any outstanding health regimes such as warfarin therapy, antiarrhythmic therapy and pacemaker checks.

You will need to inform your cruise line about any implants or pre-existing medical needs, such as oxygen or special diet, at the time of booking. Anyone with a special need or mobility restriction can pre-book wheelchair assistance at the terminal - they will help you through security and check-in and make sure you get aboard the ship safely.

## Travelling with Dementia

Cruising with someone who suffers from dementia can be daunting for all parties, even an experienced caregiver, but provided a doctor has deemed it safe for the passenger to travel, the condition doesn't have to preclude a trip. The single biggest thing you can do to ensure a successful holiday is to thoroughly research your cruise ship options and make sure to book something suitable for your group. For example, some travellers prefer smaller, more easily navigated ships with fewer passengers. On the other hand, some of the larger, more modern ships are more accessible and have a wider range of activities on offer.

Advise the cruise agent at the time of booking that the guest you are travelling with has special needs and they will be able to assess the level of help needed, assigning an accessible cabin if the guest is a wheelchair user or adjoining rooms are required. Choose a cabin close to the lifts and on or near a deck you might use the most.

Disorientation can lead to wandering, a common and serious concern for many loved ones. Newer ships have the ability to track guests with Radio Frequency Identification (RFID) tagging, GPS mapping and Bluetooth-enabled beacons which can be embedded in cruise cards, and wearable technology such as wristbands or medallions. Carnival, Celebrity, Royal Caribbean and MSC are just some of the companies that have embraced the new technology.

Elite Cruises and Vacations (*elitecruisesandvacations.com*) is a full-service travel agency that specialises in multigenerational adventures and accessibility travel. Notably, they offer dementia-friendly cruises several times a year, and caregiver respite.

## Travelling with Cognitive, Intellectual & Developmental Disabilities

Travelling abroad can be challenging for adults and children with autism, and of course their families, often because of changes in routine, overcrowding at popular tourist attractions or the general unpredictability of being somewhere unfamiliar. That being said, with careful planning, a cruise can be an amazing experience for the entire family.

Cruise lines welcome all guests with cognitive, intellectual and developmental disabilities such as autism, cerebral palsy, Down's syndrome and Alzheimer's but each guest or their carer must contact the cruise operator to discuss any special needs required during the cruise. Most cruise lines have a special services team that will work with you to meet individual cruising needs including boarding and disembarkation assistance so everyone in the party can travel with confidence and enjoy the holiday.

Picking the right cabin can make a big difference to some people with ASD. For example, if noise-sensitivity is an issue, it's best to avoid cabins close to the onboard entertainment areas and perhaps even the anchor and engine room. Royal Caribbean's 'Freedom,' 'Independence' and 'Oasis' class ships have promenade-facing cabins with soundproof windows that offer a fantastic viewpoint of some of the main attractions onboard, like the parades, without being affected by the noise. Also, choosing an inside cabin is a good idea if light sensitivity is a problem; some cruises even offer a projected 'virtual window' that can be turned off at night when you want to sleep.

People suffering from autism spectrum disorder (ASD) might find it helpful to travel with Autism on the Seas (*autismontheseas.com*), a specialised company that provides 50+ scheduled autism-friendly sailings for both adults and children each year. Royal Caribbean International, Carnival, Celebrity, Disney and Norwegian Cruise Line all participate in their program, offering priority boarding, quiet muster drills, special dietary requests and bespoke shore excursions. Royal Caribbean were the first to partner Autism on the Seas back in 2007, with the aim of developing cruise holidays for people with a wide range of special needs, including but not limited to autism, Asperger syndrome, Down's syndrome, Tourette syndrome, cerebral palsy and all cognitive, intellectual and developmental disabilities.

## Travelling with a Breathing Disorder

Cruising is generally a very good option for travellers with breathing disorders, with the only real issues arising if they are dependent on oxygen. You will need to check with the cruise lines you are considering as to what their policy is regarding oxygen cylinders and portable oxygen machines. Most cruise lines are accommodating, provided they are notified in advance.

**Oxygen Essential:** *Saga, Norwegian Cruise Lines, and Fred. Olsen Cruise Lines do not allow a liquid oxygen system onboard any of their ships.*

Set up by respiratory therapists and travel agents Celeste Belyea and Holly Marocchi, Sea Puffers (*seapuffers.com*) offer group sailings for oxygen users and will help arrange all the details of your travel for you.

> **Don't Ask:**
> *If the ship has left port can I still get on?*

## Travelling with Kidney Disease

In the past, travelling with damaged or infected kidneys was next to impossible, but recent medical advancements and the newfound availability of worldwide dialysis centres has made it entirely possible. That being said, travelling with kidney disease can still be challenging, especially due to potential travel restrictions if you are on a transplant list - make sure to discuss your travel plans with your medical specialist and determine if travelling while waiting for surgery is a good idea.

Guests requiring continuous ambulatory peritoneal dialysis are welcome to board cruise ships. However, the cruise line does not have the ability to assist or administer haemodialysis treatments. Those guests using peritoneal dialysis should have all solutions and equipment needed to perform the dialysis delivered to the vessel at least two hours prior to sailing on the day of departure. If you wish to use an independent supplier, please refer to the Rental Equipment section in 'Travel Planning Disability Resources'.

You will need to inform your cruise line at the time of booking of any renal medical equipment you intend to bring with you and confirm their policies and procedures. Discuss your special needs with the cruise agent and whether you need an accessible cabin, wheelchair assistance in the terminal when embarking or a low sodium diet.

The easiest way to undergo haemodialysis whilst on holiday is to travel with a company that specialises in renal treatment which mirrors the therapy you usually get at home. Dialysis at Sea (*dialysisatsea.com*) takes away all the stress of travelling with kidney disease, offering the comfort of knowing a trained renal care specialist team will be looking after your dialysis treatment while you are away, with select sailings on Royal Caribbean, Holland America and Celebrity throughout the year. Cruise Dialysis (*cruisedialysis.co.uk*) also provides renal treatments on a wide range of ocean and river cruise brands, including Celebrity, CMV, CroisiEurope, Celestyal and Hapag-Lloyd. As well as organising your dialysis treatment, the company also secures your cruise booking, flights and transfers.

*Following a meeting with the British Kidney Patient Association and Cruise Dialysis, NHS England have agreed to partially reimburse the cost of dialysis treatment onboard cruise ships. Dialysis Away from Base (DAFB) is only for UK residents and is designed to help pay for the cost of renal treatment while away.*

*If the majority of the ports of call during your cruise are within the European Economic Area (EEA), or a country with which the UK has a reciprocal agreement, then you can be reimbursed up to the cost of the NHS tariff. You will need to get approval from your renal team a minimum of eight weeks before you go on your cruise and you will be reimbursed once you're home, on production of treatment receipts.*

*It is important to take out comprehensive travel insurance to cover you whilst on a cruise ship as NHS England will only pay up to the cost of the renal dialysis tariff and will not pay for any other health care costs. If your cruise is outside any of the specified countries, or you dialyse in a private unit that does not have*

# Where to Start?

*an agreement with the NHS, you will have to pay for the total cost of dialysis yourself. If you or your dialysis unit require further information regarding this reimbursement then contact NHS England by emailing* england.contactus@nhs.net *or Mr Ian Wren at NHS England:* ianwren@nhs.net

Patients can use their UK Global Health Insurance Card (GHIC) – previously the European Health Insurance Card (EHIC) - within a state-run hospital for their dialysis treatment, but you will need to check first if there will be any contribution to be paid by you. Global Dialysis (*globaldialysis.com*) has a full list of renal units across the world, but you will need to find out the exact details directly from the dialysis centre.

## Travelling with a Visual Impairment

Travelling with a visual impairment can seem daunting but with a little preparation you can have a great cruise. Planning ahead is essential, think of all the things you may encounter and how you will address them and don't be embarrassed to ask for help.

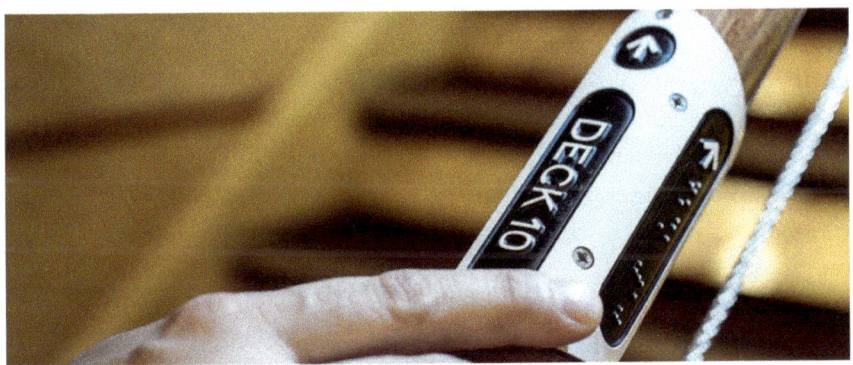

*Credit: Braille deck signage - AIDA*

Your travel planner will be happy to discuss each ship's accessibility, whether you need braille signage and elevator buttons, an orientation tour or qualified readers who will read written material such as the daily planner, shore excursions or menus. Some ships even carry audiobooks in their library. Make sure you request braille, large print literature or sign language interpreting services at the time of booking as some cruise lines such as Royal Caribbean require 60 days' notice before sailing. Also make sure you request assistance at the cruise terminal.

Certain ships have cabins that are more suited for a blind or visually impaired traveller. When booking your cruise, make sure to check what auxiliary aids are offered in the cabins that are available. The more modern ships can include visual-tactile cabin alert systems that notifies room occupants of a door knock, a telephone call, an alarm clock or the fire alarm. Cabins can also be equipped with telephone amplifiers, portable infrared or closed-captioned television. Certain ships have sign-language assistance, pagers to alert blind or impaired vision guests to ship announcements and assisted listening systems in theatres or showrooms. It is paramount that you do your research and ask the booking agent to help advise what cruise line and cabin best suits your needs.

Mind's Eye Travel (*mindseyetravel.com*) creates tours for people who are blind or visually impaired. Their service includes sighted guide assistance and help with immigration documents, boarding passes, cruise line luggage labels, embarkation and disembarkation, orientation and mobility while onboard the ship, shore excursions, braille menus (if available) and airline bookings if joining a fly-cruise. Presto Magic Travel (*prestomagictravel*) is run by Sue Slater who also specialises in cruises for people who are blind or have a visual impairment. Sue is blind herself but her mission as a travel agent is working with clients that are sight impaired. "Just because you have lost your vision, it doesn't mean that you cannot travel and experience the world through your other senses and description. I use my own personal experiences and my love of travel in helping people who are visually impaired have an amazing travel experience!"

You must advise the cruise line if you are travelling with a service dog and offer confirmation that it has been trained to a standard that allows it to travel. If you rely on a seeing-eye dog to assist you please read 'Service Dogs' for full details on travelling with a visual impairment.

## Travelling with a Hearing Impairment

One of the main concerns of those with hearing impairments is that their condition can present communication and navigational problems whilst on foreign shores; first time travellers in particular often overlook a few key obstacles, like their inability to hear tannoy announcements whilst onboard or even the ships emergency alarm. That being said, with mindful planning, cruising can be an excellent option for the hearing impaired.

> **Don't Ask:**
> It says I need a visa for India, but will Mastercard do?

One of the simplest things to do that will make for a much more successful holiday is to plan and book as much as you can ahead of time. Knowing where you need to be and when you need to be there will eliminate the need to ask for directions or listen for announcements - in fact, you can often sign up for email or text alerts so you get any important announcements directly. Alternatively, work with a specialised travel agent who can book everything for you and confirm it all in writing.

***Help Essential:*** *Download and print a notification card from the Transport Security Administration so you can subtly and discreetly inform staff of your hearing impairment. The majority of people will be happy to help in any way they can.*

When booking your cruise, check what auxiliary aids are offered by the different cruise lines and in which cabins they are available. The newer ships are more likely to have the latest disability aids to enhance your overall experience at sea. Several vessels have cabins that are hard-wired for deaf and low hearing guests including a visual-tactile alert system so the occupant will know if someone is knocking at the door, the telephone is ringing, the alarm clock is sounding or the smoke or fire alarm has activated. If hard-wired staterooms are unavailable, a portable kit might be available on request. TTY phones are available on several ships that use handy phones and text messaging allowing the guest to communicate with Guest Relations by teletypewriter.

Cabins can also be equipped with telephone amplifiers, portable infrared or closed-captioned television. Certain ships have sign-language interpreters, assisted listening systems in theatres or showrooms and pagers to alert deaf or hard of hearing guests to ship announcements. It is essential that you do your research and ask the booking agent to help advise what cruise line and cabin best suits your needs.

You must advise the cruise line if you are travelling with a service dog and offer confirmation that it has been trained to a standard that allows it to travel. If you rely on a service dog to assist you, please read 'Service Dogs'.

***Travel Tip:*** *MSC has made it a condition that guests with hearing disabilities must travel with a caregiver.*

Deaf Globetrotters Travel (*deafglobetrotters.com*) is a full-service travel agent for the deaf and hard of hearing; providing ocean and river cruises, this complete travel management service facilitates your entire trip and beyond. Deaf Land and Sea Travel (*deaflandsea.com*) also specialises in travel packages for the deaf and hard of hearing guests, and they have a certified Sign Language Interpreter on every sailing.

## Travelling Companions

Retirement no longer means watching daytime television and looking forward to a weekly outing to the bingo hall. Whether you are living with a disability or have reached an age where travelling alone could be daunting there are now other options.

### Caregivers & Chaperones

Depending on your disability, some cruise lines stipulate an able-bodied companion or caregiver accompany you on your holiday. If you live alone but require a companion, or you simply want the security blanket of knowing you have someone travelling with you that can help you deal with your particular needs or monitor your medication, there are several companies that can help.

### Able Community Care (*ablecommunitycare.com*)

Able Community Care can provide holiday carers or companions for seniors or people with special needs so they can go on the holiday of their choice. Your travel buddy can accompany you and provide personal care, medical assistance and holiday companionship. The company will do their best to find a companion that suits your preference and personality - someone who loves travel, can assist on day trips and share your adventure.

### Helping Hands (*helpinghandshomecare.co.uk*)

Helping Hands will provide a holiday care service that's fully tailored to your requirements. They can work with you, your family, your GP and professionals from a variety of other healthcare organisations to ensure your medical needs are met. The carers will provide support on your trip and will assist with all essential elements of care and take responsibility for ensuring your medication is administered correctly, allowing you to relax completely during your holiday.

### Live In Care (*livein.care/holiday-companionship-care-breaks*)

Live In Care helps you remain independent by providing a personal care service that allows you to take your holiday without cause for concern. Their essential care companion will travel with you and can stay within your accommodation so that they are there to assist with any difficulties that may arise, day or night.

**Dignity Travel** (*dignitytravel.biz*)
Dignity Travel is committed to providing easy and accessible cruises for wheelchair users and those that have difficulty walking. They understand that not everyone has someone to travel with and arrange for experienced travel companions who will assist with daily care needs, toileting, dressing, transfers and other help which might be needed. If you are travelling with a partner, they can also provide a break to the person that cares for you, or deliver additional support if needed. They work at ensuring you have a dignified, fun and adventurous travel experience.

## Service Dogs
If you have never travelled with your service dog before you will need to consider the extra logistics of undertaking any journey with your companion. First, you should seek advice from your local Guide Dogs Mobility Team or the organisation who trained your dog. If after weighing up all the pros and cons you decide to forge ahead, the law is on your side when it comes to travelling with your seeing eye companion.

A service dog is legally defined as "any dog that is individually trained to do work or perform tasks for the benefit of a person with a disability." Emotional support dogs, assistance dogs in training and pets, are not recognised as official service dogs by either the International Guide Dog Federation (IGDF), Assistance Dogs International (ADI), or by most accrediting bodies worldwide, so they will not be permitted on a cruise ship. If your disability is reliant on an animal that is not recognised as a service dog you will need to contact your preferred cruise line at least 60 days before sailing for advice.

*Bad News: If your dog fails any check or its paperwork is incomplete, it will be denied boarding. Additionally, service dogs must meet the rules of the Pet Travel Scheme when entering the United Kingdom. If you experience a problem with your documentation upon re-entry, any related costs for either the quarantine or re-export of your animal will be entirely your responsibility.*

## Cruising with a Service Dog
Any cruise ship passenger departing from the United Kingdom, or anywhere in the EU, is protected by an EU Regulation that sanctions their right to travel with a service dog if they are visually impaired, blind or deaf. However, a cruise line might refuse a booking on the grounds of safety if there are

concerns regarding the age and size of the vessel or the infrastructure of the ports being visited.

Firstly, you'll need to check how far in advance you are required to advise the cruise line's accessibility department that you'll be travelling with a service dog, as most lines differ in policy - some require as little as 48 hours' notice, while some ask for as much as 60 days. Even if you choose to book through a travel agent or specialist cruise company, it is still advisable to ring your cruise line directly to ensure there is no miscommunication and that all your needs will be addressed.

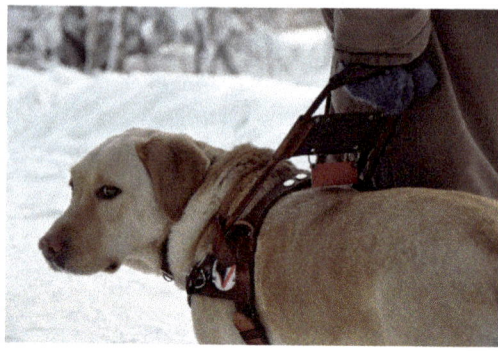

*Credit: Guide dog Opas Eevi at work - Sini Merikallio, Flickr*

**Service Dog Alert:** *Hapag Lloyd, American Cruise Lines, Ponant, Uniworld, Sea Cloud Cruises, Paul Gauguin and Star Clippers do not accommodate any animals on their ships.*

**Cruise Essential:** *Royal Caribbean is the only cruise line that allows therapy dogs onboard. Cunard's Queen Mary 2 is the only ship that carries pets, but only on select itineraries.*

**Paperwork**

At check-in, you will be asked to provide documentation proving your dog has been trained by an accredited organisation, and all dogs will need to be approved by DEFRA under the Pet Travel Scheme prior to travel so that they can re-enter the UK without being placed in quarantine. They'll also need to have a European PETS passport for any trip made outside the UK, signed, dated and stamped by an official veterinarian (for guests from the UK or EU) or official third country veterinary certificate (for guests from the U.S and other countries outside the UK and EU). In preparation, your dog must be microchipped, blood tested, immunised against rabies, have undergone tapeworm treatment and will only be allowed to travel on a DEFRA approved route. Your documented proof must be carried with you at all times.

# Where to Start?

***Essential Tip:*** *Pet Passports and Third Country Certificates must be signed, dated and stamped by an official veterinarian; this may be different than your local veterinarian and you may need to allow extra time to action this.*

Rabies vaccinations must be administered typically between 30 days and 12 months before travel, though there are exceptions in some countries. Regardless of what country your pet is travelling to, you must enter that country before your dog's most recent rabies vaccination expires.

***Vaccine Essential:*** *There are three types of rabies vaccines being administered to dogs: a one, two and three year serum. Some of the ports on your itinerary may only accept dogs that have had annual rabies vaccinations, so your dog may need a booster shot even though a two or three year vaccination has not expired.*

Most countries within the EU and the European Economic Area recognise and accept the standard PETS Passport and health certificate, but some countries have their own entry, exit and vaccine requirements, so double check that your animal meets them.

You will need an Assistance Dogs UK branded ID book that contains information about you and your dog, as well as the dog's training organisation. This can be obtained through the Guide Dogs Mobility Team or through the organisation that trained your animal. Unfortunately, the UK government has not yet issued an official certificate for service dogs that is universally recognised, but the Assistance Dogs UK branded ID book, identified by its yellow cover, will provide most companies with sufficient information as to the legitimate ownership of a service dog.

***Beware:*** *There are some trainers, organisations and agencies who promise to 'certify' your dog for a fee, but they are not worth the paper they are printed on and will not be recognised under the law.*

Although not a separate document, you will need a copy of the International Health Certificate, issued by a recognised veterinarian, that forms part of your dog's essential paperwork, along with the ID passport itself. Health certificates can usually be issued up to three weeks before you travel, but the closer to your departure date the better.

# The Autonomous Cruiser

***Vaccine Essential:*** *If travelling to Mexico your service dog is required to receive ecto-parasite and endo-parasite treatment no more than 15 days prior to arrival in port, and the vaccine must be recorded on your dog's health certificate.*

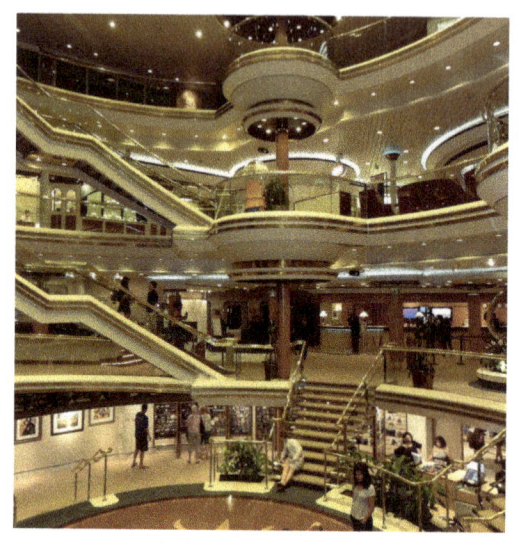

Credit: Celebrity Equinox - Stephanie C, Flickr

Take at least one duplicate copy of all your service dog's paperwork for each port as some countries might want to keep a copy for their records. Make sure to include rabies certificates, vaccination records, training certificates and your spay or neuter documents if you have them. Although this degree of paperwork might not be needed, it is best to cover all the angles in case you do get challenged by a port official.

***Blameless:*** *All documentation and immunisation requirements are established by government authorities - whatever limitations are imposed on your dog is not the responsibility of your cruise line.*

## Embarkation

Once you have boarded the ship make sure to supply Guest Relations with a copy of all your dog's documents and permits and discuss any concerns you might have. Your cabin steward will show you the exact location of your dog's relief box; the receptacle cannot be placed on cabin balconies or inside the cabin itself, but if you are unhappy about its location you can ask for it to be moved. You will also be shown where to dispose of your dog's waste.

## Accessible Areas

Service dogs are permitted to escort their owners to all public areas, including dining venues, but they must remain on a leash or harness at all times. Due to health regulations, they are not permitted in Jacuzzis, pools, splash zones or spas, nor can they accompany you on galley visits.

Your maître d' will arrange a convenient table in the dining room with nearby space for your animal. Because of rules governing food hygiene standards, you are prohibited from feeding your dog at the table, no matter the circumstances.

Most buffet venues have dedicated tables set aside for disabled passengers that also accommodate service dogs, but they must remain at the table. If you're travelling solo, a crew member will be happy to assist you in choosing your food and will bring it to your table for you so you won't need to leave your dog alone at all.

**Ports of Call**
As mentioned before, your assistance dog will only be allowed to travel on DEFRA approved routes, but you should note that it's not always perfectly clear which routes satisfy this criterion. For example, Cunard and their sister brand P&O Cruises are only licensed by DEFRA to carry service dogs on itineraries that start and finish in Southampton, including full world cruises. It's always better to be safe than sorry, so contact your preferred cruise line directly for their full guidelines on carrying service dogs on your preferred route.

***Dog Essential:*** *Tap water in foreign countries is not always processed in the way your dog might be used to, so carry bottled water for your dog to prevent an upset stomach.*

When picking your itinerary, keep an eye out for ports of call with ironclad directives in place regarding service dogs. Remember, it is the sole responsibility of the owner to consult with each port authority about their entry requirements, and for obtaining the animal's necessary permits so they can travel, visit the ports and disembark at your final destination. You will need to know the current local laws, regulations and attitudes of all the countries on your itinerary, even on DEFRA approved routes and even if you don't intend to get off the ship. Also, every country has different vaccine requirements so be sure you've addressed those. Finally, national protocol or quarantine requirements of the port might still prevent the animal being able to disembark.

***Import Permit:*** *You will need an import permit for each port of call in order to disembark with your service dog. Ignoring this directive might thwart your attempt to get off the ship.*

***Shore Excursions:*** *Foreign excursion operators can also impose their own restrictions on the carriage of your service dog, so do your best to contact them beforehand to explain your circumstances.*

If you are planning to disembark in foreign countries with your service dog you will need to arrange for treatment against tapeworm before re-entering the UK; the only exceptions are if you are travelling directly to the UK from Ireland, Finland, Malta or Norway. The treatment needs to be administered by a vet between 24 and 120 hours before you arrive in the UK and will need to be recorded in your dog's Pet Passport or third-country official veterinary certificate. It's important to check your itinerary and make arrangements with a vet in one of the countries you are visiting to get your dog treated before returning home. It's also advised that you treat your dog again within 28 days of your return to the UK. Other EU countries have their own requirements regarding treatment against tapeworm which will need to be complied with if you are not travelling directly to that country from the UK (i.e. the ship makes a call in another country first).

***Tapeworm Advice:*** *Tapeworm treatment should be arranged at the penultimate port of call before returning to the UK, just in case the final port of call be missed for any unforeseeable reason.*

The ship's crew are not obligated to look after your dog, nor can it be left unattended on the ship, so if your service animal is prevented from disembarking at a port you can only leave the ship if one of your party will stay aboard and care for your dog.

**Accessories**
Although the law does not require your dog to wear a harness or jacket, the cruise line stipulates that your dog must wear a harness at all times when not in the cabin. Some service dog owners find it helpful when travelling through airports or in ports to bring a few accessories that will automatically make people aware that their dog is a trained service animal. Service dog patches will alert passengers and crew to the fact that they shouldn't pet or distract your animal. Also, you are responsible for providing your dog with a lifejacket.

Depending on your destination you might want to take canine footwear or paw protection wax to safeguard your dog's paws from hot pavements, sand, ice and salt. If the weather on your cruise is forecast to be hot you might consider a cooling product, such as a vest, collar or bandana.

*Travel Tip:* A white cane serves as an excellent backup if you want to use the cabin bathroom or go onto the balcony without disturbing your dog.

### Food & Bedding

As the owner, you are solely responsible for providing everything your dog needs for the duration of your trip, including water bowls, a blanket or dog bed, disposable dog poop bags, wet wipes, toys, and medication (if applicable). Make sure you take enough food and treats for the entire trip, including extra in case of any delays, and for your own convenience, sealed bags of food present less of a problem with customs. It's advisable to keep your service animal on their regular diet to help prevent any stomach upsets. Dogs must be fed in your cabin and under no circumstances can they be fed food scraps in any public area. If refrigerator space is required in your cabin to store dog food or medication, request it directly from your cruise line no less than 30 days before you travel.

### Dog Toileting

Relief areas are provided on a shared basis with other service dogs onboard, and your cruise line will do its best to ensure it is as close to your cabin as possible. The 'potty box' is always a little different depending on the cruise line, but they typically measure 4'x4' with fillers ranging from paper pellets to wood shavings (sawdust). As the litter box will be smaller than what your dog is used to, ask the company that trained your animal for advice on how to implement a new toilet regime. It will be emptied and the filler replenished each day, but owners remain responsible for cleaning up after their dog.

*Nasty Habit:* If you're bothered that your dog's potty box has been placed in a designated smoking area, ask that it be moved elsewhere to avoid finding cigarette ends in the box.

### Health Issues

Your dog could become ill during your trip so it is essential that they have an excellent health insurance policy that will cover the cost of any treatment, an extended stay or repatriation. The health of your service animal is paramount so you must be aware of the limitations of cruise ships. They will not have veterinary support, nor will some ports of call, so it is important that you research exactly what facilities are available on your itinerary before you travel. It is important to note that in extreme weather, certain ports may be missed due to safety reasons, so it's always best to have multiple options. Even the best trained dog can get sick in unfamiliar circumstances, whether sailing or flying. Speak to your vet about your upcoming trip and ask what remedies they recommend you take with you in case your dog experiences diarrhoea, an upset stomach or motion sickness. You might want to make up a first-aid kit for your animal so you are prepared for any eventuality – eye wash, antiseptic wipes, bandages, surgical tape and even non-adhesive dressings may prove useful, especially on a long cruise.

**Brexit**
The UK will become a third country from 1st January 2021 and the rules for travelling to EU countries with your service animal will change. If you want to travel with your dog to the EU you should contact your vet and start the process at least four months beforehand. During the Brexit transition period, UK passengers can travel to the EU with their service dog using a current UK-issued EU pet passport. The Department for Environment, Food and Rural Affairs are in discussions with the European Commission to ensure the UK becomes a listed third country after leaving the EU, as doing so will make it easier for people to take their service dogs abroad. Any necessary changes after the Brexit transition period will depend on whether the UK becomes known as a 'listed third country' or an 'unlisted country' - the documentation needed will depend on whether the UK becomes a Part 1 or Part 2 listed country.

**Part 1 Listed Country**
Becoming a Part 1 listed country will see the rules remain very similar to their current form and will mean that you will have to have your service dog microchipped and vaccinated against rabies at least 21 days before travel, and you must protect your animal against tapeworm. You will need to apply for a new UK pet passport, but it will be valid for life as long as your dog's rabies shots are kept up to date.

**Part 2 Listed Country**
If the UK is given Part 2 listed country status it will mean you also need to get an Animal Health Certificate from an official veterinarian no more than ten days before travel, confirming your dog is microchipped and rabies protected,

## Where to Start?

and again, you will need to protect your animal with tapeworm treatment. This document will need to be renewed for each subsequent trip to the EU. On arrival in the EU, service dog owners will need to enter through a designated Travellers' Point of Entry and present proof of all the dog's medical documentation.

**Unlisted Country**

If the UK becomes an unlisted country, your PETS passport will no longer be valid for travel to the EU. As before, you will need to get your service animal microchipped and vaccinated against rabies, but in addition, your dog will need a blood sample taken at least 30 days after its last rabies vaccination. The sample will then be sent to an EU-approved blood testing laboratory, and once the blood test has been approved, there is a wait of 3 months before you can travel. If the blood test is not deemed viable, you will need to repeat the process from scratch.

You will need to obtain an Animal Health Certificate from an official veterinarian no more than ten days before travel. The certificate will be valid for ten days after the date of issue for entry into the EU and for four months from the date of issue for onward travel within the EU and re-entry to the UK. If you wish to travel with your service dog directly to Finland, Republic of Ireland or Malta, it will need to be treated against tapeworm one to five days before arriving, and the treatment must be recorded by a veterinarian on your Animal Health Certificate. Travellers will need to repeat tapeworm treatment for each and every subsequent trip.

On arrival in the EU, service dog owners will need to enter through a Travellers' Point of Entry and present proof of all the dog's medical documentation. Your service dog will need a new health certificate for each subsequent trip to the EU, though another blood test will not be required as long as your animal has an up-to-date rabies vaccination history.

As well as discussing your travel plans with your vet, you can find more information from the following organisations:

- The UK Department of Environment, Food and Rural Affairs (DEFRA) Website: *www.gov.uk/take-pet-abroad/guide-dogs*
- The Pet Travel Scheme Helpline
  Telephone: +44 (0) 370 241 1710 - Monday to Friday, 8 am to 6 pm UK time (closed Bank Holidays)
  E-mail: *pettravel@ahvla.gsi.gov.uk*

**Airline Travel**
Fly-cruises offer fantastic opportunities to sail to more exotic parts of the world without long stretches at sea, and for a few the temptation of instant sun is also a big draw, but some people are often daunted by the prospect of flying with their service animal for the first time. The good news is that airlines must allow you to travel with a service dog without charge, if the flight departs from inside the EU, except for reasons justified on the grounds of safety. (There might be additional rules to comply with if flying outside the EU.) As long as you comply with the rules of the Pet Travel Scheme, and meet the entry requirements of the cruise departure country, flying should be easy and comfortable.

*Travel Rights:* Your right to travel is protected under EU law, and by the Air Carrier Access Act regulations if it is an American carrier, or by Resolution 700 if it is a foreign IATA (International Air Transport Association) airline.

Before making an airline booking, ensure your flight is on a DEFRA approved route and accepts service dogs; if you are travelling on a non-approved route, your dog will usually be required to travel in the cargo section. Ideally you will need to inform the airline of your service animal at least 14 days prior to your flight as the crew will need to make preparations for your boarding and seat allocation. However, the staff will do everything possible to provide a flight for you and your dog if less notice is given. Airlines are entitled to ask for evidence that your dog has been trained by an organisation recognised by the International Guide Dog Federation (IGDF) or Assistance Dogs International (ADI), the accrediting bodies for service dog organisations worldwide.

Airlines will require you to have a travel companion if you are unable to put on your seatbelt, reach and don your lifejacket, apply the oxygen mask, understand safety procedures or reach the emergency exit unaided. Check with the airline, as some offer discounted prices for support chaperones.

Most airlines recognise the needs of individuals who require Emotional Support Animals (ESA) or psychiatric service animals and allow them on their aircrafts without any additional costs. Advanced notice is required and the animal needs to be able to behave in public and remain calm on the aircraft. Registration is not always legally mandatory; you may only be required to carry a letter from a licensed mental health professional detailing why you need an emotional support animal. Also, although not required by

# Where to Start?

law, it is a condition of some airlines that your dog wears an identifying jacket or harness and an ID tag. Also, you will need a recognised safety harness when travelling by air so that your dog can be secured to a seatbelt during take-off and landing, and whenever the seatbelt signs are on.

At least three days before your flight, call your airline's special assistance department and arrange for an airport escort. Anyone with a special need is entitled to support from the airport's special assistance team, which can be particularly advantageous if you are travelling alone. As well as help at check-in and through security, staff can supply braille and audio versions of all required safety demonstration documents.

Before passing through security, an assistance team member will give your dog the opportunity to relieve itself. If you leave the security area yourself, you will need to be re-screened again when returning. Mention to a security officer when you return to the security area and they should move you to the front of the screening queue.

Security personnel will not request the removal of your dog's harness, leash or collar, but they could set off the metal detector if any parts are made of stainless steel so ask for your dog's screening to be done by a hand-operated scanner. Apart from holding the leash, do not touch your dog until it has been inspected and cleared by the security team; failure to comply may require you to undergo additional screening. Security personnel will not separate you from your dog but if you experience any problems ask that a supervisor is called.

**Sight Impairment Tip:** *To reduce the chance of theft, place any small items such as your wallet, purse, loose change, keys, watch, mobile phone and sunglasses in a Ziploc bag before placing them in the screening bin.*

> **Don't Ask:**
> If I book an outside cabin, will I get wet if it rains?

Passengers with visual impairments passing through customs and security can request a witness to be present when their baggage is being searched to make sure nothing is stolen and your belongings are correctly repacked.

Once you've passed security you will be supported through the departure area before being escorted to your gate and onto the aircraft. Pre-boarding gives you time to get comfortable and settle your dog before other passengers embark, while also giving you priority over the space in the overhead storage lockers and allowing you the opportunity to discuss your needs with the cabin crew. You are entitled to pre-boarding, so if it is not offered make sure to request it.

**Relief Tip:** *Use the Working Like Dogs app (Where to Go) to help locate any American airport's dog relief area.*

Depending on your airline, your dog may be provided with floor space in the seat next to you, but some airlines will expect your dog to lay across your feet in a bulkhead row. If you have a choice of carrier it's worth exploring which airline offers the best option for you. Take a fleece for your dog to lie on to help them keep warm, and an absorbent mat which can be placed under the fleece in case of any accidents.

If you are worried about your animal getting airsick, consider limiting their food and water intake before the flight, and ask the flight crew for a few ice cubes once in the air. Make sure you carry plastic bags, absorbent granules and cleaning wipes, just in case your dog does become ill on your journey. It's also a good idea to carry bottled water (available after passing through security), a travel-size water and food bowl and any appropriate snacks.

**Rabies Laws:** *Some island states have strict anti-rabies laws which impose limits on the entrance of all animals, including service dogs. Countries with stringent regulations and prolonged quarantine confinement include the United Kingdom, Ireland, Australia, New Zealand and the State of Hawaii. Always check the regulations for each country you are visiting.*

Make sure the airline makes a note that you will need assistance at your destination airport, and again when travelling home after your cruise. On returning to the UK you will be met by a member of Animal Welfare, either on the aircraft or inside the terminal, to go through PETS checks before allowing your dog to re-enter the UK.

## Accessibility: Your cruising questions answered

More and more cruise companies are slowly but surely stepping up to their responsibility to lower (and eventually eliminate) the barriers that exist for disabled cruisers. It wasn't too long ago that a wheelchair user would have

# Where to Start?

found cruising impossible, but nowadays cruise ships provide accessible features and disability aids throughout the vessel, offering up an unforgettable travel experience. These new opportunities for disabled travellers raise a lot of questions - below are some of the most frequently asked and the answers to know before you book your holiday.

**What is EU regulation 1177/2010?**
Effective in the EU since 18 December 2012, EU Regulation 1177/2010 concerns the right of guests when travelling by sea. In a nutshell, your request to travel cannot be refused solely on the grounds of your reduced mobility or disability, and you are entitled to travel under the same conditions and costs that apply to all other guests.

However, while every effort is made to accept a booking, a request to travel can be refused if the design of the ship or port infrastructure and equipment, including port terminals, makes it impossible to carry out the embarkation, disembarkation, or carriage of a passenger in a safe and operationally feasible manner and which may have an impact on the passenger's safety and comfort.

After an assessment, the cruise line may insist that you are accompanied by a physically able companion who can assist you during your cruise. Note, this accompanying person is not entitled to free passage. If for any reason, your travel request is declined, you will be informed straightaway, and you then have the right to ask that the reason for the refusal is put in writing.

You are further entitled to assistance in embarking and disembarking the ship and help with your luggage and any specific medical equipment that you are taking. Someone will also help you to any public toilet facility, though they will be unable to help with toileting.

**How do I register my disability or medical requirements?**
If you have any disability or medical requirements, you need to inform your cruise line or travel agent at the time of your booking to avoid any possible complications. The cruise line will usually send you a medical questionnaire to complete and return, but if you book through a third party, you may have to ask that they request the medical form on your behalf.

**Are all cruise ships accessible?**
The majority of cruise ships are now mostly accessible, with the general rule being the newer the ship, the more facilities and amenities will be available,

including lifts to all floors and fully accessible dining and entertainment venues. Your booking agent will have all the relevant information at their fingertips and will ensure they marry you up with the right liner for your needs. It is, however, your own responsibility to make the cruise line aware of any special requirements you have when making your booking, and failure could result in assistance not being available when you need it. In extreme cases, because of safety or operational issues, the line might deny you boarding.

**Will I be offered help on embarkation and disembarkation?**
All cruise lines will do their best to supply a wheelchair for embarking and disembarking, just make sure you lodge your request at the time of booking. You will, however. need to bring your own mobility aid if you need one for the length of the cruise.

**Will I be able to get on and off the ship easily?**
The majority of ships now have large gangways which allow wheelchairs and scooters to embark and disembark without issue. Depending on the itinerary you have booked, a few ports of call might require the vessel to anchor in the harbour, necessitating tender boats to take guests ashore. Cruise companies have strict guidelines in place for tendering, and many might deem it unsuitable for guests that use assistive devices unless roll-on capability is available. Guests wishing to use the tenders must have sufficient independent mobility to negotiate steps and traverse a gap of up to 18" (45 cm). Crew members will be on hand to guide and steady you as you embark, but they cannot support, carry or lift guests onboard the tender for safety reasons. If you book through a specialised booking agent, they will make you aware of any tendering that might apply to any cruise itinerary you are interested in.

Apart from tendering restrictions, there will also be a few occasions when a wheelchair or scooter user may not be able to disembark the vessel because of tidal variance. Ships use a variety of gangway configurations to cope with tidal conditions, some of which are not suitable for those with mobility impairments. P&O stipulate it isn't always possible to use the short ramped low-level gangway, so access to the port may only be possible via either a long straight shore gangway fitted with self-levelling steps or, in some cases, wooden batons for foot grips. The ship may also deploy its own narrow stepped gangway, which also features self-levelling steps to take account of the tide.

Numerous ports of call provide stress-free access for wheelchairs and scooter users, however, embarking and disembarking can still be challenging for those with limited mobility. You must be aware that certain gangways may not be fully accessible for wheelchairs or scooters at the time you might wish to go ashore. Tides have a significant bearing on the sort of gangway that is used, and while a slight tidal variance is unlikely to restrict full-time wheelchair users in disembarkation, a high tide may make it impossible to go ashore.

Certain ports of call have a substantial tidal variance, resulting in a height difference between the quay and the gun-port doors, making the gangway too steep for the safe passage of wheelchairs or mobility scooters. These ports include, but aren't limited to: Bilbao, La Coruña, Le Havre, La Rochelle, Lisbon, Zeebrugge, the Canary Islands, Hamburg, Boston, Halifax, Portland, Quebec, Darwin, San Francisco and Mumbai. The ship's daily planner will have restrictive tidal times displayed for a particular port and announcements are usually made advising passengers of the times to avoid when embarking or disembarking the vessel. In certain circumstances, it might mean a wheelchair or scooter user cannot alight the ship at all.

## What sort of cabin should I book?

Wheelchair-accessible or modified staterooms are available on most ships but they are in extremely high demand, so you should book well in advance if you're unable to enjoy a standard cabin. Be careful in checking what each cruise line is offering and that it is suitable for you to avoid any hiccups whilst onboard. The term 'wheelchair-accessible' usually means it's been designed for purpose, often with wider doorways and a roll-in shower. On the other hand, 'adapted' means the cabin has been modified based on its original specifications, which could pose a problem to a full-time wheelchair user, as accessible cabins are generally larger than standard rooms to allow for wheelchair manoeuvrability. If your wheelchair is custom-made or larger than a standard model, make sure you advise the booking agent so they can allocate a cabin that will be suitable.

## Can I book a standard cabin?

The short answer is yes, but only if you're absolutely sure a standard cabin will meet your individual needs. It is unlikely that a wheelchair will fit through the threshold as a standard entry doorway is typically only 22" (56 cm) across and mobility equipment is not allowed to be stowed in passageways outside your room. You must also take into account that the cabin will not be large enough to navigate in a wheelchair - some cabins have an 8" (20 cm) lip into the bathroom and a 4" (10 cm) lip into the shower stall, and a 7" (18 cm) threshold to get onto the balcony. In fact, some standard cabins have a bath rather than a shower.

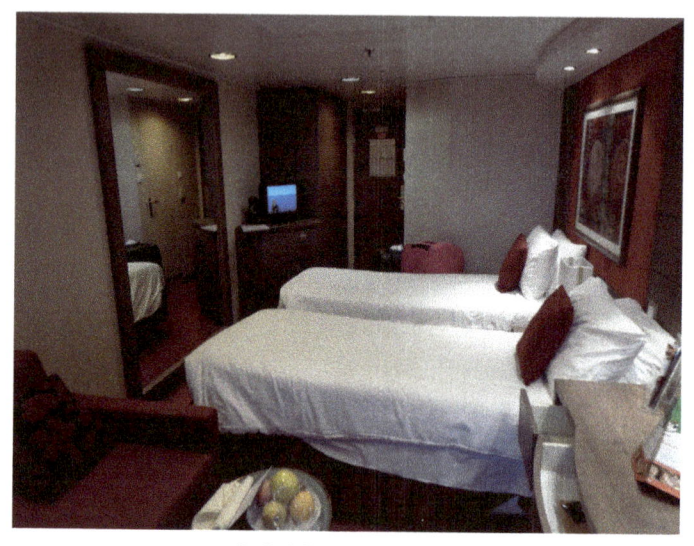

Credit: MSC Magnifica Cabin 11134 - CovBoy2007, Flickr

## What equipment is in an accessible cabin?
A fully accessible cabin will be barrier-free, allowing a wheelchair easy access to and from the bathroom, the balcony (if applicable) and of course the room itself. They will typically feature a roll-in shower, pull-down shower seat or bench, grab bars to assist with balance, lowered sink and vanity area and lowered wardrobe hanging rods. Portable visual and hearing kits will also be available on request.

## What are ADA kits?
Americans with Disabilities Act (ADA) compliance kits are usually found in hotels, ships and hospitals to help support the deaf and hearing impaired. A cabin or room should include a text telephone (TTY) to access the phone, a signal to indicate the phone is ringing, a handset amplifier to boost the sound, a door-knock sensor, an alarm clock with a bed shaker and smoke detectors with visual or audio notification.

# Where to Start?

## What if there are no suitable cabins that can accommodate my electric scooter?

If you are advised that there are no suitable cabins for an electric scooter available on a specific itinerary or ship, consider taking a collapsible manual wheelchair (if it will meet your needs) that can be safely stored within your cabin.

## Do any of the cabins have hospital-style beds?

Specialised beds are not fitted on ships as standard, but you can hire one in advance and it will be delivered and set up in your cabin ready for your arrival. Check out the 'Travel Planning Disability Resources' in the Directory for a full list of mobility equipment suppliers.

## Can I travel alone if I use a wheelchair or scooter?

If you are able to care for yourself then there is no reason why you can't travel alone, but you need to bear in mind that the ship's crew, although supportive, are unable to help you in moving about the ship or assist with personal care. If a guest is unable to care for their own basic needs and requires help with dressing, eating or administering medication, they must have a travelling companion with them.

## Will the ship provide specialised equipment?

Your booking agent will advise you as to what your chosen vessel can provide in the way of equipment. Most accessible cabins have shower stools or chairs, raised toilet seats and bath seats. If you need a commode, bed blocks or a hoist, you are invited to bring your own or to arrange for them to be delivered to the ship by contacting an independent supplier, such as those listed in the 'Travel Planning Disability Resources' section in the Directory.

***Mobility Essential:*** *If you plan on bringing your own hoist onboard you need to check it is compatible with the ship's electrical supply.*

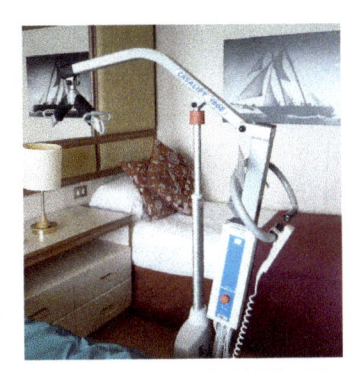

*Credit: Mobility at Sea*

### What sort of wheelchair can I take onboard?
Most cruise lines accept gel, dry cell, sealed lead acid or lithium-ion battery operated wheelchairs, but it is your responsibility to check with your booking agent before you travel that your wheelchair is allowed onboard. Collapsible wheelchairs can be taken into most cabins, but you should ensure that the width of your chair, when collapsed, will fit through your cabin door.

*Mobility Essential:* *If you fail to book an approved cabin, you will not be able to bring your electric wheelchair or scooter on board.*

*Mobility Essential:* *It is imperative that you book a cabin large enough to store your wheelchair or scooter when not in use, as equipment cannot be left in corridors or stairwells because of health & safety issues.*

### Can I hire a wheelchair once onboard?
Although you will see a large quantity of wheelchairs used during embarkation and disembarkation, it is the cruise line's ground staff, and not the ship, that provide wheelchair assistance. Cruise ships don't operate an onboard wheelchair rental service though most carry a few extra chairs in case of a medical emergency, but they will not be given out for individual use so you'll need to travel with your own or hire one from an independent supplier.

### Can I bring a Segway onboard?
Cruise lines do not accept Segways, trikes and similar non-standard, powered mobility aids on board. If you are unsure if your mobility aid is accepted, you should contact the cruise line directly.

### Am I able to charge my electrical mobility aid in my cabin?
Most ships have either 110- or 220-volt outlets depending on the vessel's nationality, however, some of the newer builds offer both. If you check that your charging equipment is compatible with the ship's electrical supply and bring the relevant converter or adaptor, there is no reason you can't charge your equipment in your cabin.

*Medical Essential:* *All guests taking electrical medical equipment on board will need to bring their own extension leads with them (surge protectors are not allowed).*

*Mobility Essential:* *The bigger the cruise ship, the further you will be travelling each day, and it is easy to underestimate how much battery life you will use. Charge your equipment every night to avoid any problems.*

### Does the ship have a medical facility?

Every modern cruise ship has a fully equipped medical centre that is designed to meet the care of its passengers. There is usually at least one fully trained and licensed doctor and two nurses on board, with the exact number dependent on the size of the ship. Newer vessels have sophisticated medical facilities featuring diagnostic and lab-test equipment, cardiac monitors, defibrillators, digital x-ray equipment, nebulizers and oxygen. The infirmary mainly treats minor complaints ranging from stomach upsets to flu-like symptoms, but the staff are also trained to perform life support if needed.

Although the centre is not open around the clock, the staff are on standby 24/7. The operating hours will be posted in your ship's daily planner with most guests seen on a walk-in basis. Appointments will be given if ongoing treatment is required.

If a condition presents as serious, the medical team will stabilise the patient and refer them to an onshore hospital once the ship is in port, or in extreme cases evacuated by helicopter to shoreside facilities. Specially trained care teams exist onboard and ashore to assist passengers and their families in the event of a traumatic incident or experience.

The pharmacy will stock basic first-aid essentials, such as painkillers, cough and cold remedies and bandages, but they are also equipped to deal with gastrointestinal and respiratory conditions and they carry life-support drugs. For those on regular medication, make sure you pack ample supplies because the ship might not be able to meet your prescription needs should you run out, and some medications can be difficult or impossible to find in port.

Fees for treatments can be costly so you should make sure you have taken out the highest level of medical insurance before you travel to cover every eventuality. The medical centre's fees will automatically be applied to your onboard account, but shoreside hospitals will need to be paid in cash.

### What happens if I get seasick?

Most ships offer seasickness tablets at Guest Relations or the medical facility, but most don't carry wristbands or motion sickness patches. If you are prone to motion sickness, it is best to bring your own remedies on board with you.

In severe cases, an injection can be administered in the medical facility (fee applies), but this is not suitable as a preventative measure.

### Can I drink the onboard tap water?
Shipboard tap water is drinkable but may have a different taste to what you are used to. Bottled water, though expensive, is available on all ships and is sometimes included as part of a drink's package.

### Can I bring my own oxygen supply?
The ship is not equipped to provide guests with oxygen other than on an emergency basis in the ship's medical centre. Cruise lines usually permit guests to bring their own oxygen equipment onboard with them, but a lot will not permit liquid oxygen. Make sure that you check with the cruise line as to what is allowed and if you have to use one of their approved suppliers.

### I use an electrical feeding pump, can my liquid feeds be stored?
Most lines will be more than happy to provide extra refrigerated storage if required.

### How should I dispose of medical waste?
Most cruise lines will, by request, supply a sharps container in your cabin, and your room steward will be happy to provide any red bags for the safe disposal of any medical waste while you are onboard. Please note, soluble pouches must not be flushed into the plumbing system, place them into a sanitary bag (available from your steward) and throw in the waste bin.

### Can I receive dialysis while on the ship?
Cruise lines welcome guests who require continuous ambulatory peritoneal dialysis, however their medical staff do not have the ability to assist or administer haemodialysis treatments. Those guests using peritoneal dialysis at home should have all solutions and equipment needed to perform the dialysis delivered to the vessel at least two hours prior to sailing on the day of departure. If they do not arrive before the ship's departure, you will be unable to sail as ships do not carry dialysis fluids or equipment. Independent advice on travelling with renal conditions can be obtained from the National Kidney Federation (*kidney.org.uk*). Check with the cruise line operator for more information on their dialysis policies and procedures.

Patients can arrange to have their treatment done in port through Global Dialysis (*globaldialysis.com*), who work in partnership with dialysis centres across the globe. With a network of more than 16,800 centres in 161 countries, cruise passengers have found it easy to source a centre to dialyse while on holiday through their service.

**Dialysis Warning:** *You run the risk of missing a treatment if your ship has to bypass a port because of bad weather.*

The UK Global International Health Card (GHIC) helps patients to access state provided healthcare in all European Economic Area countries but it is not accepted on cruise ships.

Several companies provide dialysis treatment with Dialysis at Sea the largest provider on cruise ships in the world. Since their debut in 1977, they have helped thousands of dialysis users experience a cruise to a wide range of destinations throughout Europe, the Caribbean, Asia, South America and Australia. Other companies include Cruise Dialysis and Dialysis-Cruise, who provide their services on select itineraries with a number of different cruise lines including Celestyal Cruises, Hapag-Lloyd, and CroisiEurope.

### Can I buy distilled water on the ship?
Many of the leading cruise lines are able to provide you with distilled water for use with any medical equipment, though they might impose a small charge.

### What is Dialysis at Sea and how does it work?
Dialysis at Sea provides dialysis services onboard select cruises with Celebrity Cruises, Holland America and Royal Caribbean International, with treatment parallel with your usual land-based unit and medical regimen. Each cruise will sail with a renal specialist team consisting of a nephrologist, dialysis nurses and certified technicians. The dialysis takes place in the ship's medical centre, with two beds/chairs per room, usually between the hours of 6 am and 2 pm. Appointments are allocated on a first-come first-served basis, and your slot will stay the same throughout the cruise.

**Why do Disability at Sea prices differ from those offered directly by the cruise line?**
The prices advertised by Disability at Sea may differ from the cruise lines' because they have medically contracted rates and are subject to variable fees. These rates are per cabin and include the cost of their medical staff, technicians, trucks, supplies, and equipment, as well as other additional fees. The company must also carry extensive medical liability insurance for the cruise lines to allow them to provide this specialised service.

**Are we able to book just the treatment through Dialysis at Sea?**
Patients and those travelling in the same cabin must book their entire cruise through Dialysis at Sea Cruises.

**Does Dialysis at Sea offer travel insurance?**
They offer travel insurance which covers pre-existing conditions through CSA Travel Insurance. The price is based on the total cost of the cruise and the age of the travellers.

*Medical Essential:* The US insurance industry is very different from that in the UK. Make sure you buy comprehensive travel insurance that covers you for all pre-existing medical conditions and medical equipment before you book.

**Does insurance cover my dialysis treatments?**
All dialysis providers require bookings to be paid in full prior to your travel date, with treatment costing a flat rate dependent on the length of the cruise. Patients will be provided with an itemised statement of the treatments received so that a claim for reimbursement can be submitted on your return home.

Unfortunately, Medicare and Medicaid have never covered dialysis costs on a cruise as they are American companies and most ships are not US registered. However, there are other supplemental insurance companies that will reimburse a percentage of the cost of dialysis, so it is best that you contact your own insurance carrier and discuss your options.

Following a meeting with the British Kidney Patient Association, NHS England has agreed to make a contribution towards the cost of dialysis treatment onboard cruise ships, subject to certain conditions. The patient must be from England and will need permission from their renal team before travelling as they will ultimately help to recover costs on their return to the UK but they will still need comprehensive travel insurance in place as any additional medical costs would be the patient's responsibility. You will qualify for partial reimbursement per the National Tariff, on receipt of proof of payment, if a country has formal healthcare agreements with the NHS (e.g. those covered under Article 56 or those countries who have bilateral agreements with England) or the majority of ports visited are within the European Economic Area. For cruises outside of these countries you will be responsible for paying the total cost of your dialysis treatment.

Adults and families affected by kidney disease who are unable to pay for the full cost of a holiday can apply to the British Kidney Patient Association (*britishkidney-pa.co.uk*) for a grant. To check your eligibility and apply, please contact your renal unit social worker or a member of your kidney care team.

### Will I be suspended from the transplant list if I go on a cruise?
You could be taken off the transplant list if you travel outside the UK where returning the Transplant Centre could be problematic. You will need to discuss this with your renal team and ensure that the donor coordinator is aware you will be away and where you will be.

> **Don't Ask:**
> *Do the outside cabins have extra blankets?*

### How far in advance should I book my cruise with Dialysis at Sea?
Dialysis appointments and cabins aboard ships are limited, so book as early as possible to ensure that what you need is available. Dialysis at Sea can take up to 16 patients per cruise and the dialysis times are allocated on a first-come first-served basis. Cabins generally go on sale 18 months to two years in advance.

### Are the visually impaired provided for?
Most modern cruise ships incorporate braille signage throughout their public areas, including on lift buttons, and they can also provide large-print or braille menus on request. P&O, Cunard and Princess stock a selection of talking books in their libraries, and Holland America utilises Window-Eyes computer software that can read text on the internet to those with vision impairments.

# The Autonomous Cruiser

### Can I take my service dog onboard?

Several lines allow service dogs on board, but as with most things, this needs to be arranged in advance, usually at least 30 days prior to your cruise's departure. Guests must provide the cruise line with copies of the dog's International Health Certificate and current vaccination records, showing that all shots, including rabies, are up-to-date. Some ports of call will not allow dogs to disembark at all, so guests should check with all ports of call on their itinerary for any special requirements that may be in place. Guests are responsible for bringing their dog a lifejacket and all the food and medication they might require. For more information, see the 'Service Dogs' section.

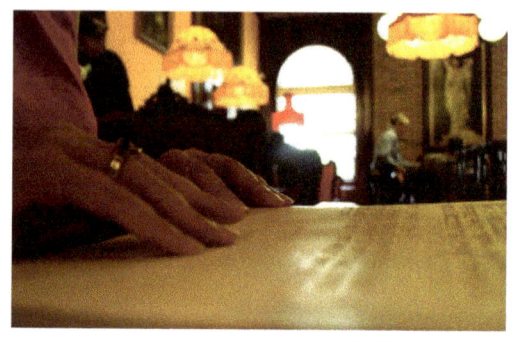

*Credit: Romanlily, Flickr*

**Disability Essential:** *Emotional support dogs are not recognised as service dogs on most cruises and are often not allowed onboard.*

### Are the hearing impaired catered for?

Cruise lines have designed several of their accessible cabins for hearing impaired guests, including ground-breaking equipment such as vibrating alarm clocks and doorbells, telephones, and smoke detectors and fire alarms with indicating-light systems. Cabins without these facilities still feature alert kits which can be fitted to any stateroom and include visual-tactile smoke detectors, door-knock alerts, wake-up systems and telephone alerts. Most cruise lines have closed-captioned televisions in all cabins across their fleet and a sign language interpreting service.

### I'm a diabetic; will I have a problem taking my needles through security?

You'll have no problem taking any needles you need onboard, but you should carry a letter from your doctor confirming that you have diabetes and require insulin, and keep all prescription medication in its original packaging. If you have an insulin pump fitted under the skin, just advise any security officer that you are wearing one and that it cannot be removed.

**Do cruise lines provide for passengers with Autism Spectrum Disorder (ASD)?**
Royal Caribbean has been leading the way in supporting passengers with ASD since 2007 when they became the first certified 'Autism Friendly' cruise line, providing a flexible children's program and autism-friendly low-volume films, among other things. They list everything in detail at *royalcaribbean.com/autismfriendly* and also have a free downloadable social story booklet, which acts as a wonderful keepsake of your cruise.

Royal Caribbean might be the frontrunners, but other major cruise lines have also followed suit and do their utmost to meet the needs of autistic passengers. For a trouble-free holiday, contact Autism on the Seas (*autismontheseas.com*), who have partnered with Royal Caribbean, Celebrity, Norwegian, Disney and Carnival to provide autistic-friendly sailings throughout the year. Their staff will accompany you on your cruise to deliver amazing travel experiences.

**I have Sleep Apnea; can I take my continuous positive airways pressure (CPAP) machine with me on the ship?**
There is no reason a CPAP machine can't be accommodated for, but you will need to check with your cruise line that the ship's electrical system is compatible. You might feel more comfortable renting a suitable machine from a reputable supplier (*ukcpap.co.uk*)(*britishsnoring.co.uk*) who will not only ensure you have the right device for your needs, but will also provide extra masks and filters for your trip . Remember, there is a shortage of plug outlets in cabins so pack a long lead extension cord to make sure you can place your machine optimally. Most of the major cruise lines will provide distilled water for your machine, but this is something their staff can advise you on when you call to notify them about your particular needs.

**Does the ship's excursion office provide accessible tours?**
Cruise lines will provide accessible tours at selected ports wherever possible. The excursion brochure usually indicates whether a given outing has an activity level deemed mild, moderate or strenuous to give you a vague idea of how accessible they are, but you should consult with the staff at the excursion desk for assistance when purchasing tours to make sure they're suitable for you. If the trip requires you to access a vehicle yourself, you or your caregiver are responsible for collapsing a wheelchair or scooter and placing it on the bus.

***Mobility Essential:*** *You need to ensure staff are aware of your actual needs. Wheelchair users have booked tours in the past, only to find that they were expected to be able to climb the steps into the tour bus themselves.*

***Tour Essential:*** *If your shore excursions are operated by minibus, there will usually be no storage space for mobility scooters or wheelchairs.*

If you booked your cruise through a specialised travel agent, they should be able to recommend local accessible tour agents in each port. Independent accessible tour companies will even offer a guarantee to get you back to the ship before sailing, so you don't have to worry about being left behind. These firms are specialised and have everything in place to meet your needs and provide an enjoyable day. These tours can all be pre-booked and a representative of the company will be waiting quayside for you and your companions on the day of a tour. There may be additional costs, but they will have more sightseeing options and flexibility than the ship's tours, and if for any reason you need to cancel or the ship has to miss the port, most companies will offer a no quibble refund.

### What if there is an emergency on the ship?
If you have a disability or are mobility impaired and feel as though you may need extra help in an emergency situation, you must advise your cruise line at the time of booking. In the unlikely event an emergency does present itself, members of the crew will be dispatched to guests needing assistance getting from their cabin to their muster station.

To comply with worldwide emergency procedures, lifts are not used in an emergency. Instead, evacuation chairs are used to transport guests down sets of stairs if needed. Guests with motorised aids will need to transfer to a standard wheelchair or evacuation chair if they need assistance due to the additional weight and the subsequent risk of injury to the guest or crew member.

### Do people die at sea?
Several decades ago, it wasn't unusual to hear horror stories concerning a death on a ship. It was thought that if large quantities of ice cream appeared on the menu, it was because the freezer was needed to accommodate a body. Contemporary cruise ships are now legally required to carry a small morgue that can house three to six bodies (varies by ship size) to accommodate the estimated 200 passenger deaths a year.

Cruises of three or four months can usually only be afforded by retirees, with an average age of 75, and for a ship dominated by septuagenarians, a few deaths are to be expected. The majority of cases are the result of natural causes.

The ship's care team will help the deceased's next of kin with repatriation, contacting their insurance company, arranging travel and working with local authorities. On a long cruise, the body will be offloaded at the next port if the country is willing to accept the charge and issue a death certificate before repatriation. If the incident occurs on a shorter trip, the body might be kept in the morgue until it reaches the return port.

**Can I scatter ashes at sea?**
You are permitted to scatter ashes in international waters – 12 miles out to sea from any port of call – but not all cruise lines allow guests to do so in open waters, so you will need to check with the cruise line operator before making any firm plans.

Scattering a loved one's remains at sea is a growing cruise trend, and lines like Marella offer a Social Host to help you make arrangements for the scattering ceremony, as will P&O, Cunard and Carnival, who perform over 200 services each year for families.

There are no strict laws governing scatterings at sea although in most cases, a Death Certificate and a Cremation Certificate are required. You could simply release the ashes straight into the sea, or you might consider using a biodegradable salt urn specifically designed to float and slowly dissolve into water. Ashes don't affect the quality of the water but do not throw materials such as wreaths, ribbons, or balloons into the ocean as they might contain metal or plastic parts and they pollute the water and can be a danger to the wildlife.

## Disability Apps

*An abbreviation of 'application', an app is a piece of software designed to perform a specific task on your mobile device, such as a smartphone or tablet. In just a few short years they've become a phenomenon, and nowadays there's an app for almost everything, with the majority available for both Android and iOS devices. Below is a short list of some of the most tried and tested apps for people with disabilities.*

**Travel Smart**
This handy travel app provides a potentially life-saving database of police, ambulance and embassy numbers for just about every country on any itinerary. Other useful features include live access to UK and US travel warning notifications, a seven-day weather forecast for your selected location, a currency converter, a basic translator for every national language and a list of national country holidays.

**Doctor Care Anywhere**
This app lets you arrange a virtual consultation with a UK trained doctor no matter where you are in the world. They'll offer support and advice, and will help you access the medication you need by way of a private prescription delivered to a local chemist, whether at home or overseas.

**mPassport**
This app connects you to care doctors and specialists, hospitals, dentists, chemists and embassies worldwide. You can then request appointments, file a claim, find a medication's availability or its generic and local brand name, and you can even translate medical terms and phrases using the app's audio feature.

**iTriage**
An app created by two ER doctors that helps you locate your nearest hospital, emergency room, urgent care clinic, imaging centre, GP surgery and chemist, and includes maps and directions to their facilities. You can also access emergency hotlines and medical advice lines, and you can even look up the waiting time at select hospital emergency rooms and urgent care facilities. You can also search for medical symptoms, diseases, conditions, procedures, medications and drugs.

**Ask a Doctor**
This app gives you instant access to a database of more than 15,000 reliable doctors worldwide. You can ask health questions, attach photos of symptoms or send your latest laboratory results, and you'll receive a reply in a matter of minutes.

# Where to Start?

**CareZone**
This app helps you manage prescriptions, medications and keep track of any instructions your doctor may have issued you after diagnosis, treatment and discharge. Track your symptoms, weight, changes in diet, glucose, blood pressure, oxygen saturation, mood changes, medication reactions, bowel movement, etc., and share detailed information with medical and professional services.

**LookTel Money Reader**
Just point your mobile phone at a currency note and this amazing app will instantly recognise it and speak the denomination in real-time, enabling users with visual impairments to easily identify and count bills, whether paying them out or receiving them. The app supports 21 of the most popular currencies, and the voiceover feature is provided in several languages, including English.

**KNFB Reader**
This text-recognition app is invaluable for blind, dyslexic and users with a vision impairment; it accurately converts any printed text, whether emails, documents, books, labels or memos, to speech or braille (via a connected braille display) at the touch of a button.

**TapTapSee**
This app is designed especially for the blind and visually impaired and allows you to take a picture or video of almost anything and the voiceover function will identify it verbally. This fabulous app can recognise any 2 or 3-dimensional object from any direction within seconds.

**Color Blind Pal**
This app is packed with powerful features to help people who are colour blind see the colours of the world around them. The app offers three modes: the first gives a description about the particular colour, the second corrects for colour blindness, and the third is a simulation experience in which the user sees the screen as someone who is colour-blind would.

**uSound**
Developed by hearing and sound specialists, this personal amplification smart audio system helps people with hearing impairment and boasts many similar features to that of a high-end hearing aid.

### HearingOS – Hearing Aid App
By attaching headphones to a digital device, this app lets users amplify (per ear) the sounds around them, with three frequency bands tuned towards speech understanding and the option to heighten foreground or background sounds. *('Hear Max: Super Hearing Aid & Sound Amplifier' is a similar app that works on Android).*

### RogerVoice
This ground-breaking app works in over 100 languages worldwide and uses voice recognition to convert voice to text, so the deaf and hearing impaired can 'hear' phone calls. Call anyone and get a real-time transcription of the conversation. The call's recipient doesn't need to have the app or a Smartphone themselves.

### Relay UK
This simple app helps deaf, hard-of-hearing, and speech-impaired people make phone calls to anyone using the national relay service. Just download the app, link your phone number and it's ready to use. You pay nothing for the service, just the cost of the phone call itself.

### Spread Signs
This app provides the largest dictionary of sign languages, with over 200,000 signs in 19 different languages that help you to learn individual letters, whole words and phrases.

### Medisafe Pill Reminder
A life-changing drug management tool that keeps all your medical information in one place. Receive personalised medication alerts, drug interaction warnings, prescription refill reminders, doctor appointment prompts and automatic time zone detection. You can even nominate a family member, friend or caregiver to receive notifications if you forget to take your medicine. The app also boasts a health journal with 20+ trackable health gauges, such as weight, blood pressure and blood sugar levels for various medical conditions, including HIV, Crohn's disease, diabetes, hypertension, cancer, anxiety, depression and multiple sclerosis.

### Diabetes Pal
A diabetes management app that helps track, analyse and share your blood glucose level, medication, and food data manually and automatically. There

is a built-in logbook that is updated with a single tap to display trends over a selected period, including your blood glucose average over time, averages based on meal tags, and breakdowns of your highs and lows.

**Glucose Buddy**
This comprehensive diabetes management app tracks and records blood sugar, insulin, weight, blood pressure and A1C levels. Monitor your blood sugar and carbohydrate intake hourly and log your meals using the substantial food database.

**Carbs & Cals - Diabetes & Diet**
This app contains over 3,500 food and drink photographs with the carbohydrate, calorie, protein, fat & fibre values clearly displayed above each image.

**Wheelmap**
Available in 32 languages and with more than two million sites, this invaluable app helps you find and rate wheelchair-accessible shops, restaurants, cafes, toilets, parking lots, bus stops, clubs and public transport anywhere in the world. Anyone can help evaluate a venue according to its wheelchair accessibility using a simple traffic light system, so you can trust that the ratings are genuine and written by like-minded people who have used the facility themselves.

**WheelMate**
Another fabulous tool that offers an instant overview of the nearest wheelchair-accessible toilet facilities and parking spaces worldwide. With over 35,000 locations across 45 different countries, this app is powered by wheelchair users who have verified every single site themselves, ensuring its accuracy.

**accessaloo**
Created by Disabled Accessible Travel, this accessible toilet finding app addresses an essential part of living with reduced mobility. With information on transfer space, turning circle, support rails, ramps and changing facilities, the app is invaluable and unique in

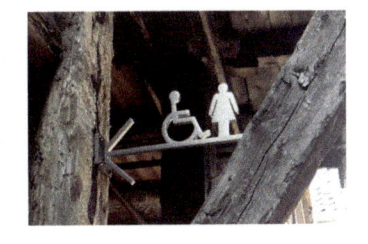

# The Autonomous Cruiser

that it also offers visuals of each toilet so you can judge whether the facilities will suit your specific needs. You can also add new or update existing facilities to extend the database.

### Flush – Toilet Finder & Map

This essential tool provides the quickest and easiest way of finding a nearby public bathroom. Simply open the app and it will display the nearest toilets to you, giving clear directions on how to find them. With over 190,000 bathrooms in its database, you are sure to find one wherever you are, plus you can filter the search results for toilets that are wheelchair-accessible, require a key, or that charge for their use.

### Access Now

This great app identifies accessible sites around the globe. Search for specific locations, filter the map to find places with specific accessibility features, and if the information isn't already there you can add it yourself and contribute to the worldwide community.

### Access Earth

A community effort that makes travel easy and equal, and encourages more people to take on a new adventure. The app's database finds places based on the accessibility criteria that will suit your special needs. Simply select a place to eat, drink, sleep or sightsee in the area you want to go and the venue's page explains the features available such as step-free access, wide doors, ground floor rooms or accessible bathrooms.

### Uber Taxis

This useful cab-hailing service provides fast, reliable rides in minutes and is available in more than 630 cities worldwide, day or night. The app pinpoints your location so your driver knows where to pick you up, and you will be sent your driver's picture and vehicle details, and you can even track their arrival on the map.

Uber has two solutions aimed at helping disabled passengers. Uber Assist or UberX is available for people with general disabilities, service dogs, and foldable wheelchairs. For non-foldable chair users, Uber Access has vehicles that are fully wheelchair-accessible. Check *uber.com/cities* to see if Uber is available in the city you want.

# Cruise Choices

Once you've decided that you want to book a cruise there are several things you need to think about when it comes to planning a holiday appropriate for your group. The first, of course, is what type of cruise you should book:

> **Don't Ask:**
> *Does the ship make its own electricity?*

- **Mini cruises:** Mini, taster or preview cruises are offered by several cruise lines to tempt first timers into trying life at sea by providing the same amenities, food options and entertainment available on their longer cruises, but without the same time or financial commitment. Seasoned travellers also often book these two- or three-day getaways to go duty-free shopping or sample the many European Christmas markets available in December.
- **No-fly cruises**: A no-fly cruise is perfect for those that can't or simply don't want to fly. The last few years has seen more UK port sailings than ever before and the days of having to travel to Southampton are a thing of the past. With more regional sailings than ever, locals have the benefit of a close-to-home getaway. Fred. Olsen offer multiple departure points across the UK, with popular cruises to Norway, Greenland and the Canary Islands. Of course, Southampton is still home to the big brand cruise lines, such as Royal Caribbean, Princess, Celebrity and P&O.
- **Fly-cruises**: Exactly what it says on the label, fly-cruises are the perfect way to explore distant lands in a limited amount of time. Flying to an exotic location allows you to maximise your time spent exploring the surrounding areas without having to endure extended time at sea. Plus, if you have booked a cruise from the Caribbean or the Amazon, you will also have the advantage of enjoying a warmer climate from the moment you step off the plane. A fly-cruise might be the perfect opportunity to book a few extra days holiday either side of your cruise to fully explore your home port.
- **All-inclusive cruises**: Luxury brands such as Azamara Club Cruise, Regent Seven Seas and Silversea offer all-inclusive getaways as standard which can include business-class flights, transfers, unlimited drinks, Wi-Fi, shore excursions and gratuities. All-inclusive deals do vary widely - some lines even include free parking, specialty dining, a drinks package and no gratuities. They can represent great value

for money, but do your research before committing yourself to make sure the deal will work for you; for example, you may have a drinks package included in your cruise fare, but if you find out that your favourite tipple is not included and incurs an extra cost, you'll very quickly spend more than you bargained for.

- **River cruises**: For those that don't want to risk sea sickness or don't fancy a lot of sea days, a river cruise can be a perfect holiday and a great way of exploring some of the most beautiful waterways and cities in Europe. Usually smaller and more intimate than a standard ship, a river cruise gives you a front row seat to beautiful landscapes, world-famous vineyards and fairy-tale hamlets that the bigger cruise ships cannot access.

- **Expedition cruises**: These cruises typically focus on exploration and adventure, visiting natural habitats and specialist locations. Enrichment talks are delivered by experts in the fields of ornithology, photography and geopolitics. Usually carrying a complement of Zodiacs (*inflatable boats*), passengers are rewarded with amazing beach or polar landings.

- **Special events and themed cruises**: Today's market offers themed cruises aimed at almost every special interest, from antiques and art to astronomy and cookery, the list is truly endless. Special event themed cruises are often based on a major festival, celebration or sporting event, some of which could even include your ticket to the event itself. These unique sailings have the added bonus of an enhanced activity program that might include seminars, tutorials, celebrity workshops and special shoreside tours. If you have a particular interest and would like to go on a themed cruise, check out those already on offer at *themecruisefinder.com* or sign up to several cruise lines' emailing lists.

- **Cargo, container & freighter ship voyages**: These sailings are primarily used to transport cargo, but they do carry a limited number of passengers who eat, live and interact with the captain and his crew. These cruises are about the journey, not the destination, and one has to bear in mind that the itineraries, dates, duration and ports of call are not binding: they can be, and often are, altered at any time. While container ship travel might not be for everyone, it does offer up a new type of adventure which is a little off the beaten track.

- **Repositioning cruises**: Throughout the year many cruise lines move their ships from one side of the world to the other to take advantage of better weather and a buoyant market. Instead of travelling across the globe with an empty ship, the cruise lines offer the one-way journey at a greatly reduced fare to make up for fewer destinations and more sea days. They are often advertised as transatlantic or oceanic crossings and the fare can include the cost of the flight.

- **Back-to back cruises**: Back-to-back cruising is a popular option that simply means taking two consecutive cruises in a row on the same ship. Each leg is handled separately so you will be required to settle your onboard account from the first sailing and pick up your new cruise card during the turnaround. If you wish to leave the ship and visit the home port, you will be issued with a 'transit card' if your cruise card is not ready, ensuring you bypass the check-in lines when you want to re-board. You will usually need to clear immigration on changeover day, but the process varies according to your cruise line and the laws in place in the disembarkation port. On some cruise lines, back-to-back passengers will only have to meet in a designated area to get clearance without actually having to leave the ship, while others will escort you into the terminal to clear immigration, after which you will be free to re-board your ship. If you have managed to book the same stateroom for both cruises, you will be able to leave your luggage in your cabin - if not, you will need to re-pack your cases ready for your steward to store until your new cabin is available.

- **Adult-only cruises**: Some of the more popular cruise lines have adult-only ships or dedicated sailings that are exclusive to grownups. Older ships tend to cater to the over 21s as families tend to opt for one of the newer builds with extensive resources aimed at children. The larger liners do, however, have private, adult-only spaces so there will always be a chance to get away from it all. In fact, you may even be able to visit adult-only beaches, bars and restaurants if your cruise line docks at their own private island.

- **Voyages**: Several cruise companies offer longer sailings that involve a lot of consecutive sea days to reach distant destinations. P&O and Princess have regular trips from the UK to the Caribbean, which typically take over a month. Extended days at sea are the perfect way to unwind before experiencing the excitement of landing in exotic shores. Other popular long-haul destinations include Alaska, Hawaii and the Far East.

- **World Cruises**: The ultimate travel experience and one that used to only be available to the wealthy, but with so much competition, prices are now more reasonable than you might think. World cruise itineraries vary between cruise lines, but they generally range between 90 and 120 days. If you can't afford to be away for that length of time, you could always opt for just one of the world cruise 'legs', which can range from two weeks to a month.

# European River Cruising

Some of the most beautiful rivers and waterways in Europe can only be accessed by canal or longboat, posing many problems for the mobility challenged. Accessible cruising is much more difficult on river cruises because, by design, the vessels are much smaller than cruise ships. River cruise operators would love to be able to provide total accessibility, but with low bridges and tight locks to navigate, each vessel is restricted to a maximum build size. As such, river cruising is not best suited to those who use a wheelchair, but it may be appropriate for passengers with other disabilities and mobility impairments.

Two of the biggest obstacles for wheelchair users are the limited access on gangways and the crew's restriction from being able to personally attend to passengers who have mobility challenges. Accessing a modern-day cruise ship is easier to manage at a dedicated cruise terminal with level access and lifts, but the same is not true for riverboat landing piers where gangways have to be used. They are problematic because they are generally narrow, ridged and invariably placed at a steep angle when water levels rise. Less able passengers must have a caregiver or travel companion with them who is willing and able to help where needed.

Watch out for the terminology 'wheelchair-friendly' - it does not necessarily mean that a wheelchair lift is available. Also, though a cabin might be deemed 'adapted', it doesn't necessarily mean you can navigate the whole stateroom by wheelchair. For instance, a lot of cabin bathrooms are not fully accessible, so you need to be realistic about whether a journey along a river is really the right cruise for you.

*Mobility Essential:* Wheelchairs will not fit through most cabin doors on a river cruise, so only standard-sized collapsible chairs are accepted onboard, and they

## Where to Start?

*must be stored in your cabin. Electric wheelchairs or scooters are not permitted, with the exception of cruises on MS Viola and Prins Willem Alexander.*

River cruising has grown in popularity enormously over the last few years, and where once your vessel could berth by the town it was visiting, now the waterways are saturated with traffic looking to moor. River ships all share docking ports in Europe, and during your cruise it is likely your ship will be docked next to one or two other vessels, two or three abreast (known as rafted moorings). On these occasions, a neighbouring vessel may temporarily obscure the view from your stateroom. If your ship happens to be moored furthest from the landing pier, disembarking could involve walking across gangways that link the ships together (usually on the Sun Deck or Atrium level) before having to traverse a set of stairs to get ashore. It is unlikely that a cruise line operator will be able to advise you in advance as to whether or not you will encounter these rafted moorings.

**Mobility Essential:** *Wheelchair users will need to be able to get off the ship without their chair, and it will need to be light enough to be lifted on and off the ramps if you want to take it ashore.*

Another alternative type of docking might see you berth at an industrial port, often a fair distance from the town you wish to visit, meaning a shuttle bus will be needed. Note, there is no guarantee that it will be accessible to wheelchairs.

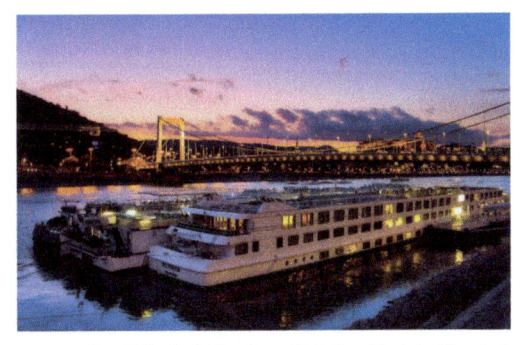

*Credit: Rafted Moorings - Krisztian Korhetz, Unsplash*

As with any cruise, the ports tend to be the highlight of your experience. It's best to choose your river cruise itinerary carefully as Europe's older towns and cities aren't the easiest to traverse in a wheelchair, owing to the cobbled streets, steep inclines, winding lanes with no dropped curbs and cafes and shops with a stepped entrance. UNESCO World Heritage Cities are often the most challenging as the sites are protected and don't allow for any modern additions, including ramps or lifts.

# The Autonomous Cruiser

The historic waterways of Europe offer easy access to all the major cities and towns that adorn it, meaning some of the most popular attractions are very close to the landing piers used by river cruises. In this sense, Viking has an advantage over its rivals in that they have their own docks at prime locations in most major cities, making it even easier for the mobility challenged to travel independently.

### *River Cruising Mobility Essentials:*

- *Getting on and off the ship can present a challenge, as gangways are narrow, ridged and steep. As such, it is not possible for a wheelchair user to embark the ship in their chair.*
- *Unlike an ocean cruise, a lot of gangways have rope steadiers rather than a solid handrail.*
- *River cruises are low in the water so they can easily pass under bridges, however, this means the top deck, typically the Sun Deck, is often only accessible by stairs.*
- *The storing of mobility aids can be a problem as most cabins are too small to accommodate a wheelchair or walker. River cruise lines stipulate that any equipment would need to be collapsible and stored in the closet or under the bed as floor space needs to be kept clear.*
- *All river cruise lines stipulate that an able-bodied companion must accompany a physically challenged guest, including wheelchair users, and assist them throughout the cruise.*
- *The majority of tour excursion operators do not supply an accessible coach or bus, meaning they typically don't have an accessible ramp and guests will need to be able to negotiate the vehicle's steps and store their mobility aid themselves.*
- *Tour or shuttle buses may not be able to accommodate the transportation of wheelchairs, scooters, and at times, walkers. If a wheelchair is deemed necessary for use ashore, then guests are recommended to explore independently.*
- *Tours are often included in your cruise fare but you are under no obligation to participate. Those that do should be able to walk unassisted and navigate flights of stairs, cobblestones, unpaved areas and the occasional steep incline. Most historical sites are not completely accessible by wheelchair or scooter.*

# Where to Start?

- *Each guest would need to be able to evacuate the ship unaided in the event of an emergency.*

If you are a permanent wheelchair user planning your itinerary, it might be better to select a cruise with fewer ports of call so you can stay onboard and enjoy the stunning scenery from a perfect spot on deck. If you prefer to explore, a trip through the wine-growing regions of Southern France is ideal as it stops in Macon, Lyon and Avignon, which can all be explored without a shuttle transfer.

**River Tip**: *Be prepared for any eventuality. Shallow water can halt your sailing in its tracks. On a recent Russian river cruise, water levels were so low that passengers were transported to the local attractions by a coach, however it was not suitable for wheelchair guests.*

As with ocean cruising, expectant mothers are usually only allowed to sail if they will be less than 24 weeks pregnant by the end of the cruise. A doctor's letter or medical certificate is required stating the estimated due date, that mother and baby are both in good physical health, fit to travel and that the pregnancy is not high-risk. River cruising generally doesn't provide medical facilities because of the close proximity to ports and hospitals in Europe. Doctors are typically only seen on Russian itineraries but there is usually a first-aid trained staff member onboard and the Cruise Director will have a list of hospitals, doctors and chemists for each port of call.

River cruising is definitely not for everyone, especially those that have difficulties with their mobility. However, if you decide you can tackle the restrictions, stand for short periods and can climb a few steps onto a tour bus, then it can make for a fantastic holiday.

**Don't Ask:**
*Does the ship work better at sea level or in the mountains?*

## Old vs New

Cruising was not always as popular or widespread as it is today, starting with the advent of mail and cargo transport, with ships not catering to passengers until the late 1800s. Immigrants were added to the manifest but they were hidden away in steerage, where they grabbed what little sleeping space they could and were left to their own devices when it came to sourcing food. It is hard to

## The Autonomous Cruiser

believe now that the industry nearly met its demise in the advent of the post-war period, losing popularity in the wake of ships being seized by military forces and used as troop carriers. Cruising lost its way until the advent of the much-loved television programme *The Love Boat*; possibly the most bizarre marketing tool of the time, Princess Cruises' *Pacific Princess* and its much-loved character cast inspired people with their stories of life aboard the seas.

Cruising the seven seas was always an elitist's luxury, with only the wealthiest clientele able to actually afford an ocean voyage. It wasn't unusual to see film stars and royalty rubbing shoulders in a ship's card room. Elizabeth Taylor, Ginger Rogers, Laurel and Hardy and Walt Disney have all left their footprint across the teak decks. While cruising has changed radically in the past decades, the silver-rinse brigade often yearn for the lost elegance of cruising, where the dress codes were strictly enforced and ball gowns and tuxedos floated across the dance floors in time with the orchestra.

Silver service in the dining room or on your balcony has almost been eradicated. Leather-bound menus lovingly showcased Russian Beluga caviar before you retired to the library for a cognac and cigar; now menus' typeface is so small that it is hard to read the chef's options and a magnifying glass is needed to make anything legible. While one can't moan at the celebrity chefs who have created the more exquisite menus for the fussiest of epicureans, you now have to pay extra for the privilege of sampling their Michelin wares.

Well-appointed libraries were one of the ship's star attractions but even they are fading into oblivion, fighting for space against rows of computers. The smartphone and kindle generation see no need for the printed word and some ships have eradicated the area altogether, making way for more 'thrilling' zones, with some cruise lines morphing their ships into mammoth floating resorts where the onboard experience is just as significant as the destinations.

Staterooms of the past were almost uncomfortably small compared to the mega-liners of today, some such as Norwegian Cruise Line offer garden villas with private gardens and sun decks. Even the standard cabins offered now have been hit by the technology bug, seeing LED lighting, flat-screen televisions, minibars, electronic safes and internet ports, and they don't even use a key. Instead, you are issued with a credit card-sized sea pass that offers no indication of which way up it goes, with some having to feed the lighting system as well - not only does this inevitably lead to leaving your card in the wall slot when you exit the cabin, but on several occasions, the 'key' doesn't even work. Of course, the blame is put on you because your sea pass has touched your mobile phone and become demagnetised. The fact that you don't even own a mobile phone doesn't help the situation, but eventually you are issued with a new card. Another trip to reception because that doesn't work either. You then have to stand outside the cabin door and wait for maintenance, who finally arrive only to find that the batteries needed replacing in the lock. You don't get all those problems with a proper key!

Gone are the days of a tour excursion brochure that was posted to your home address twelve 12 weeks before your departure, allowing you to leisurely look at what the itinerary offers in way of destination experiences. Now, you have to endure the frustration of trying to access the 'Manage My Booking' area online. When you finally find the tours being offered you have to click back and forth to find what you need. After coming back from a quick bathroom break the system has logged you out and you have to start over again. It is a hateful process that takes away the sheer joy of dipping in and out of a picture-laden booklet.

Some people of a certain age don't own a computer let alone the printer needed to obtain your e-ticket and luggage labels! The days of gorgeous tags arriving in the post used to evoke excitement that the holiday was fast approaching, but now you are among the lucky few if your luggage doesn't go astray because the paper label has been ripped off. Hours later when you realise you haven't received your bags, a search-and-rescue mission is initiated to try and unite you with your precious belongings.

Apps are being introduced so that the ship's daily planner, entertainment, menus and excursions are at your fingertips, probably marking the end of paper versions being delivered to the cabin each night. To cap off the whole experience, the Guest Questionnaire is now sent out digitally one or two days after your return home. While it makes sense to avoid the ship's senior officers being able to doctor the bad points before it is seen by Head Office, not offering a paper version for those that don't do email isn't fair either.

Those passenger vessels of old have become resort destinations - 2014 saw the first official smartship with the introduction of Royal Caribbean's Quantum of the Seas. Brimming over from bow to stern with next-generation technology, one has to wonder where it will stop.

Before the advent of the smartphone, e-reader, laptop or tablet, people couldn't wait to turn their back on the workplace to enjoy a well-earned break. Now, they can't wait to take the office with them. Apparently a big selling point nowadays, Regent Seven Seas Cruises recently announced that

# The Autonomous Cruiser

it was doubling the internet bandwidth size across their fleet, meaning faster surfing for those that want to stay in touch and share their travel experience with family, friends and business associates at home.

There is little argument against the implementation of stabilisers and bow thrusters, though some would say they love feeling the swell of the sea beneath them. The larger ships are limited in the ports they can berth at and the thought of offloading 5000 people by tender is terrifyingly tedious, not just to you but also the locals who shudder at the thought of being flooded with more foreigners than the port can handle.

What once appealed to only the elite, senior and retiree with stable incomes now appeals to younger age groups and the family market, with the Caribbean topping the polls as favourite destination. The benefits to cruising remain: unlimited luggage, a safe environment, amenities remain open unaffected by delays, and you wake up in different countries.

In order to grasp a hint of those glory days, one has to opt for a smaller sailing vessel that upholds the traditions of the past, like those offered by Regent Seven Sea, Crystal, Oceania and Silversea, where the beauty of the cruise is the peaceful days lounging at sea. However, most of these brands have a good selection of staterooms catering to wheelchair users and the hearing and seeing impaired, and with only a few hundred guests onboard the service is personal and the crew will bend over backwards to help but unfortunately, they carry a hefty price tag for the luxury of an element of the past.

The negatives with small ships are in the facilities they offer the disabled especially at the budget end of the scale, Fred. Olsen are not really designed for a permanent wheelchair user and the adapted cabins are not equipped with any of the features such as bed-shakers, flashing lights or an emergency button that a deaf or visually impaired guest might require. All Marella's ships have accessible cabins and cater for the visually impaired and hard of hearing but guests need to be able to walk up the gangway themselves when embarking or disembarking.

**Non-Disability Cabin**

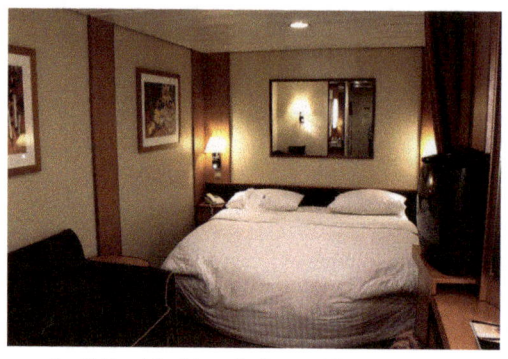

Credit: Royal Caribbean Radiance of the Seas Cabin 3045 – Thank You, Flickr

Smaller numbers mean smaller queues and you won't just be a number on the ship's manifest. There will be outside deck seating options and quiet spaces to reflect in. The crew will not only know your name, but your drinking and dining habits, and they will remember it year after year.

You will be more likely to dock throughout your itinerary and not be held ransom over the weather cancelling a port. Being able to stroll off the ship gives a great sense of freedom and you gain hours in the port of call instead of the time wasted queuing for a tender, a process that of course has to be repeated to get back on the ship. The number of tenders launched, are limited by the port authority and trying to get 5000 people across the bay, can take as much as three hours.

Although not for everyone, traditional cruising will enforce dress codes more rigorously than the super-liners, have a real orchestra for after-dinner dancing and have dance hosts at your disposal. Each offers smaller, more intimate surroundings, fewer gadgets, less technology, and although there are children to be found onboard, they are considerably less in number than on the mainstream cruise lines.

Old vs new, tradition over technology, the decision is yours.

## Dress Codes

> **Don't Ask:**
> Do all the decks go to the same port?

The age-old question of "what should I wear?" has to be answered quite frequently when it comes to packing for a cruise, and for some it is a fashion minefield. In order to attract a younger and more diverse clientele, many cruise lines have relaxed their stringent dress codes, no longer insisting on black tie every night but instead introducing new, more relaxed themes, like Cunard's 'Semi-Formal Nights', Oceania's 'Country Club Casual' and Celebrity's 'Evening Chic'.

Azamara Club Cruises have even completely strayed from the customary dress code and has adopted an overly relaxed regimen. Formal nights are no longer enforced, instead they encourage their clientele to adopt a 'resort casual' dress code, where the only criterium is a pair of shoes and a cover-up in the dining room.

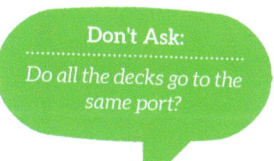

There are, however, several cruise lines that have chosen to stick with more traditional dress codes. The 'Three Queens' that make up Cunard's fleet have been defining luxury ocean travel for more than 175 years and still operate a class system. There might not be mention of first, second or steerage class, but the division is there, excluding certain guests from eating in the Queens or Princess Grill, or from visiting the private lounge or sun deck. Ladies are expected to wear cocktail dresses and men to wear dinner jackets each night, except formal nights when the ship is awash with tuxedos and ball gowns.

Information on each cruise line's dress code will be available in their brochure, on their website, and within your final cruise confirmation documents, giving you an indication of what to expect when you arrive on board and helping you plan what to pack for your trip. Typically, cruises of six nights or more will have at least three casual, two elegant and one formal evening, but you can always choose to opt-out and eat in the buffet restaurant for a more casual dining experience on any evening. In general, cruise ship dress codes only apply in the evenings, with most restaurants, bars and theatres adopting the policy from around 6pm. The ship's daily planner advises on what the dress code is that day, and when and where it will be enforced.

The bottom line is, if you don't want to dress up every night or adhere to strict dress codes, then you should not book a cruise line that enforces them - research a cruise lines' official dress code policy before making a decision.

## Where to Go?

It's up to you whether you pick your destination first and then look for the best ship that can take you there, or if you want to pick the perfect ship first and see where it goes. Both methods are perfectly viable provided you research the accessibility of the ports, otherwise you might find you spend more time on the ship than the places you'd hoped to visit.

Norway offers snowy peaks, fabulous vistas, pebbled beaches, cultural outings, husky rides, great food and wonderful shopping, albeit at a price. You wouldn't recommend it as a budget destination as it's among the most expensive countries in the world because of high taxes and high salaries, but the beautiful landscape of mountains, forests, beaches, islands and lakes, and the friendliness of the locals, make it worthwhile. Norway can be quite difficult to navigate for permanent wheelchair users during the winter season because of thick ground snow and the likelihood of tendering, but if you are the type that likes to stay on the ship then it may still be a good option because the scenery is stunning. The Northern Lights are typically only visible in the winter so make sure you have the appropriate snow tyres for your wheelchair with you. Summers see the snow melt and the more popular cities of Bergen, Stavanger and Oslo become very wheelchair-friendly. Olden offers accessible red bus tours and trips to the glaciers, while Tromsø's Villmarksenter offers dog and reindeer sledding for wheelchair users and even arranges accessible transport to their husky centre.

The Caribbean islands offer tropical heat, stunningly beautiful beaches, balmy rainforests, fabulous scenery, great food and quirky shopping. The warm waters offer fishing, sailing, scuba diving, snorkelling, kite surfing, boat trips, turtle, and stingray swims; in fact, they offer every type of water-related sports you can think of. Most of the popular islands are wheelchair-friendly if you stick to the main towns, with flat paths and restaurants and shops with ramped access. Unfortunately, the Caribbean isn't renowned for having accessible public buses, but the locals generally offer a good selection of fully accessible tours. However, there are some islands that are hard to recommend for disabled passengers, though they can still be options with good planning. Dominica has steep hills, rough terrain and terrible pavements, if any at all, Grenada has very narrow pavements, where they exist, and Jamaica is extremely hilly with steep wheelchair ramps; you would definitely need to book an independent accessible tour as most of the key sights are several miles from the cruise ports. Doublecheck the number of tender landings on each itinerary and avoid Grand Cayman and Belize if you are not able to travel over on the small boats.

European cities offer vibrant, trendy destinations you must visit for the great street life, café culture, bars, dining, fashion and shopping, not forgetting the stunning architecture and sightseeing opportunities at some of the worlds best UNESCO sites. Most European cities have made great strides in making public transport, museums and key attractions accessible - a lot of them have websites, such as *barcelona-access.com*, where you should be able to find all the information you need. Barcelona is one of the best ports for those with mobility issues, and the wheelchair ramped T3 port shuttle, known locally as the Blue Bus, runs in a continuous loop from all seven of the cruise terminals to the Christopher Columbus monument, a minute's walk to La Rambla Boulevard (Las Ramblas). If you decide you don't want to explore independently, there are plenty of disabled transport and accessible tour companies to choose from such as *accessibletravelnl.com*. As well as accessible walking tours in Amsterdam, they offer cocktail shaking workshops, private canal cruises and guided tours for the blind and visually impaired.

# The Autonomous Cruiser

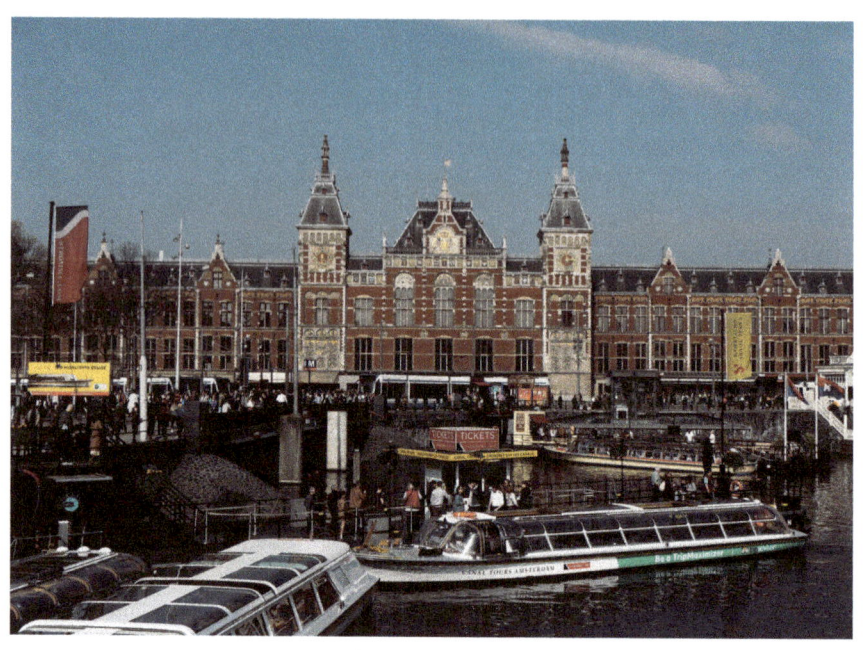

*Credit: Amsterdam canal cruises- Kanan Khasmammadov, Unsplash*

temples and unusual shopping opportunities at some of the best markets in the world. You can trek into the hills, swim in dozens of waterfalls, zipline through the jungle, experience a gibbon safari, sail on a traditional junk, take lessons in cookery or visit indigenous tribes. The scenery offers national parks, volcanoes, geologic formations, historic walking areas, mountains, bridges and sacred sites. Hong Kong public transport is one of the most accessible in Asia, with 90 of the 93 MTR stations offering lift or ramped access from the street to the main concourse and portable ramps to access the trains. In Singapore and Kuala Lumpur, the majority of key attractions are disabled and wheelchair-accessible. At the other end of the scale, Cambodia has crumbling and fractured pavements, pitted roads and staircases so steep they can even be hard for able-bodied travellers to traverse, plus, accessible toilets are practically non-existent unless you pop into a luxury hotel or the main airport. Although there are some toilets that resemble ours, others are squat toilets with no toilet paper in sight (just a nozzle spray) so take a travel pack of tissues. Most have no flushing system, just some water and a scoop. Cambodia isn't on its own, and the same applies to parts of China, Vietnam and Myanmar.

## Where to Start?

***Travel Tip:*** *Arm yourself with good destination guidebooks and the addresses of the embassy and local tourist boards in the countries you plan to visit.*

One of the big selling points on any ship is their excursion program, but finding accessible tours can often be difficult. Some cruise lines are now trying to address the situation but read the description of each tour and the small print as there are sometimes discrepancies. For example, Carnival's website boasts a selection of wheelchair-accessible tours, but on further investigation, it transpires that very few are actually step-free. The majority do not provide an accessible tour bus, and you'll be required to climb several steps into the vehicle. 'The Scenic Salem & Historic Witch Museum' is advertised as wheelchair-accessible, but in the small print it notes "Wheelchair-accessible transportation can be provided for this tour, but it is not guaranteed."

Royal Caribbean International and Celebrity Cruises offer accessible excursions that will accommodate scooters, wheelchairs and walkers but they are only available in certain destinations. If there are none on offer on an upcoming destination, the ship may still be able to make private arrangements through a land operator but it is best not to wait until you get onboard the ship before asking them to do so as it is not always possible. Small-group tours aim to provide an in-depth holiday experience with accessible vehicles with ramps or lifts, manageable attractions with flat or ramped access, step-free routes, disabled-friendly bathrooms with doors wide enough for wheelchairs, and an experienced tour guide familiar with special needs.

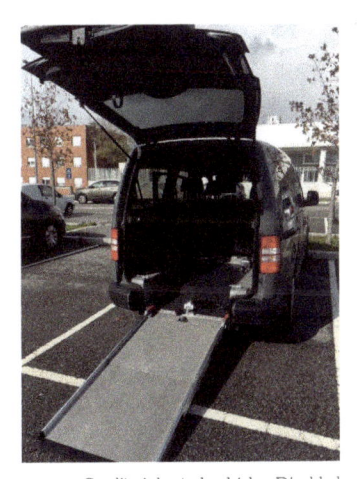

*Credit: Adapted vehicle - Disabled Accessible Travel*

P&O and sister company Cunard send out an 'Accessible Shore Experience' guide to all guests who are full-time wheelchair users and tours can be booked up to one day prior to sailing. Not every destination offers accessible vehicles, but P&O will provide pertinent details including accessibility around the port, taxi information, distance into the main town, disabled-friendly toilets, step-free places of interest and where the nearest shopping areas are. A disability questionnaire is sent out at the time of booking, and depending on how far in advance you booked your cruise will

# The Autonomous Cruiser

depend on when the accessibility excursion guide is sent to you, the earliest being twelve weeks before departure.

**Celebrity City Guide:** *Tailored exclusively to Royal Caribbean, Celebrity Cruise and Azamara Club Cruise passengers, this self-guided city tour app allows you to pinpoint all the must-see points of interest using GPS and an offline-map without any roaming costs.*

MSC has partnered with Accessible Travel Solutions and has recently launched custom accessible tours for guests with all types of mobility restrictions in 20 destinations across the Caribbean and Mediterranean. These excursions have been created with careful consideration for safety and accessibility, guaranteeing disabled-friendly transport, step-free tour routes, run at a slower pace and accessible restroom breaks are planned during the experience. Wheelchair users must be able to self-propel or have a companion accompany them.

**Tour Essential:** *Accessible tour excursions need to be booked with your cruise line in advance, the sooner the better as minimum numbers need to be realised if the tour is to run. Independent excursions will run however few book - the choice is yours.*

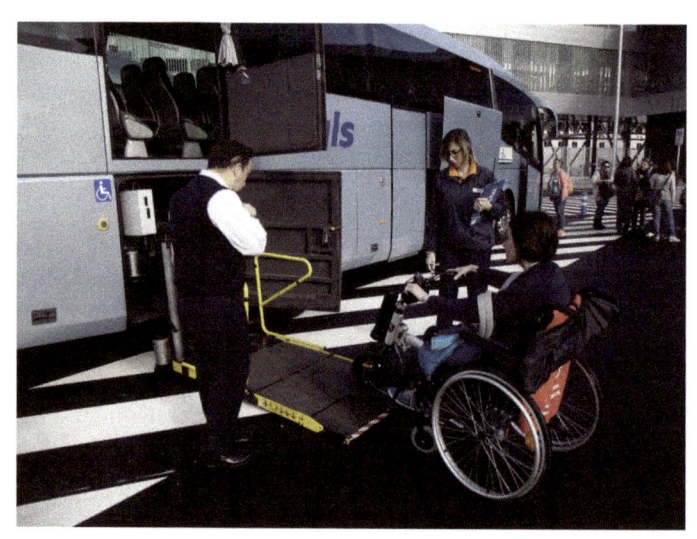

*Credit: "Adagio Tour" accessible shore excursion – Costa Cruises*

## Where to Start?

Silversea is taking their guests closer to the authenticity of its destinations, showcasing their history, culture and natural beauty with the introduction of accessibility-enhanced shore excursions. Having recently forged a new partnership with Accessible Travel Solutions, Silversea has introduced accessible tours designed especially for its disabled and senior guests in 9 destinations throughout the Caribbean and Central America, with additional shore excursions in the Mediterranean. The programs will offer step-free access, vehicles equipped with ramps or lifts, disabled-friendly restrooms and expert guides experienced with special needs guests.

Thanks to an initiative promoted by Costa Crociere Foundation and the Italian Multiple Sclerosis Association (AISM), Costa Cruises has launched 'Adagio Tours" on their flagship *Costa Diadema* which offers guests with impaired mobility the ability to participate in shore excursions on Mediterranean cruises. At every port of call, at least one group shore excursion will be offered that is accessible to everyone, including guests with impaired mobility, at no extra cost. The list of tours currently includes visits to the cities of Genoa, Marseilles, Barcelona, Palermo, Rome, Palma de Mallorca and Cagliari. 'Adagio Tours' have been developed with the help of 15 women with multiple sclerosis who have considered the needs of all guests with permanent or temporary mobility impairments, and the elderly, who want to enjoy their chosen destinations at a slower pace, with more time to discover. Neil Palomba, President of Costa Cruises, is hoping the initiative can be extended to other ships in their fleet shortly.

Looking out for a deal is probably at the top of every holiday makers 'to do' list, so bear in mind that cruise lines regularly relocate their ships to other regions to take advantage of better weather and market activity, and there is usually a price drop for these one-way sailings, to avoid sailing with empty cabins. Usually termed transatlantic or transpacific voyages, repositioning cruises aren't as attractive to the majority of cruisers as there can be long stretches at sea, fewer port visits and it will mean a flight back. That being said, cruise lines usually offer an enhanced entertainment schedule to compensate for the extra sea days, and the cruise fare might include your flight home.

Cruise lines can afford to offer up tantalising deals by heavily discounting the fare to make the sailings more appealing to the majority of passengers who usually prefer port-intensive itineraries. The lower price is partially offset by a higher revenue onboard the ship as passengers will typically spend more in the casino, bars, shops and photographic department during a sea day than if they are ashore in port.

# The Autonomous Cruiser

Clearly this list is not complete by any stretch of the imagination as there are literally thousands of itineraries to choose from - it is your mind's eye that you need to tempt. The important thing to take from this is that thorough research into the accessibility of the ports is paramount. If you picked your destination first, now's the time to grab some cruise brochures or go online to see which cruise lines and ships visit the ports you are interested in

## Bucket List

*Gibraltar, United Kingdom*: Hobnob with Barbary Macaques on the rock.
*Bergen, Norway*: Ride the funicular up to Mount Fløyen for the best views of the Norwegian UNESCO World Heritage city.
*New York, USA*: Sail in past the Statue of Liberty, the colossal neoclassical sculpture on Liberty Island.
*Moorea, French Polynesia*: Not a power cable in sight on this tiny white sand beach island paradise.
*Komodo Island, Indonesia*: Grab a Kodak moment with the largest lizard on Earth, named after its island.
*Phuket, Indonesia*: Grab a longboat to James Bond Island, the film location of The Man with the Golden Gun.
*St Petersburg, Russia*: Winter Palace, Church of Spilled Blood, Peterhof Palace, the Hermitage, St Catherine's, the Faberge Museum, the list is endless.
*Halong Bay, Vietnam*: Weave through the limestone islands in a private junk visiting the floating villages.
*Green Island, Australia*: Take a helicopter to this natural wonderland on the doorstep of the Great Barrier Reef.
*Dublin, Ireland*: Raise a glass at the famous Guinness brewery.
*Naples, Italy*: Step off the ship, and you are only steps away from L'Antica Pizzeria da Michele, the best wood-fired Neapolitan-style pizza in the city.
*Whitsunday Islands, Australia*: Have a romantic picnic on Whitehaven Beach, a spectacular uninhabited private beach.
*Gardens by the Bay, Singapore*: Don't miss the light and sound show in the giant vertical gardens. Awesome.
*Lisbon, Portugal*: Take the Glória funicular up to São Pedro de Alcântara viewpoint.
*Exuma, Bahamas*: Take a dip with the famous swimming swine in the pristine turquoise waters of Pig Island.
*Santorini, Greece*: Ride the cable car to the capital Fira adorned with white-washed houses and blue-domed buildings.
*Îleŝ du Salut, French Guiana*: Explore the prison ruins on the site of the

infamous Devil's Island penal colony guarded by hundreds of monkeys.
*Hong Kong, China*: Take a cable car ride to the Peak for the most beautiful vistas of the city.
*Sydney, Australia*: Climb the iconic Sydney Harbour Bridge and get a bird's eye view of the city's famous Opera House.
*Paris, France*: Book an exclusive lunch on the first floor of the Eiffel Tower for exceptional panoramic views of this Parisian city.
*Tallinn, Estonia*: Step back into medieval Old Town in this gorgeous UNESCO World Heritage City.
*Venice, Italy*: Hire a private gondola and cruise the intricate network of canals at night.
*Seville, Spain*: Take a horse and carriage ride past the magnificent 15th century Gothic cathedral and its famous bell tower La Giralda.
*Akureyri, Iceland*: Take a private Golden Circle tour to Godafoss Waterfall and the stunning Blue Lagoon.
*Aqaba, Jordan*: Visit the lost city of Petra and bask in the blushing red-rose coloured rock formations.
*Valencia, Spain*: Don't miss the annual Las Fallas firework and pyrotechnic festival

## Hateful Grumbles
*Port Said, Egypt*: Industrial port in the middle of nowhere.
*Rodney Bay, St Lucia*: Unpleasant hawkers touting drugs.
*Langelinie Pier, Copenhagen*: Wheelchair user's inability to cross the road at the port.
*Manaus, Amazon*: Constant muggings walking to the Opera House.
*Kuşadası, Turkey*: Relentless pressure to buy from vendors.
*St Maarten, Caribbean*: Six ships docked spewing bodies over this small, once idyllic island.
*Trinidad, Caribbean*: Unsafe atmosphere with pickpockets and begging.
*St Petersburg, Russia*: Tacky souvenir shops shoving Matryoshka dolls down your throat.
*Roatan, Honduras*: Riddled with violence even in Coxen Hole.
*Quintana Roo, Mexico*: Drug trade is a major threat.
*Prague, Czech Republic*: The Žižkov Television Tower is hard-to-love soaring to 216 metres and spoiling this city's gorgeous skyline.
*Ponta Delgada, Azores*: Two volcanos and a Burger King!
*Cairo, Egypt*: McDonald's among the pyramids! Not a pretty sight.
*St Lucia, Caribbean*: Hateful smell of rotten eggs at the Pitons.

# The Autonomous Cruiser

*Gibraltar, United Kingdom:* Duty-free liquor and cigarette shops vying for space up the high street.

*St Petersburg:* Russia: Visiting the Hermitage Museum on Monday morning to find it closed!

*Barcelona, Spain:* Isn't the price of a cruise expensive enough without Barcelona's new tourist tax.

*Fort-de-France, Martinique:* Seedy cargo terminal, long walk to town and closed on Sundays.

*Venice, Italy:* The stench of the canals.

*New York, USA:* The windowless AT&T Long Lines Building is a shocker. Tom Hanks cited it as being the most frightening building in New York, and he isn't wrong.

*Hamilton, Bermuda:* Regardless of what the itinerary says, ships larger than 700 feet long are unable to dock in Hamilton and detour to either King's Wharf or Heritage Wharf at the Royal Naval Dockyard. A bus ride to Hamilton takes an hour, and for the most part, the capital is closed on Sundays.

*Belize City, Belize:* A place to gather to discuss going somewhere else. Litter is strewn on every street corner.

*Las Palmas, Gran Canaria:* Standing tall in Las Palmas is the AC Hotel, resembling a Dalek without its arms. Talk about an eyesore.

*Nassau, Bahamas:* Dirty, dangerous, crime-riddled and unfriendly. Heavy military and police presence do not deter the locals trying to force-feed you their merchandise. Unless you pay the high-end price to visit Atlantis, stay on the ship.

*Amsterdam, Netherlands:* Why build metal-enclosed urinals and not put a urinal in them?

## Most Dangerous Cruise Ports

The U.S. State Department and travel-security experts list these destinations as posing a real danger that can threaten the loss of life or freedom. Incidences include victim drugging, gang violence, gunpoint thefts, kidnapping, terrorist attacks on tourists, machete attacks, murder and rape.

*Tunis, Tunisia.*
*Roatán, Honduras.*
*Mindanao, Philippines.*
*Jakarta, Indonesia.*
*Dhaka, Bangladesh.*
*Margarita Island, Venezuela.*
*Izmit, Turkey.*

# Where to Start?

*Aden, Yemen.*
*Acajutla, El Salvador.*
*Puerto Quetzal, Guatemala.*
*Nassau, Bahamas.*
*Manila, Philippines.*
*Port Harcourt, Nigeria.*

## Tendering at Sea

With more and more super-liners on the high seas than ever before it isn't always possible for your ship to berth in a port of call, sometimes because of the sheer weight of port traffic but often because the vessel is simply too big.

In these instances, your ship will anchor just offshore and small boats typically carrying 100 people at a time, will transport passengers free of charge to the quayside. While some passengers see tendering as an added adventure, others feel put out and get downright cross at the prospect.

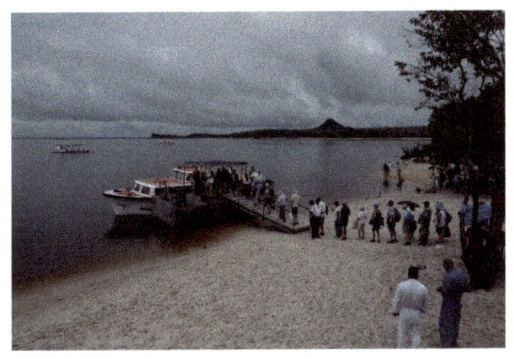

*Credit: Tender Alta Du Chau, Amazon*

Advantages of tenders:
- They offer a chance to visit small ports that larger ships cannot dock at
- They offer a great vantage point for taking photographs of your ship

Disadvantages of tenders:
- The process leads to congestion on the ship's stairs and lifts due to long queues of people waiting to disembark
- The time spent queueing and tendering can lead to a significant loss of time in port
- Some passengers can be more prone to sea-sickness on the smaller boats
- Tender ports can be cancelled because of rough seas

# The Autonomous Cruiser

When booking your holiday, check each cruise's itinerary first. Tender ports are often indicated by a small anchor or asterisk next to the port name. While it is possible to ensure your itinerary doesn't include any tendering, on occasion, even though you may be due to berth quayside, unforeseen circumstances might deem it necessary to anchor offshore.

Cruise lines require all guests wishing to go ashore to be sufficiently and independently mobile enough to be able to negotiate a small number of steps and traverse the gap between the ship's platform and tender unaided. Crew members are always on hand by the tender to help steady you as you access the vessel, but they are not allowed to support, carry or lift passengers for safety reasons. The exception to this rule is children, and as long as a parent or guardian can carry or pass them safely across the gap, they will be allowed to go ashore.

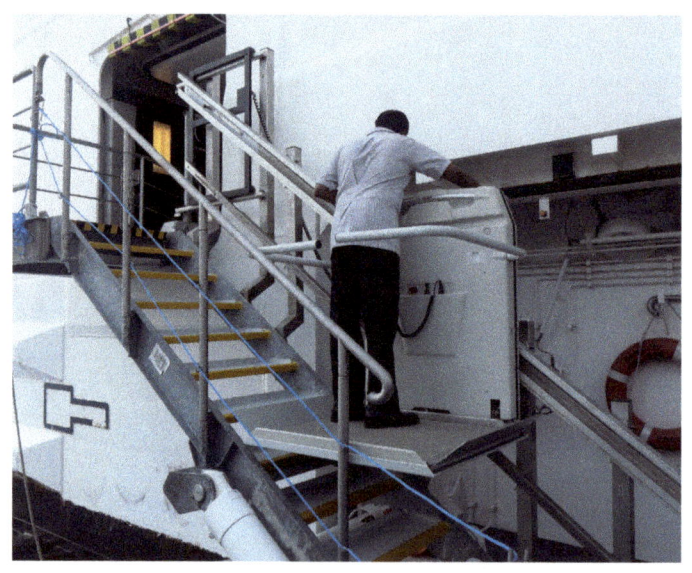

*Credit: Tender lift Celebrity Eclipse*

## Mobility Issues

A cruise might seem the perfect choice for people with special needs, especially compared to some of the obstacles associated with flying. While most cruise companies have spent small fortunes making their ships accessible, one key area has consistently been overlooked. On most cruises, guests with assistive devices who are unable to walk a few steps by themselves will be unable to board tenders and disembark at specific ports. The only real exception, especially for an electric wheelchair or scooter user, is on tender boats that have 'roll-on' capability; these are available in a few ports, and every effort is made to secure them when they are available.

***Tender Tip:*** *Princess, Celebrity, Holland America and Royal Caribbean do their best to accommodate guest's wishes, and some have installed accessible tender lifts to make the process easier.*

Guests must have sufficient mobility to be able to negotiate as many as 24 steps, typically 8" high (20 cm) down to the tender platform and traverse a gap of up to 18" (46 cm) between the ship's platform and the tender unaided. Certain cruise lines insist guests prove they can step across a certain distance by way of a mobility test before they are allowed to access the tender.

Guests who have collapsible manual wheelchairs may be able to disembark, but they or their travelling companion or caregiver will be responsible for assembling and disassembling the mobility aid. In these instances, the crew will attempt to assist where practical, provided no individual part weighs more than 20 kg (44 lbs).

***Tender Hiccup:*** *Even if the ship is scheduled to dock at a pier, it can change to tendering.*

Crew members are not allowed to lift or assist a guest in or out of a tender, so, with very few exceptions, guests with assistive devices who are unable to board the tender boat independently will be precluded from going ashore. Also, unless the equipment can be disassembled, electric or motorised mobility aids cannot be taken on standard tenders.

Holland America is one of just a handful of companies that allow wheelchair users on their shore tenders, providing a special boarding ramp and scissor lift so that wheelchair passengers can go ashore. Another is Celebrity, whose brand-new Edge and Apex offer their state-of-the-art Magic Carpet moving platform that has hugely improved the tendering process, especially for wheelchair users - an electric stairlift will take your chair down to the Magic Carpet and from there you roll onto a ramp over to the tender.

If the tender crossing is deemed difficult because of weather, swell, current or tidal conditions, a ship's officer may decide it is not safe for wheelchair users to board a vessel. Although disappointing, the decision will have been taken to ensure everyone's wellbeing, in accordance with maritime health and safety laws.

***Cruise Essential:*** *Cruise lines will not issue a refund or credit for missed ports because of tender restrictions.*

If getting off at a particular port is your main reason for booking a specific itinerary, it is best to check with the cruise company if tender restrictions are in place for those with limited mobility before booking.

***Weighty Problem:*** *Holland America states that "scooters and wheelchairs which are more than 100 lbs. (45.3 kgs) without the battery are not allowed to be transferred from the ship to tender and/or from tender to shore."*

## Where to Go From?

When it comes to choosing where to sail from, UK-based cruisers have two main options: you can sail out of one of the many great cruise ports around the UK itself, or you can choose to travel to another country, often by air, to catch your cruise.

## UK Cruise Ports

Cruising from the UK offers a wide range of top destinations and is a wonderful experience if you want to avoid flights and the trauma of trying to get through an airport unscathed. You don't have to weigh your luggage to the exact milligram or check that its dimensions will satisfy the airline's requirements, and you don't have to throw away lotions and potions because of current rules and regulations.

Forget about delays, cancelled flights, lost luggage, turbulence, plastic food, lousy hygiene or naughty brats that kick the back of your seat; there is definitely a better option. Simply drive to the port of your choice and offload your bags before parking your car and walking to the terminal - that's it, you're on holiday. The ship's eateries and bars will already be open and ready for you to enjoy. There is no sitting in a cramped departure lounge for hours on end because the plane has developed a fault or the porters are on strike. Plus, you are allowed to take as much luggage as you want as long as it will fit in your cabin.

**Don't Ask:**
*Can I water-ski off the back of the ship?*

# Where to Start?

See the section in the Directory for full details on all UK Cruise Ports and their facilities.

## Armed to Fly

### Fly-cruises

If you are flying to meet your cruise ship there are several things to bear in mind that don't factor into cruising from the UK. Flying with a disability, restricted mobility or a special need can be an unnerving experience, so it is essential that you know what help and support is available at the airport, so your journey is as stress-free and comfortable as possible. Special assistance is available to those with a hearing, visual, phycological, physical or temporary disability, those with an illness and the elderly.

Your airline must allow you to travel with a service dog if the flight departs from inside the EU, but there might be additional rules to comply with if flying from outside the EU. You can enter any UK airport with your service dog, but you must bring a harness when you travel by air, so that your dog can be secured when the plane takes off and lands. For further details, see 'Service Dogs'.

*Mobility Essential:* *The Civil Aviation Authority requires service dogs to be accredited by Guide Dogs for the Blind or another approved organisation.*

The law was changed in July 2007 with regards to flights from all EU airports in a way that ensures airlines and tour operators carry passengers regardless of their reduced mobility. Regulation (EC) No 1107/2006 stipulates that an airline reservation or aircraft boarding can only be denied for justifiable safety concerns or if the transport or boarding of a disabled traveller with special needs or reduced mobility is physically impossible, due to the size of the aircraft or its doors. If you are

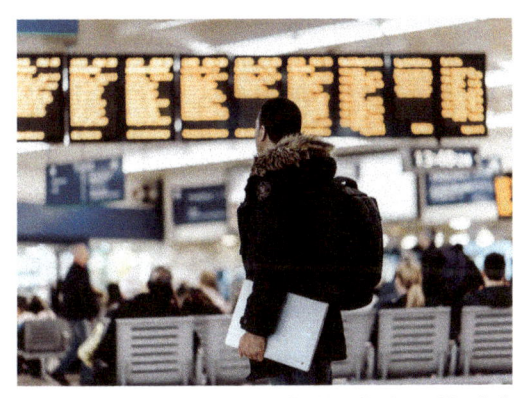

*Credit: Anete Lusina on Unsplash*

refused a reservation, an acceptable alternative must be offered. If boarding is denied having been given a reservation, you must either be provided with a full refund or a different flight route. Airport authorities are obliged to provide assistance without extra cost to the traveller concerned. Other provisions under this regulation came into force on 26 July 2008, including:

- The airport authority is obligated to ensure that every passenger receives the necessary support and assistance from their arrival at the airport right through to boarding the aircraft.
- Airlines are required to transport wheelchairs, medical equipment or service dogs free of charge on flights within the EU.
- Airport authorities and airlines must provide staff training, so those providing direct assistance to people with disabilities and reduced mobility recognise and understand how best to meet their needs.
- All airport staff should undergo disability equality and awareness training.

Regardless of whether you booked your flight through a cruise company, commercial airline or travel agent, you must inform them of your disability, special needs and any additional requirements as fully as possible at least 48 hours prior to travelling. The information will then be attached to your booking and will give airport staff time to make any special arrangements you will need upon arrival at the airport. If wheelchair assistance is requested, it should be available at your departure and arrival airport.

It is usually best to choose the fastest and most direct flights you can, even if the fare costs more. The money you could save by taking an indirect flight is not usually worth the angst of trying to negotiate changing planes and hoping your luggage and medical equipment make the same flight as you. The more your equipment is handled, the more chance there is of it getting damaged or lost. If you book multiple flights independently and one (or more) suffers a delay you could miss a connection and in turn your cruise, as the ship will not wait for late arrivals unless flights have been booked through the cruise line itself.

**Airport Essential:** *Bring your Radar key as the airport may have separate disabled toilets.*

## Where to Start?

Every UK and European airport should, by law, have their own special assistance team who are there to help guide you through the airport, all the way to your allocated seat on the aircraft. You should find assistance buttons throughout the airport to help you get help if needed, and you will also be given help with accessing the bathrooms in the terminal and on the aircraft, but you will be required to look after your own toilet needs, as airport staff and cabin crew cannot provide such support. Your destination airport will offer help deplaning, retrieving your luggage and will give general support in helping you reach your destination.

U.S law requires airlines to provide adjoining seats for a disabled traveller and their caregiver. In contrast, EU legislation simply requires air carriers to do everything possible to ensure a person with a special need is seated next to their companion, but it's not always a given - it may be best to pre-book your seats, even if there is a small charge but check the terms for doing so as different transport carriers have varied policies.

***Seating Tip***: *Passengers can request a specific seat to accommodate their particular needs. Use seatguru.com to review the aircraft's seating plan so you can determine the best place for you to sit on the plane and then request it at the time of booking. Because of safety regulations, you will not be allocated an aisle seat if you are blind or visually impaired. Speak to the airline personally if you need a seat with moveable armrest.*

eGO.net is an excellent website with a guide about the special needs, disabled facilities and parking services at each of the UK's 26 most popular airports, including who you should contact and how far in advance you need to book special assistance before travelling.

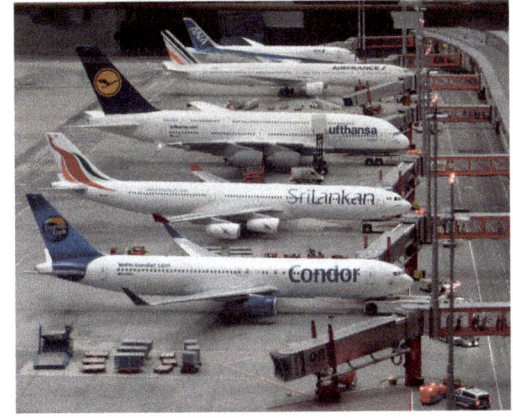

*Credit: Pixabay, Pexels*

Flying can block your ears, especially on take-off and landing. Most people experience pressure in their ears when there is a change in altitude, and if left, it can prove uncomfortable or even painful. There are several easy solutions with chewing sweets or gum the most popular. Yawning on take-off and landing is another remedy while some passengers use 'earplanes', a specialised earplug which uses filters to help regulate air pressure. Lastly, there are two equalisation manoeuvres that are effective, the Valsalva which is usually done by closing your mouth, pinching your nose shut and attempting to blow out and the Toynbee, done by pinching your nose and swallowing.

## Wheelchair Advice

Airlines are legally obliged to carry disability equipment free of charge, and you are allowed to take either a manual or electric wheelchair, or a scooter, when you fly, but you must inform your airline beforehand. You will need to provide them with the make, model, weight, measurements and whether it uses wet (acid) or dry cell batteries to ensure it can be taken in the aircraft's hold safely. If you use an electric wheelchair, take the batteries out of your mobility aid yourself and place a small piece of electrical tape on both ends of the connector. Airline staff are extremely vigilant when storing batteries during a flight, especially wet cell (acid) batteries. By disconnecting them yourself, there is less chance of the baggage handlers damaging your equipment in their attempt to detach the batteries from the chair, which they have to do to conform with airline safety. Airline policies vary hugely, so check whether you are allowed to use your own wheelchair on the flight and what procedures have to be met.

Attach clear instructions to your power chair as to how to handle it, including how to deactivate the power, how to set the free-wheel mode and how to lift it safely. Use Google Translate if you want to write your instructions in your destination's language, and if possible, laminate the information so it is rainproof.

### *Do medical devices count towards my luggage allowance on a fly-cruise?*

*The usual limit of one carry-on bag and one personal bag does not apply to medical supplies and or assistive devices (including service dogs and their equipment). Passengers with disabilities may carry medical equipment, medications, and assistive devices as an additional item of luggage. Under current law, airlines are not allowed to charge passengers excess baggage fees for medical equipment on commercial airlines, though the request does need to be made at least 48 hours in advance of travel to the airline and the cruise line.*

Wheelchair users are likely to be asked to transfer to another chair on check-in so that their own wheelchair can be loaded onto the plane. Ask the member of staff to 'gate-check' your wheelchair - this means a tag will be attached that tells the baggage handlers at your destination to immediately bring the wheelchair to the door of the aircraft, rather than wait for it in baggage claim. Even if you are not permitted to remain in your wheelchair once on the aircraft, you can ask if it is possible to take your chair through right to the cabin door. Once you've boarded the plane, your wheelchair will be placed in the hold. Before the aircraft begins its descent, remind the cabin crew that you will need your wheelchair immediately after you exit the plane.

Make sure your wheelchair is serviced and in good working order before your trip, so any potential problems show up before your holiday. Trying to fix a problem or replace parts can be impossible in the middle of an airport or abroad, but it may still be worth taking some basic tools along in your checked luggage - a screwdriver, hex key, duct tape, inner tube, tyre repair kit, adaptor plug and transformer could prove invaluable.

Put your own labels on your chair, including your name, flight number, destination airport and cruise ship, so that in the event it does get lost you are more likely to be reunited with it. You might consider buying a GPS or 'Tile' tag. Take several photos (from multiple angles) of your wheelchair before you fly so that you can prove its pre-flight condition if it's lost or damaged. EU legislation requires airports to provide a temporary replacement; this won't necessarily be on a like-for-like basis, while yours is repaired or replaced. Sadly, several airlines hide behind the Montreal Convention when they damage disability equipment, and limit compensation to approximately £1200 whereas anti-discrimination laws in the US dictate they pay the full cost.

**Special Declaration of Interest:** *'Reduced Mobility Rights' campaigner Roberto Castiglioni advises travellers booking a flight, with mobility equipment that exceeds the liability limits, to make a 'Special Declaration of Interest' pursuant to Article 22(2) of the Montreal Convention, in the delivery of your luggage. The latest you can implement the declaration is at check-in when handing over your equipment to the airline. Similar to an insurance policy it covers the transport of goods worth more than the limit set by the Montreal Convention. Every air carrier has to provide this but some charge a supplementary fee.*

It is prudent to secure any loose or moveable parts on your mobility equipment so that they are less likely to get damaged during the journey. Remove any accessories such as straps, bumpers, footrests, and seat cushions, and carry them on the plane with you.

Passengers with special needs are usually invited to pre-board the aircraft, but if you are not offered the option, ask for it. Some airlines will allow you to fly in your wheelchair, but the majority will need you to transfer to an airline seat. If you are unable to move down the aisle of the aeroplane unaided, an airport transfer chair will be provided, and a staff member will manoeuvre you to your designated seat number. Some airports also use sling straps to lift travellers into their seats. If you have any concerns, it's important to talk to the airline staff before your flight. If the aircraft is not connected to an 'airbridge', an Ambulift or scissor lift may be used.

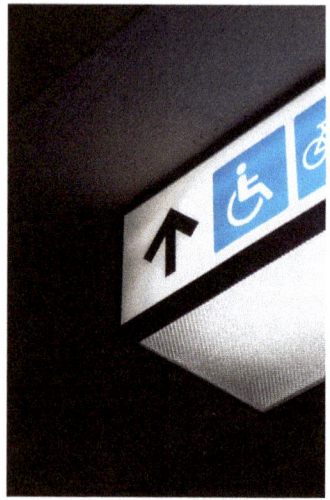

Credit: Charles Deluvio, Unsplash

**Research Essential:** *Research the airline, specifically about what facilities, seating plans and services they can provide. Confirm your preferred means of communication and whether you need information in large print or braille. It is your responsibility to ensure all travel personnel are informed of your requirements at every stage of your journey.*

Typically, disabled people do not need to get medical clearance before flying, however, some airlines may ask for evidence of your fitness to travel, mainly to better understand your ability to attend to your own personal needs. If you do need evidence, ask your doctor to provide a letter outlining your medical condition, details of any difficulties that could occur while travelling and what assistance you might then require. It is standard practice for some airlines to ask you or your doctor to complete a Medical Information Form (MEDIF) so the correct support is in place during your time at the airport and during your flight - it will only be valid for one trip and can only be used on the flights and dates shown on your ticket. Habitual travellers with a stable impairment may be able to apply for a Frequent Travellers Medical

Card (FREMEC), which will enable the airline to keep a permanent record of your specific needs on file so that you won't have to repeatedly fill in a form and make arrangements every time you fly.

Because of increased security at airports, you must check with your airline provider as to what documentation you should bring to prove your need to carry medication, and what containers your medicines should be carried in. It may be necessary to carry a letter from your doctor stating your need for the medication just in case you lose it or need to get more, especially if you are visiting a country with strict drug controls - you should always be ready to show this letter to customs officers.

Ask your doctor if your medical condition makes you vulnerable to circulation problems when flying as narrow seats and limited legroom can increase your risk of blood clots if you already suffer from restricted blood flow to your feet. To lower the risk of oedema, blood clots or deep vein thrombosis, wear compression socks which work by applying gentle pressure on your legs, ankles and feet to help blood flow. Move around the aircraft as often as possible, and while sitting in your seat do some simple exercises like shrugging your shoulders, flexing your feet, looking over your shoulder and shaking your hands back and forth as these all help blood flow. Avoid restrictive clothing, uncross your legs, keep hydrated and abstain from alcohol before and during the flight.

***Passport Essential:*** *If you are recently married and are booking a fly-cruise as your honeymoon, make sure the booking is made under your maiden name so that the name on the flight documents matches your passport. If, on the other hand, you are booking a honeymoon several months after the wedding then you will have ample time to change the name on your passport.*

## Travelling to the Airport

When making your way to the airport, the single most important thing is to allow plenty of time for your journey. If you live a long way from the airport, are travelling during rush hour, or need to park the car and are relying on an airport shuttle, it's best to allow yourself extra time just in case something goes awry. Factors like traffic jams, road closures, flat tyres, passport control, snaking security lines and distant departure gates are all things that can delay and stress you out before you even get to your airline seat. Also, travelling during peak holiday periods and on bank holidays can easily add an hour to the queue at security. You also might need to allow extra time if you require wheelchair assistance or need to check medical equipment into the hold.

If you have booked a fly-cruise or have a long journey, think about leaving a day early and staying somewhere nearby. There is a good selection of hotels near every port so enjoy a leisurely dinner, sleep off any jetlag and arrive at the terminal relaxed and ready to go.

Most airlines advise you to arrive at the airport at least three hours before an international flight and two hours before a domestic or European flight. Doing so should give you ample time to check your luggage, get your seat assignment and boarding pass, and make your way through security. Some airlines even allow you to check in the night before if you have an early morning flight.

Several airlines offer you the option of checking in online, which is both convenient and can save you time once you reach the airport, as you will only be required to deposit your luggage in a designated area instead of having to queue up to drop it off. Make sure to follow any guidelines though, as some will only require you to show confirmation on your phone, while others instruct you to print your boarding card (some insist on a specific format). Failure to comply can result in a charge of more than £100 if the airline has to print it for you.

> **Don't Ask:**
> *If I fell overboard and no one knew, would the ship come back for me?*

## Coronavirus (Covid-19)

2020 saw the world brought to its knees by a virus that is totally unprecedented. Coronavirus has affected all businesses especially the travel industry but as lockdown eases, countries are starting to reopen for tourism. There are now fewer options when it comes to flying as the demand for air travel plummeted and airlines scaled back their services. Having said that, several airlines have announced their plans to resume their flights abroad from 1 July 2020 although the UK Foreign and Commonwealth Office is still warning UK nationals against non-essential travel. Self-isolation could be obligatory for anyone entering the UK, whether by plane, train or ferry, and the 14-day rule could also be in force in several other European countries. Protective measures are either already under consideration or have already been implemented at airports worldwide and although it can present a challenge, it is for the safety of everyone. Airports have undergone a transformation with plastic protective screens, one-way floor markers that will manage flow and enforce social distancing, free masks and gloves, hand sanitiser stations, and temperature scans. Staff will wear masks and personal protective equipment in 'passenger-facing areas' at check-in and security.

Self-service check-in stations are being encouraged to lessen queues so before arriving at the airport, print your boarding card and luggage labels ready for the automated bag drop. Contactless fingerprint ID, biometric scanning focusing on face recognition, thermal cameras, and touchless data entry are all being trialled to protect airport staff from close contact with passengers and virus detection dogs are being brought in.

Safe distancing is the key and boarding gates are being redesigned to avoid congestion and seating configuration has been reduced and rearranged to give passengers more space. Large carry-on luggage won't be allowed so as to reduce congestion in the aisles during boarding. Several airlines have suspended or limited their in-flight food and drink service so there is less interaction between passengers and air crew, but holidaymakers can still bring their own supplies onboard. Aircraft carriers have enhanced their cleaning programs by sanitising their aircrafts with a fogging machine that coats and sticks a high-grade disinfectant to all the surfaces that passengers come into contact with as well as issuing sanitising wipes. HEPA filters are used on the majority of US airlines which implement an air change in the cabin every 3 minutes.

Destination countries will all follow slightly different guidelines with rapid testing on arrival in certain cities. It is best to check online before your travel date to see if any new changes have been put in place at the airport. It may be advisable to contact your airline before you leave home for any updates to the status of your flight.

As confidence returns to the tourism market, these measures could be eased back but as with other precautionary security measures of the past, this new way of flying could be here to stay.

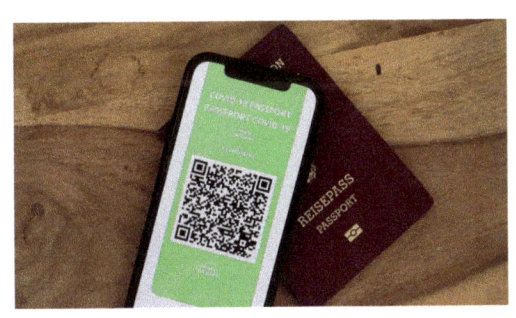

*Credit: Lukas, Unsplash*

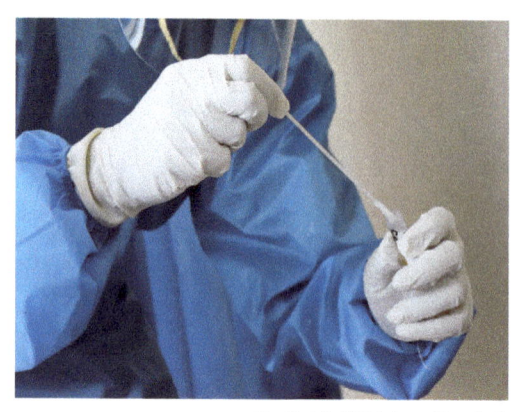

Credit: Mufid Majnun, Unsplash

## Airport Guides

Some airports, such as Manchester and Heathrow, have produced fabulous guides detailing step-by-step procedures in place at the airport. The guides cover checking in, security, baggage help and boarding the aircraft. These guides feature easy to understand text and illustrations covering everything you will need to know. *https://www.heathrow.com/at-the-airport https://www.manchesterairport.co.uk/help/passenger-guides/*

The Airport Guides Network is an excellent independent resource created to help you find everything you need when travelling to, from and around the most popular UK airports, including travel links, travel money, airport parking, car hire, maps and directions. *https://www.heathrow-airport-guide.co.uk*

The UK Airport Guides website provides in depth coverage and information on the thirty main UK Airports, including routes and timetables for buses and trains, taxis, driving directions, airport shops, bars and restaurants, long and short stay and disabled parking facilities, airport telephone numbers, UK weather, and live flight arrivals and departures. *https://www.ukairportguides.co.uk*

## Car Park Assistance

If you are planning to leave your car in one of the airport's parking bays while you are away, you must notify your chosen parking company of your disability when you make your booking so that staff are on hand to make sure your experience is stress-free. If the company doesn't have a dedicated staff member that can escort you to the terminal, ask that they contact the terminal's special assistance team to meet you at the car park and escort you to your check-in desk. Assistance buttons can usually be found close to the disabled bays, allowing you to call for support yourself if necessary.

The 'Blue Badge Scheme' is recognised throughout the UK and all car parking companies have disabled parking bays located near to the exit or shuttle bus pickup and drop off point. These parking spaces will provide the extra room needed to offload you and a wheelchair safely.

## Delayed or Missed Flight

Flights get delayed, connections get missed, ferries can be cancelled because of bad weather and road accidents can cause gridlock on the motorway. Airlines are usually unsympathetic if you miss your flight, but advise the check-in agent that you have a connecting cruise and they will do their best to help you. You should contact the cruise line or your travel agent immediately so that they can advise the ship. If your plane has been delayed and there are quite a few cruise passengers booked onto the same flight, the cruise line will do their best to wait, but it is dependent on how long the delay is. Failing that, your agent will advise you which cruise port to fly to so you can join the ship.

## Checked Luggage/Carry-on Bags

Airlines have become extremely strict over the last few years when it comes to overweight luggage and they will either impose a hefty fee to carry it, or you will be required to remove items until the case weight conforms to policy. Size and weight limits vary between airlines, so ensure you check the restrictions specific to your flight before you get to the airport. Don't forget medical equipment is not classed as extra luggage. Some airlines allow you to check in an additional suitcase, but you'll want to pre-book this as it is much cheaper online than if you pay at the airport. Airlines also impose size and weight restrictions on your carry-on luggage, the rule of thumb being that it has to be stored under your seat or placed in the overhead locker.

*Valuable Tip:* *Don't pack any valuables in your checked luggage, especially medical equipment that you can take on the plane, as insurance companies won't pay out for lost, stolen or damaged items if you check them in.*

Don't forget the 100 ml liquid restriction and ensure all liquids, creams, lotions, gels, pastes, perfumes, contact lens solutions and toiletries over the allowance are packed in your suitcase. Put all your medication, travel documents, glasses, keys, jewellery, camera, laptop, and any other important items in your hand luggage.

Make sure to attach clear labels onto each piece of luggage, including your carry-on. It is also prudent to place a label with your name and contact number into the luggage itself just in case the outer label gets detached. Unfortunately, airport luggage theft isn't uncommon, so ensure your cases have a reliable theft deterrent attached. Padlocks are easy to break into, instead, use numbered or unusually coloured zip ties as it is unlikely that a thief will have the exact replacement colour to hand. An alternative is buying Tamper-Evident luggage seals or security tape, which will ensure the integrity of your luggage.

**Security & Customs**

If you are a full-time wheelchair user, you will be able to remain in your chair during security checks, and you may wish to make one of the security team aware of any specific medical needs before a search is undertaken. If requested, security staff will take you to a quieter area so the search can be carried out with additional privacy. You must advise security staff if you feel uncomfortable or if you are experiencing pain during the process.

Passengers who have 'hidden disabilities' should carry an ID card or documentation, especially if you have a pacemaker, implanted defibrillator or metal device such as an artificial joint, and make security staff aware of where they are located. Ask for a pat-down inspection rather than going through the metal detector if it will affect you in any adverse way.

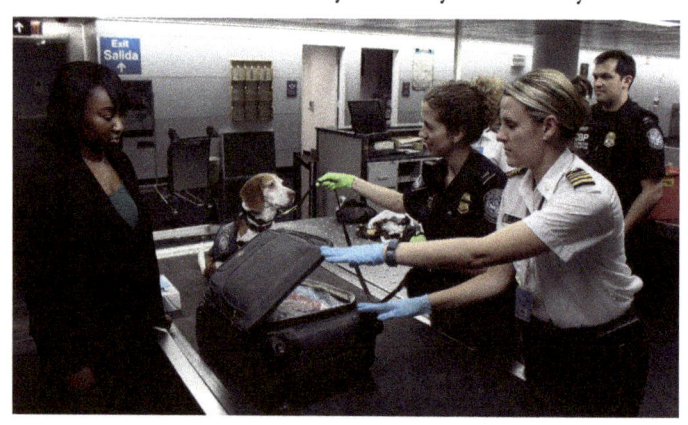

*Credit: CDC, Unsplash*

# Where to Start?

***Travel Tip:*** *Depending on your disability, security may still require you to remove your shoes to go through the screening process, so make sure they are easy to remove.*

## Special Needs

### Flying with Pre-existing Illness
Thousands of people with pre-existing medical conditions are now able to travel safely, provided that the necessary precautions are considered in advance. The World Health Organisation suggests "Those who have underlying health problems such as cancer, heart or lung disease, anaemia and diabetes, who are on any form of regular medication or treatment, who have recently had surgery or been in hospital, or who are concerned about their fitness to travel for any other reason should consult their doctor or a travel medicine clinic before deciding to travel."

In every instance you will need to inform the airline at the time of booking about any pre-existing condition, whether you are taking medical equipment onboard the aircraft, are travelling with a service dog or need oxygen or a special diet.

Medical alert bracelets enable fast identification for people with a number of chronic conditions including diabetes, epilepsy and heart patients who might be unable to communicate their illness to others. Wearing a medical ID bracelet alerts medical personnel of a specific medical or allergic condition and can help prevent misdiagnosis, unwanted drug interactions and treatments that can pose a threat to a patient's medical status.

Anyone with a disability or mobility problem is entitled to help from the special help team at the airport, whether at check-in, with wheelchair assistance, when going through customs, with guidance to your seat on the plane or with help in stowing your luggage.

### Flying with Prescriptions and Medication
Please refer to the relevant section in 'Before You Go'.

### Flying with Epilepsy
Patients with controlled epilepsy can generally enjoy air travel safely provided they are conscious of the potential seizure threshold-lowering effects of dehydration, delayed meals, hypoxia and disturbed circadian rhythm. Some

people's seizures are triggered because of excitement, anxiety or fatigue, and this can happen because of a long flight or jetlag. Inform your airline when making your booking so the cabin crew can accommodate you during the flight.

## Flying with Diabetes

You will need to contact your airline before you travel to discuss the medical equipment you need to take on the aircraft, especially if you use a wireless insulin pump or continuous glucose monitor, as the electromagnetic interference could interfere with the plane's communication and navigation systems. You might be required to disconnect your equipment (disable pairing or Bluetooth) during take-off and landing and treat your diabetes with an insulin pen, and test your glucose levels manually with a standard blood glucose meter while in flight.

***Airplane Mode:*** Once onboard your aircraft, check the policy about the use of personal medical electronic devices that communicate via Bluetooth. If it is allowed you can still take a blood glucose reading by enabling the airplane mode on your device.

Diabetes patients are exempt from the 3.4 oz. liquid rule for medicines, fast-acting carbs (e.g. juice), and gel packs to keep insulin cool; simply obtain a letter from your doctor stating that you have diabetes and require insulin and that you need pumps, syringes and needles aboard the aircraft.

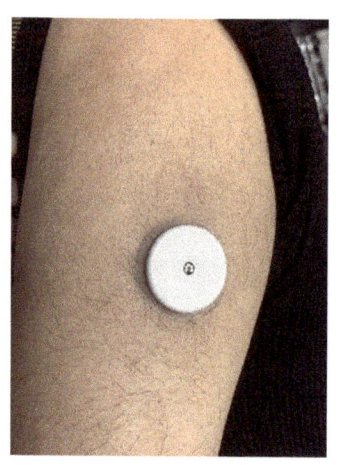

*Credit: Continuous Glucose Monitor - Vee & Mark Sweeney*

***Diabetes Passport:*** The credit card-sized Insulin Passport is used to keep an up-to-date record of the type of insulin, syringes and pens that you use. It also contains emergency information on what to do if you become ill or found unconscious and can be obtained from your doctor, diabetic practice nurse or chemist.

***Don't Forget:*** The UK Civil Aviation Authority (CAA) and Airport Operators Association

*(AOA) have sponsored the new Medical Awareness Card, which is offered as a free download from caa.org and covers insulin pumps and continuous glucose monitoring systems for those with type 1 diabetes. Regulations allow passengers with these medical devices to ask for an alternative security screening process.*

Notify security staff that you are wearing an insulin pump or continuous glucose monitor and opt for an alternative screening method, such as a pat-down, instead of going through an x-ray machine, as the electromagnetic waves could stop your equipment from working properly. Passengers should never be asked to remove a medical device from their body for a security screening. If you are carrying a spare device in your carry-on luggage be sure to remove it, as it should also undergo an alternate security screening process, such as a hand search.

If you require medication or have a dietary restriction, you and your doctor should work out an individual schedule for mealtimes, taking into account the length of your journey and any change in time zones. You should be able to order a special in-flight meal through the airline that will better suit your needs, and it's wise to carry a bag that you can keep near you with your insulin, glucose tablets and snacks like fruit, raw vegetables and nuts to prevent episodes of hypoglycaemia.

If your travel plans include time zone changes, make sure to keep a note of exactly when your insulin is due. The National Diabetes Education Program suggests keeping your watch on your home time zone until the morning after arriving at your destination. It's also a good idea to set an alarm on your phone for an alert, though beware that it doesn't switch to your new time zone automatically. If you are concerned, speak to your diabetes care team before you travel.

***Diabetes Essential:*** *Changes in air pressure within an aircraft cabin can cause bubbles to form in your insulin, and the accompanying upsurge can cause an unexpected insulin delivery if wearing a pump. Check with your insulin provider whether to disconnect your device before take-off and landing. If you administer your insulin manually, tap out any bubbles before injecting to ensure dose accuracy.*

## Flying with Heart Disease

According to the British Cardiovascular Society, "most people with heart and circulatory disease can travel by air safely without risking their health.

However, you should always check with your GP or heart specialist that you are fit enough to travel by air, particularly if you've recently had a heart attack, heart surgery or been in hospital due to your heart condition."

The choice of destination may be pertinent as the heart has to work harder in hot and cold weather extremes so you might want to consider a destination with a moderate climate. Discuss your travel plans with your doctor so he or she can tailor advice based on your personal circumstances. You will need to carry a letter from your cardiologist or doctor outlining your condition and if you have an implantable device. You will need to include copies of your medical history, repeat prescriptions, any clinical notes, most recent ECG results, scans or confirmation of any liquid heart medications such as glyceryl trinitrate that you need to take onto the aircraft as well as confirmation that you are fit to fly. Your doctor will also need to indicate if your heart condition is stable, the small reductions in oxygen levels on the aircraft shouldn't present a problem, however, your doctor may still prescribe supplemental oxygen for the flight.

If you are flying with a cardioverter defibrillator (ICD), pacemaker or insertable cardiac monitor, carry your device identification card with you and inform the security team that you have a device inserted. Identification cards can be downloaded for free at *heart.org*, or are available on *amazon.co.uk*. Heart devices such as a stent or pacemaker can pass through the screening detectors safely without setting off the alarms and without harming your equipment. However, don't allow a handheld detector to be passed directly over your device as they don't always react well and can deliver an inadvertent shock to the wearer. If you have any concerns, ask for a hand search.

***Rest Assured:*** *It is perfectly normal to be anxious if travelling with heart failure for the first time. Plan ahead and allow plenty of time at the airport so you don't feel rushed as stress is more likely to ruin your holiday than anything else. If you decide on a fly-cruise, ask for help with luggage to avoid lifting anything heavy and if possible arrive a day early and schedule a rest day.*

***Medication Tip:*** *It's safe to use your glyceryl trinitrate spray while on the aircraft.*

One of the biggest risks facing people with heart disease when flying is deep vein thrombosis. Sitting for long periods increases the risk of swelling in the legs and the chances of developing a blood clot. Consider wearing compression socks on the flight and, where possible, walk up and down the aisle when the seatbelt signs are off. If this proves difficult, move your ankles in circles for several minutes every hour. Also, avoid alcohol and drink plenty of fluids to keep hydrated.

## Flying with Dementia

If a doctor has deemed it safe to travel then flying with someone who has dementia doesn't have to preclude a trip, but you will need to be realistic about what to expect. Travelling abroad can be daunting for all parties, but with the help and support of the airport team, you should be able to travel with confidence. Always carry a doctor's letter outlining the condition and ask your GP if it would be appropriate to prescribe a mild sedative before flying, and make sure to go over all your travel plans several times with the person under your care.

Try to avoid arriving at the airport too early as the shorter the waiting time, the better the chances of avoiding disorientation and irritability. Ask the airline staff to allocate the passenger a middle or window seat so that you can sit between them and the aisle and prevent them from getting up unnecessarily. Make sure they wear an ID badge around their neck with your flight information and contact details as it is common for a person with dementia to wander about and get lost.

One particular challenge of dementia is that it is often an invisible disability, and confusion, anxiety or fear can be perceived as rude or aggressive behaviour to those unfamiliar with the person. A good percentage of the UK's leading airports now offer support for those travelling with dementia, with the introduction of wristbands, lanyards, factsheets and pins. A simple identifier might be enough to prevent unnecessary problems at security or throughout the airport in general. The process of having to remove shoes, belts and open hand luggage at security can create confusion and paranoia. Make sure to go through security behind your companion; doing so means you'll be able to assist them if they encounter a problem, whereas if you've already gone through the screening process before them, you won't be allowed to go back to help.

Look for a companion or family bathroom so you can easily assist your ward before heading to the boarding gate. They are more likely to be in the main airport's hub rather than at a boarding gate depending on the size of the terminal. Most aircrafts have one bathroom larger than the others so ask one of the flight crew to point it out to you.

It might be worth investing in an airport lounge day pass which has comfortable seating areas and a calm and relaxing atmosphere; especially beneficial if the flight is delayed or cancelled. If you have time to kill an alternative is to look for an empty boarding gate en route to yours that can offer extra space and a quiet atmosphere.

Dr Gianetta Rands, Specialist in Dementias and Mental Capacity at Re:Cognition Health, suggests that "flights with current cabin environments may challenge mental and physical health due to reduced air pressure and lower humidity. This can cause dehydration, hypovolaemia and reduced peripheral circulation thus meaning the body and brain receives less oxygen than usual, and could accentuate the cognitive difficulties experienced by the person with dementia."

> **Don't Ask:**
> *Can I fish off the ship?*

Triggers such as a crowded aircraft, cabin pressurisation, seatbelts that are seen to restrict movement, sensory overloads such as bright lights and loud noise can all cause unexpected behaviour in a person with dementia. Take snacks and noise-cancelling headphones and a music player with favourite tracks in hand luggage as once onboard the aircraft they can make the flight more comfortable, alleviate any anxiety and offer less distractions.

The Airport Parking Shop has an excellent web page called 'Flying with Dementia: The Need for Dementia Friendly Airports' with information that covers destination guides, travel tips and details of the assistance available at the UK's leading airports.

## Flying with Cognitive, Intellectual & Developmental Disabilities

UK airports have done a lot to make air travel easier for people with autism spectrum disorder (ASD), with quiet routes and areas within the airport, and online guides to help you prepare effectively. The first step to a successful flight is to inform the airline and let them know you are travelling with someone with special needs. Make sure to have a doctor's letter allowing the patient to fly and giving permission to take their medication or equipment aboard the plane. It's a good idea to carry an 'ASD Attention Card' so airport staff are made aware of the condition; if you can't get a hold of one, some airports will provide you with a lanyard for the same purpose. If you don't need any special assistance, then you might want to check-in online and print your boarding card so as to skip the queues and go straight to security.

Travelling through an airport, particularly going through security, can be daunting not only for people with ASD, but also for their companions or caregivers. The most impactful things you can do is to stay as calm as possible so that your angst doesn't transfer to the person you are travelling with, and let security staff know of any behaviour that might make your companion particularly uncomfortable. Also, putting together some visual aids to familiarise them with the security screening practice can go a long way to easing their anxiety on the day of your flight. Travelling with comfort aids like ear defenders, sensory headphones and textures, fidget spinners and weighted blankets can also help your journey go more smoothly. Alternative Airlines has a useful web page offering tips on ASD travel preparations. *alternativeairlines.com/flying-with-autism*

The Arc's Wings for Autism/Wings for All (Wings) program gives families the confidence to take to the skies by providing an airport 'rehearsal', as well as a presentation on the aircraft features and in-flight safety protocols. Put together a visual chart of photos, diagrams or maps of the airport, aircraft and destination, or watch videos so as to familiarise them with the flying process.

Gatwick Airport has produced an autism-friendly visual guide that offers an in-depth understanding of processes which can be applied to any airport. *gatwickairport.com/globalassets/passenger-services/special-assistance/autism-guide.pdf*

## Flying with a Breathing Disorder

If you're dependent on oxygen you will need to check with your chosen airline as to the requirements of taking your equipment or medicine onboard, as each airline has its own policy regarding oxygen cylinders. In most cases, a letter from your doctor will suffice, but some airlines will insist that they fill in the airline's medical form informing them of, among other things, your fitness to fly. Some airlines also have specific seating requirements, such as passengers who use a portable oxygen concentrator not occupying an exit row seat. It should be okay to take a CPAP machine onboard as hand luggage, but again, always check with your airline before you travel, and make sure to carry a copy of your prescription.

You should ensure that your equipment is in good working order and that you have enough batteries in your carry-on case to power it for the duration of the flight, plus 50% extra to allow for any unexpected delays. Also, make sure the battery terminals are covered or taped to prevent them from coming into contact with other metal objects, which could cause a spark and ultimately a fire.

## Flying with Kidney Disease

Travelling with kidney disease can be challenging, and you may be subject to certain travel restrictions if you are on a transplant list, so be sure to discuss your travel plans with your medical consultant and determine if flying while waiting for surgery is prudent. They might want to consider your destination carefully and advise you to avoid long flights.

Passengers are able to take a peritoneal dialysis machine onboard as hand luggage, but because of their size, a home dialysis machine will usually need to be stored in the hold as checked luggage. As long as you are carrying the correct documentation to prove you are exempt from liquid regulations, the airline will allow syringes and dialysis fluids on the aircraft. If you have been given a special low sodium diet to follow from your doctor, you can pre-order a special inflight meal from the airline and pack natural snacks to eat between meals to avoid processed foods sold onboard.

## Flying with a Visual Impairment

A sight impairment isn't always visibly apparent and can present communication and navigation challenges with others unaware of the struggles you can come up against when travelling. Flying with a visual impairment can be an intimidating prospect, but with a little preparation, you can have a smooth and easy journey. Planning is essential: think of all the obstacles you may encounter and how you will address them, and don't be embarrassed to ask for help at any point of your journey.

As with all special needs, you will need to inform the airline of your requirements as far in advance of your departure date as possible (at least 48 hours), especially if you are travelling with a service dog, wheelchair, medical equipment or if you need help through security and onto the aircraft. Ensure that you also request assistance at your destination airport so that a member of staff will meet the plane and walk you to the gate of a connecting flight or through customs and to your pick-up point. If you are travelling with a service dog you will also need to offer confirmation that it has been trained to an acceptable standard that allows it to travel safely by air. For further details, refer to the 'Service Dogs' section.

Passengers needing special assistance will need to check-in at the airline desk and not online or at a self-service kiosk. Before checking-in your luggage it's wise to make it easier to find at baggage claim: affix it with tactile bump dots (made of plastic with a self-adhesive backing), attach an audio luggage locator that you can control via a controller, or wrap it with neon-coloured tape so you can easily describe it to someone helping you collect it.

Airports are full of unfamiliar territory, wandering and confused travellers, and carelessly placed luggage. As such, it might be best to ask for wheelchair assistance even if you don't usually use one, as terminals are cavernous and difficult to navigate at the best of times, and the distance from check-in to the aircraft can be extremely long. The handler will whisk you through security and to your gate without you having to traverse the obstacle course yourself.

**Seating Tip:** *Aircraft safety regulations stipulate that aisle seats are not allocated to the blind or visually impaired. If you do have any specific seat requirements, such as needing a moveable armrest, speak to the airline personally.*

A lot of airports don't make audible announcements, but if you have already spoken with your airline about special assistance then a member of staff will inform you if there is a flight delay or when it is time to board your aircraft. KNFB Reader is a multiplatform app that converts any printed text, such as terminal maps, flight departure boards and menus, into audible speech which can be read aloud or turned into braille that you can read on a compatible braille display. The app doesn't even require an internet connection, so you can activate it anywhere.

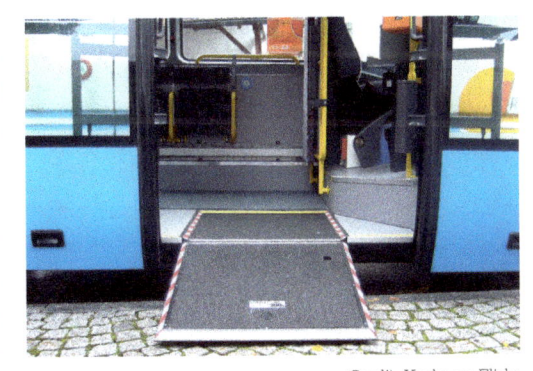

Several airports worldwide, including Heathrow and Gatwick, now offer Aira, an app which connects travellers to a trained agent for advice on navigating through the airport, help reading flight screens, assistance finding gate numbers, accessible toilets, shops and restaurants

*Credit: Kecko on Flickr*

within the airport, and even help identifying luggage. The free, on-demand app provides blind and visually impaired passengers with the confidence to move through the airport.

Visit the Transport Security Administration website and print and fill out their wallet-sized disability notification card before arriving at the airport, as it can provide a discreet way of informing officers at the security checkpoint of your sight loss. Your hand-luggage, walker and white cane will be passed through the x-ray scanners. If you can't walk through the scanners without your cane, let security know and they will either provide a physical pat-down or return it once it has been scanned.

Once onboard your aircraft, the cabin crew will be more than happy to help you throughout your flight. If you use a white cane that does not fold, they will secure it in an overhead locker for you. They will be happy to help open bottles or cans, read the menu before the meal service, identify food and explain where it is placed on the tray, unwrap and cut up your in-flight meal and help you in filling in an embarkation form. If you require the toilet during your flight, press the call button located above your head and someone will escort you to the nearest facility and then assist in taking you back to your seat.

**Safety Tip:** *Most airlines provide a personal safety briefing for blind and vision-impaired passengers before take-off. If you would prefer the safety instructions in braille, request it at the time of booking.*

No matter which overseas port your ship is sailing from, make sure you research what facilities and services are available in the area. If you are staying in a hotel the night before getting on the ship, find out if there is a shuttle bus available, or if not, what ground transport can take you from the hotel to the port. Uber is excellent for travellers with a disability, but they are not available in every city.

### Flying with a Hearing Impairment

Hearing impairments aren't immediately apparent to others and can present communication and navigation challenges when travelling, especially to foreign shores. Planning and implementing as many arrangements as possible prior to your flight is essential and will make your journey much easier.

What can be a simple exercise for the average person can be overwhelming for travellers with an inability to hear important information and announcements, make or confirm reservations over the phone, understand accented speech or local terms, use a mobile phone in a public place, hear warnings or safety announcements on the aircraft, or hear fire alarms during an emergency.

Consider making your reservations online and sign up for email or text confirmations and alerts so you have instant access to any important announcements about delays or cancellations. Alternatively, work with a travel agent who specialises in working with the hearing impaired and request that all arrangements are confirmed in writing. Download your airline's app so you can review your reservation, check-in early and access your boarding card. For health and safety reasons, those with hearing loss are prohibited from flying in an exit row, so be sure to check your seat location when checking-in. Consider reserving an aisle seat so you can more easily communicate with the flight staff whilst onboard.

As with all special needs you will need to inform your airline of your travel plans at least 48 hours before your flight, especially if you require assistance to guide you through the airport, through security and onto the aircraft. Advise your airline if you are travelling with a service dog at least 14 days before your flight and offer confirmation that it has been trained to a standard that allows it to travel safely by air. For more details on travelling with a service dog, see the 'Service Dogs' section.

The majority of UK airports have specialised assistance personnel who are trained in basic sign language skills, so it is important to contact the airport's help desk to request this service and verify that it can be offered upon your arrival. If, for whatever reason, the help is unavailable, using a self-check-in kiosk can help sidestep the difficulties of communicating with the airline staff at the regular check-in counter. Visual noticeboards listing arrivals, departures and gate numbers are readily available throughout the airport, so you don't have to worry about missing an announcement over the tannoy. Most of the airport's public address systems do, however, include audio induction loops which will amplify and enhance the sound quality and reduce background noise if you use the 'T' (Telecoil) switch on your hearing aid. Alternatively, you can also request that someone inform you personally as soon as your flight is announced, if it is delayed or if your gate number is changed. If you're worried about not being able to find an electronic noticeboard when you need one, the FlightTrack5 and FlightTracker apps essentially transform your smartphone screen into a flight board, with more than 3000 airports and 1400 airlines covered worldwide.

When passing through airport security you are not required to remove your hearing aids, but the Transport Security Administration (TSA) recommends that you advise a security officer that you're wearing them before the screening process begins. Visit the TSA website and print and fill out the wallet-sized disability notification card before arriving at the airport as it can provide a discreet way of informing officers at the security checkpoint of your hearing loss. Security scanners won't harm your hearing aids or other personal listening devices, but it may be a good idea to lower the volume as scanners can occasionally cause excess noise in your hearing aids.

Once at the departure gate, tell the airline staff that you have a hearing impairment and need to be notified in person when it's time to board the aircraft. You will usually be offered pre-flight boarding, giving you time to go over the safety procedures with one of the aircrew before other passengers start boarding. Ensure that the cabin attendants are aware of your special needs so you are alerted to any important announcements made before, during and after the flight; most of the standard announcements, such as the information and safety videos, will have subtitles on most airlines. Before take-off, the flight staff will ask for all electronic devices to be turned off. This directive does not apply to hearing aids unless they feature an FM system. It might be tempting, but try not to take your hearing aid out during the flight so you are still able to hear any in-flight announcements or directives.

Before leaving home for your holiday, pay a visit to your audiologist and make sure your hearing aids are in good working order.

Although hearing aids are available from the NHS as a long-term loan, getting them privately can cost hundreds, if not thousands of pounds, so if you have a spare take it with you in case of damage or breakage. Bear in mind that hearing aid batteries and tubing might not be easy to buy in the countries you're visiting, so take extras and pack them in your carry-on luggage, along with a converter if they are rechargeable. Most hearing aids are vulnerable to damage from moisture, so if you are visiting hot and humid climates be sure to pack a dehumidifier. Lastly, pack a protective waterproof case and cleaning kit to keep your hearing aids safe and well maintained.

**Pre-flight Checklist**

- In all cases, you will need to inform your airline of your special needs at least 48 hours in advance. Discuss any specialised equipment you need with you, such as portable machines, batteries, respirators or oxygen. Some airlines won't accept wet cell (acid) batteries or oxygen cylinders. You will be required to provide the airline with details on the make, type and weight of your equipment.

- You should carry a doctor's letter explaining your condition, any medical notes, EKGs, prescriptions, scans or anything else you might deem necessary to help make your journey comfortable and stress-free.
- Ensure that you take ample medication with you and that it is allowed in the countries you are visiting - all medication should be kept in its original packaging. Always keep a copy of your prescription and dosage in case you lose your medicine while abroad.
- It is obligatory to travel with an able-bodied companion if you need help eating, using the toilet, or cannot get to an emergency exit unaided - cabin crew are not allowed to provide such assistance. Failure to meet these conditions might mean you will not be permitted to travel.
- Make sure you take out specialist insurance that covers your pre-existing conditions and any equipment you are taking with you, including full replacement cover, repairs and the hire of a temporary replacement.

## Return Journey

If you need to book a flight for the same day you disembark the ship, make sure it's not early in the day. Even though your scheduled docking time might be as soon as 6 am, the vessel will need to be cleared by customs which can be a lengthy process. You'll also need to factor in the time required to disembark the ship, collect your luggage, clear customs, and make the journey to the airport, which you'll need to arrive two to three hours before your flight. The time adds up quickly even with a smooth departure, not to mention the possibility that the ship docks late due to adverse weather conditions. For all these reasons, it's best to book your flight for the late afternoon or early evening, if not the next day.

> **Don't Ask:**
> *Are there kids on the adult-only cruises?*

Passengers should prearrange any specific help they require with the assistance services at the airport at least 48 hours before travelling home. This will ensure that the support is available as soon as you arrive at your departing airport and when you land back at your home airport.

## Lost/Delayed Luggage

There are a few things you can do to reduce the chances of losing your luggage, or minimise the repercussions if it does happen. For example, using a luggage locator or a luggage 'tile' will massively improve your chances of locating a lost bag quickly. If your baggage is delayed, have the cruise line liaise with airport officials on your behalf and arrange for your bags to catch up with you. If you're travelling with someone else, pack a change of clothes in their bag as it's unlikely both of your cases will go astray. Finally, it's worth taking photographs of all your luggage before leaving home as it will be easier for the ground crew to locate lost bags this way and also acts as proof of their condition before your flight.

**Transfers**

Booking a fly-cruise will include a shuttle transfer from the airport to the pier, which you can secure at the time of booking through your cruise representative, travel agent, or online personaliser before your cruise. The round-trip service will also guarantee your shuttle bus seat from the cruise port back to the airport on the day of your departure. If you choose to book your flight independently, you'll have to provide your cruise line with your flight details before purchasing your transfer; occasionally the transfers are included in your fare, but usually there will be an extra cost involved. A uniformed representative of the cruise line will meet you at baggage claim if arriving on a domestic flight, or outside of customs if on an international carrier and ensure your safe and timely transfer to the ship. Note that, though you might get through immigration quickly, you may have to wait for other passengers to come through or arrive on another flight before the shuttle will leave for the ship. If there are several of you travelling together it will be quicker, and often cheaper, to simply catch a cab from the airport's taxi rank. If you do use a taxi, make sure to know your ship's exact docking location (some cities have more than one cruise port) and inform your driver accordingly, otherwise you run the risk of being dropped at the wrong place with no

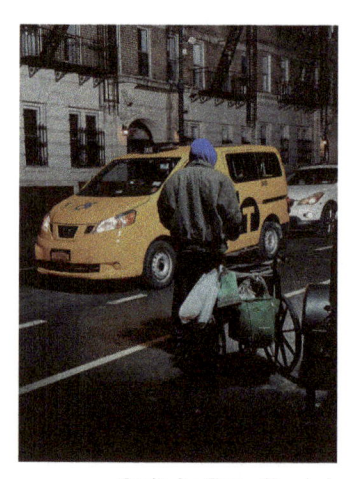

*Credit: Jon Tyson, Unsplash*

easy way of getting to the correct port or dock. Uber is a good option if it's available, as your destination is entered through your phone so you won't have any communication problems if you don't speak the language. They are typically cheaper than a regular taxi, offer accessible vehicles and arrive fairly quickly.

**Doublecheck:** *Accessible lift or ramped transportation may not be available from the airport or embarkation port you are using. You will need to inform the cruise line of your needs in advance so they can offer an alternative arrangement if at all possible.*

If you have booked accommodation for a pre- or post-cruise stay, most major hotels have their own airport transfer services that will also drive you to your port on the day of your cruise. The shuttle may be included in the price of your hotel room, but the fee is usually reasonable if not. When you check-in to the hotel, confirm the times the shuttle is running to the cruise port, as some only offer a limited service.

## In-flight Tips

- Wear loose clothing and comfortable shoes as feet tend to swell.
- Wear knee-length compression stockings to avoid swollen legs and to reduce the risk of thrombosis, which is always a risk when flying, especially if in the air for more than four hours.
- Avoid blood clots forming by avoiding alcohol, drinking plenty of water, exercising your calves and stretching your legs as much as possible.
- Chewing gum, sucking a sweet, swallowing, yawning or blowing your nose will relieve air pressure in your ears.
- Avoid wearing contact lenses as aircraft cabins can often dry out your eyes and make the lenses uncomfortable.

## Pre- or Post-cruise Accommodation

With practically every fly-cruise it is possible to add on a few days either side of your cruise to enjoy your embarkation port. Be specific about your accommodation requirements – ask for whatever you need to make your stay comfortable and ask for written confirmation of everything that's promised to you. Your cruise agent or tour operator should be able to advise you on the suitability of most hotels, but you can also call the hotel or resort directly to speak to someone more familiar with their rooms and services. Some questions particularly worth asking are:

# The Autonomous Cruiser

## Bedrooms

- Can the hotel offer ground floor accommodation or can you be near a suitable lift?
- Is the bedroom door wide enough and does it open outwards or inwards?
- Do the bathroom facilities suit your needs: is the room large enough, is there a roll-in shower, are there grab bars?

## Facilities and wheelchair access

- Is there ramped or step-free access to all the main areas of the hotel or resort?
- Is a lift available that will be suitable for your wheelchair or other equipment?
- Are charging facilities for electrical equipment, such as a wheelchair, available in the room?
- Can any equipment you need, such as backrests, bathing equipment, hoists, ramps or mattresses be hired locally? Local disability groups might be able to provide rental information.
- Can your dietary requirements be met?
- Are there facilities for service dogs?

## Car use

> **Don't Ask:**
> Has the Captain been trained?

- Although there has been no official disclosure from the Government post-Brexit, the Blue Badge Scheme should still be recognised throughout the EU, so take yours with you if you intend to hire a car.
- Many countries have adapted vehicles available for hire, but make sure you know the licence requirements, driving laws and road conditions of the area.
- If hiring a car, make sure the company is fully aware of your needs and check the level of insurance they offer.
- In many areas, accessible vehicles might not be available. If this is the case, try to book a taxi in advance, but be sure to state your needs to ensure they can accommodate you safely.

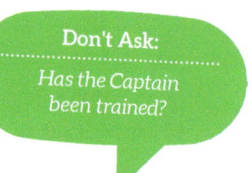

Where to Start?

## Armed to Fly Apps

*If you are among the thousands of passengers considering a fly-cruise, these apps might help make your journey a little easier.*

**App in the Air**
After entering your flight number, this free app will keep your entire journey organised from start to finish, including showing you your check-in times, boarding times, take-off and landing times, any delays and your gate number. You can set up notifications to keep track of any changes to your flight or gate number so you will know before arriving at the airport.

***Did You Know:*** *It can take up to a day to readjust for each time zone you cross when travelling by air.*

**Hopper**
This award-winning gem of an app trawls through millions of flights and analyses the data, notifying you of the cheapest time to book your flight. Grab a deal quickly and securely, right in the app with just a swipe.

**iFly Airport Guide**
A must for frequent travellers, offering information on more than 700 airports, including a list of which restaurants are closest to your gate, whether or not there is Wi-Fi, local parking rates and locations, on-site banks and ATMs, and what your transportation options are once you've reached your final destination.

**LoungeBuddy Lounge Access**
This app gives you access to airport lounges around the world in seconds. Look up the hours of operation, location, ratings, reviews, photos, amenities, access requirements and guest privileges for more than 2000 lounges.

**Rome2rio**
Searches any city, town, landmark, attraction or address across the globe to find you thousands of multi-modal routes on flights, trains, buses, ferries, rideshares or rental cars. Whatever your preferred mode, they get estimated prices, journey durations and booking details from over 5000 companies in more than 160 countries.

**TripIt**
This pocket travel agent pulls together your travel information from your confirmation emails for flights, hotels, transfer reservations, car rental, and event bookings and converts them into a single itinerary that can be shared on social media.

**TravelerBuddy – Trip Planner and Flight Checker**
Check your flight status, including delays and cancellations, gate changes, local weather, currency exchange rates and customs regulations. Get information on any travel risks, visa requirements, and necessary passport validity. Edit your travel plan either on your phone or web app and print and share your itinerary. You can even navigate to places such as a hotel address with their offline built-in maps.

## Who to Go With?

Deciding which cruise line, and more specifically which ship, to book is one of the biggest decisions you have to make when planning your holiday. There are a host of things to consider to make sure you choose a ship that's suitable to your group's needs, but with so many options on the market, you are sure to find something that will work for you.

British travellers had a raw deal up until a few years ago because most ships catering to the UK market were older and thus the onboard facilities for the physically challenged were sadly lacking. Now that the more modern American cruise lines have started regular seasonal sailings out of Southampton, things are getting better for the UK cruiser. Carnival Cruises, Celebrity Cruises, Disney Cruises, Holland America Line, Norwegian Cruise Line, Princess Cruises, Regent Seven Seas and Royal Caribbean International are frontrunners when it comes to the disabled facilities onboard their ships as they work to Americans with Disabilities Act (ADA) standards. Most also have specially trained staff for physically and mentally challenged guests.

There is little point in considering a Fred. Olsen cruise from Liverpool, Rosyth or Leith if you use a wheelchair or scooter, as you will be physically unable to board the vessel; unfortunately, neither port has an overhead air-bridge or a sloped gangway (with angle subject to tidal conditions), so passengers must be able to manage a stepped gangway with minimal assistance.

# Where to Start?

Fred. Olsen and Saga specify that unless the overseas ports have an overhead air-bridge, wheelchair-bound passengers may not be able to disembark.

If you are looking for naturism, then cruise with Hapag Lloyd or Aida which both have designated topless areas or choose a nudist cruise with a company like Bare Necessities or Shoes Only Travel.

It's best to arm yourself with the brochures of the lines you are considering and check their websites, as most lines have pages dedicated to special needs and accessibility. For those with impaired sight, a travel agent should be able to provide all information in large print or braille, on disc or memory stick, as an audio file or in an email.

One of the most important things to consider is the size of the ship that will suit you - there are more than 350 vessels to choose from, with sailings on super yachts that carry around 60 people all the way up to the mega-resort-style ships that can carry more than 6000 passengers, and of course everything in between. The larger the ship the longer the distance to walk or wheel. Your decision should be based on, among other things, the facilities you want onboard, how busy you want the public areas to be, and whether or not the ship will be able to dock in your preferred ports, bearing in mind that smaller ships are less likely to require tenders. While many ports provide easy access for wheelchairs and scooters, due to various conditions (steepness of the gangways, tendering, weather, tidal and sea conditions, and shore-side facilities) anybody using assistive devices may be precluded from getting on or off the ship.

*Credit: Mobility at Sea*

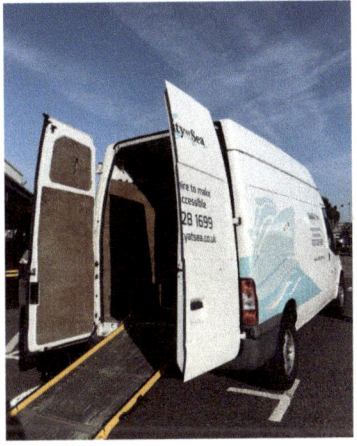

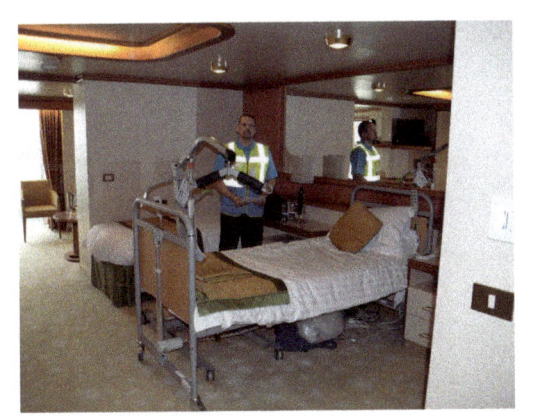

*Credit: Mobility at Sea*

Before discounting a cruise line or ship because it doesn't have the specialist equipment you need as standard, check if you can 'order' what you need, either directly through the cruise line or through a specialised supplier such as Mobility at Sea. Note, if you book equipment independently, it is your responsibility to have it delivered and picked up from the ship.

For full information on the disabled facilities available onboard different cruise lines, see the 'Disabled Facilities on Your Favourite Cruise Lines' section in the Directory. Before making your final decision, check out *cruisecritic.co.uk* and *worldofcruising.co.uk*, the best websites for unbiased reviews written by cruise experts.

What follows is a few cruise line recommendations for various groups, tastes and interests, designed to whet your appetite - of course, there are many more options out there.

## Best for Romantics

If you've just met a new partner, have recently rekindled an old relationship, want something special to celebrate your 30th anniversary, or want to book a honeymoon, a cruise can be the perfect way to share an unforgettable romantic experience together.

*Passport Essential: If you intend to get married and want to book a cruise as your honeymoon straight after, make sure the booking is made under your maiden name so that your name on the cruise documents match the one that is in your passport. If on the other hand your honeymoon is several months after the wedding then you will have ample time to change the name on your passport.*

### Seabourn

This cruise line prides itself on offering the crème de la crème of cruise experiences, with the Odyssey offering a nearly 1 to 1 crew to passenger ratio. All five ships offer luxurious amenities both inside and outside the suites, intimate spaces, couplesT massages, elegant dining and sprinkled rose petals on your bed. Seabourn is committed to providing accessible accommodations for all persons with disabilities. (*seabourn.com*)

### Windstar

Windstar's fleet of intimate sailing and power yachts offers luxurious touches, attention to detail and port-intensive itineraries. Queen-sized beds, luxury linens, flat screen TVs with DVD players, fresh flowers and fruit await your arrival. Enjoy intimate candlelit dinners for two by the pool or sample 5-star dining at a time to suit you. Star Breeze, Star Pride and Star Legend each have four accessible suites equipped for disabled guests. (*windstarcruises.com*)

### Azamara

*Azamara has three intimate ships with port-intensive itineraries, offering fabulous shoreside adventures. Book the 'Nights in Private Places' package for sole use of the aft spa deck together with your own private butler who serves champagne and canapés followed by a sumptuous candlelit dinner. Float in the thalassotherapy pool and spend the night nestled in your loved one's arms on the canopied daybed stargazing. Azamara welcomes all guests with special needs, including those that use dialysis or oxygen. Wheelchair-accessible cabins are available, as well as cabins equipped for the deaf or hard of hearing, and the blind or visually impaired. (azamaraclubcruises.com)*

## Best for Weddings

There is a wealth of lines offering customised wedding packages if you want to renew your vows or plan your dream wedding - most offer a vast array of options, which can turn a basic package into a full-blown spectacular affair. Upgrades can include unique photography and videography services, including a 'Trash the Dress' photoshoot, hors-d'oeuvres, specialty menus, live entertainment, fresh flowers, aisle runners and even a fresh rose arch.

Some ships offer 'Embarkation Weddings', which takes place on the ship before it sets sail so you can celebrate with family and friends who are not sailing with you. 'A Wedding at Sea', on the other hand, requires all guests to sail with you. 'Onboard Destination Weddings' are offered when the ship is docked at a particular port, with the ceremony taking place onboard, while a 'Destination Venue Wedding' happens off the ship, either on a beach or a similar beautiful location.

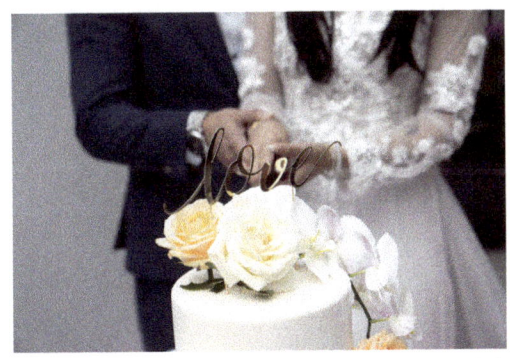

Credit: Wedding Dreamz, Unsplash

# The Autonomous Cruiser

*Cruise Essential: Most cruise lines offer ceremonies at sea, but not all of them are legally binding – some may just be symbolic.*

British law dictates that for weddings to be legal the ceremony must be held in a publicly accessible space, so if you want to get married while actually sailing, be sure to choose a cruise line registered in a country that permits marriages at sea. Companies such as Princess Cruises, Royal Caribbean, NCL, Cunard, Celebrity Cruises and P&O Cruises have their ships registered in the Bahamas or Bermuda, allowing them to offer this service, with the captain in full regalia overseeing proceedings. In order for a captain of a ship to perform a marriage at sea, he must also be a judge, a justice of the peace, a minister or an officially recognised officiant, such as a notary - check with the cruise line if you specifically want the captain to perform your ceremony.

## Celebrity
*Shoreside nuptials, vow renewals and wedding ceremonies performed by the ship's captain, Celebrity is there to help you celebrate your special day. If you want to splash out, consider a deck ceremony under a stunning canopy with billowing white drapery and your choice of flowers. Packages can include a Bridesmaid Tea Party, a Cigar and Cognac Party, and even a Test the Waters Pre-Wedding Consultation and Tour. All Celebrity ships, except Xpedition-class, are fully accessible. (celebritycruises.com)*

## Norwegian Cruise Line
*Whether you want to renew your vows or plan the perfect wedding ceremony, your own experienced wedding planner will be on hand to talk you through their a la carte options and help you plan the perfect day, whether at sea, harbour-side in Santorini or in Hawaii with the dramatic mountains of Kokee as your backdrop. Onboard ceremonies are officiated by the ship's captain on Breakaway, Getaway, Epic and Escape. NCL is committed to providing accessibility on their ships for all persons with disabilities, and a meeting with a staff member is arranged for the guest on embarkation day who will see to their special needs throughout the cruise. (ncl.com)*

## Princess Cruises
*Dream it and Princess is happy to make it come true, whether you want your wedding on the ship, a beach or atop a glacier. 'Tie the Knot' weddings can be held harbour-side or ashore and turn your special day into a lifetime of memories. If*

you want to get married off the ship then you can opt for a garden, beach, chapel or glacier setting depending on the destination. State-of-the-art technology allows you to broadcast the ceremony via webcam to friends and family at home, and the 'Honeymoon Wishes Registry' offers friends and family an easy way to give you an unforgettable gift. All ships are fully accessible. (*princess.com*)

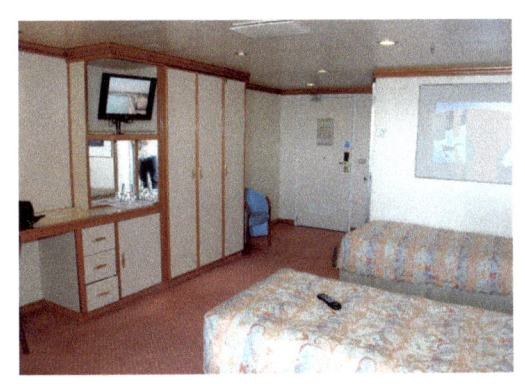

Credit: Disabled Cabin, Grand Princess - Mike McBey, Flickr

## Best for Luxury Offerings

### Crystal Yacht Cruises
*A distinctive cruise line offering touches of the grandeur of the past on their incredibly high-tech yachts, with cabins loaded with state-of-the-art technology, feather beds and plush duvets. Exceptional dining is complemented by an extensive wine cellar offering up a culinary adventure. The envy of many cruise lines is the Umi Uma & Sushi Bar (formerly Silk Road), world master chef Nobuyuki 'Nobu' Matsuhisa's only restaurant at sea. The ship is laden with the finest crystal, stunning china and exquisite table linens, and the attention to detail is second to none. Designed to be disabled-friendly, the Serenity has eight accessible cabins and the Symphony has 4, all with roll-in showers, grab bars, foldable shower benches, handheld showerheads and lowered sink and vanity units. Also, the ships have ramped access to most public areas and decks. (*crystalyachtcruises.co.uk*)*

### Regent Seven Seas Cruises
*Originally built for royalty, this luxury line's prices might be extortionate, but they include pre-cruise luxury hotel stays, accessible balcony suite accommodation, fine dining, onboard premium drinks, exclusive shore excursions, Wi-Fi and gratuities. Regent also lays claim to having "the most luxurious ship afloat", their $450*

# The Autonomous Cruiser

million-dollar Regent Explorer, where a suite will set you back a jaw-dropping £10,000. The Explorer has 375 exceptional suites, all with marble bathrooms and oversized balconies, offering Veuve Clicquot or Jacquart Champagne, L'Occitane bath amenities and plush bedding and furnishings. The onboard fine dining is sublime, with breakfast offering a self-service caviar bar and with dinner in the main restaurant served on Versace designed plates underneath the main focal point that is the hand-blown Murano glass ceiling. Regent Seven Seas welcomes passengers with all disabilities, with wide corridors for wheelchair manoeuvrability, automatic doors and access throughout the ship. Also, all staterooms are equipped for deaf and blind guests. (*rssc.com*)

## Scenic Luxury Cruises & Tours

An army of staff and a butler for each guest are on hand to satisfy all your needs aboard the Scenic Eclipse, the world's first 'Discovery Yacht', a floating sanctuary of six-star opulence and world-class comforts. Each suite is furnished with king-size beds, luxury linens and a varied pillow menu, while sweeping sea and landscapes greet you throughout the cruise from your suite's secluded terrace. Their all-inclusive policy includes a pre-departure hotel stay, return flights, transfers, ten dining venues, premium branded beverages, shore excursions, Wi-Fi, gratuities and use of the onboard seven-seat submarine and helicopter. There is one suite with modified facilities on-board the Eclipse, with additional grab bars available on request. There are lifts on board, however they do not service the Marina platform, which is only accessible by approximately 12 steps. (*scenic.co.uk*)

## Seabourn

Seabourn is redefining ultra-luxury cruising with the advent of the all-suite Ovation, the brand-new sibling ship of the Encore. The beds in the oceanfront suites are decked out in the finest Egyptian linens, with king-size feather and down pillows and a luscious all-season duvet. Bespoke furnishings, walk-in wardrobes, flat-screen TVs, high-end stereo systems and a complimentary in-suite bar all deliver five-star delights. Dining options include The Grill by Thomas Keller, The Restaurant, and Sushi, whose menu features caviar along with a selection of maki rolls, sushi and sashimi. Don't miss Seabourn's Signature 'Caviar in the Surf' beach event, where officers stand waist-deep in the sea and serve caviar and champagne off a surfboard. Now offering its own private jet service to transport its passengers to and from ports of call, this cruise line really has pushed the boat out. Seabourn is committed to providing accessible accommodations for all persons with disabilities. (*seabourn.com*)

# Where to Start?

## Best for Spas

### Celebrity Cruises
The Spa on Celebrity Edge and Apex offer a holistic wellness journey like no other. The revolutionary new ships are designed to create a closer connection between you, the sea, and the breath-taking world beyond. With more than 22,000 sprawling sq. ft. for guests to renew, restore, and reinvigorate, their nature-focused approach unites every experience throughout your wellness journey. Combined with state-of-the-art technology, The Spa has incorporated these natural therapeutic features into all the spaces, therapies, and experiences they offer. The Spa Clubs all have the unique Persian Garden, offering an excellent range of aqua-therapy experiences. All Celebrity ships, except Xpedition-class, are fully accessible. (*celebritycruises.co.uk*)

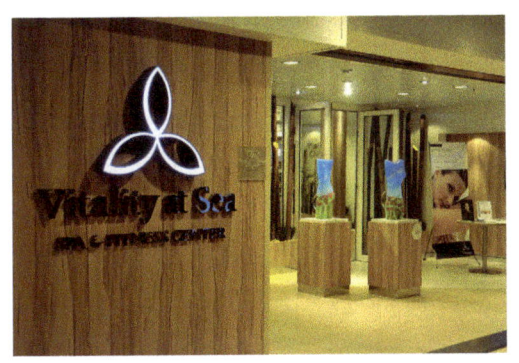

*Credit: Royal Caribbean, Allure of the Seas - John Ostrom, Flickr*

### Marella Explorer
Britain's oldest health spa resort has taken to the sea. Champneys' two floating spas feature on Marella Explorer and its sister Marella Explorer 2 and offers a full treatment menu including refreshing facials, body wraps, massages, manicures, acupuncture, as well as a salon, wellness centre, made-for-two suites and treatment cabins with hot tubs and stylish relaxation rooms that boasts comfortable beds complete with endless sea views. The newly refurbished Marella Explorer has seven outside and one inside accessible cabin with wet rooms. All located on Deck 5, they are conveniently next to reception and a bank of lifts. (*tui.co.uk*)

### Regent Seven Seas
Enrich your travel with Serene Spa & Wellness, a globally inspired, tranquil haven of health, beauty and wellness. Relax and restore aching muscles, moisturise and rejuvenate your skin, and both strengthen and elevate your body and mind as you engage with a variety of holistic treatments and services that have been thoughtfully developed to promote mental and physical rejuvenation. Indulge in massages, body

*wraps, facials, manicures, hair services and more, including exclusive treatments created especially for Regent Seven Seas Cruises. The company welcomes all disabilities and all ships have adapted cabins with 180 degree turns in public areas for wheelchair manoeuvrability, automatic doors and access throughout the ship. All staterooms are equipped for deaf and blind guests. (rssc.com)*

### Viking Cruises
*Scandinavian designed wellness spas aim to enhance the quality of life inspired by the Nordic way of living. As you would expect from a spa themed around ancient Nordic culture, the LivNordic Spa offers hot and cold bathing experiences to stimulate the circulatory system and a magic snow grotto where snowflakes sprinkle magically from the ceiling. Nordic ash wood connects the relaxation areas including thalassotherapy pools, hot tubs, heated tile loungers and a fabulous open fireplace. Although Viking do not offer accessible cabins, guests can bring a travel-sized collapsible wheelchair onboard and several of their ships have lifts. (vikingcruises.co.uk)*

### Virgin Voyages
*Scarlet Lady's Redemption Spa is decked out with luxurious touches that aim to dazzle. From its underwater cave featuring a hydrotherapy pool, cold plunge pool, jacuzzi, quartz beds, authentic hammam steam room, thermal zone, mud and salt rooms to its tailor-made treatments, you will come away feeling renewed, restored and reinvigorated. The ultimate in pampering, the treatment rooms are complemented by the Dry Dock Salon (hairdressing services), Stubble and Groom (barbershop), Blow Dry Bar, Male Pedicure Spa, and the Mani-pedi Spa. At night this gorgeous wellness complex transforms into a dancing lounge with live DJ music. The ship is fully accessible. (virginvoyages.com)*

### Best for Disability
The following cruise lines all welcome service dogs provided the necessary documentation is completed - see 'Service Dogs' for full details.

### Carnival
*Every ship in the fleet provides accessible features to enhance the cruise experience for guests with disabilities, including early boarding and wheelchair assistance during embarkation and disembarkation. Onboard facilities include step-free routes to most areas of the ship, diagrams of accessible routes, cabins, restaurant*

## Where to Start?

seating and public toilets, accessible tables at all dining venues and wheelchair-friendly lifts. The main entertainment venues have dedicated seating areas for wheelchair guests and assistive listening headsets.

Carnival offers several categories of cabin for the disabled with wider 32" doorways, generous turning spaces, accessible wardrobe rails and bathrooms with roll-in showers, grab bars and shower seats.

The vision and hearing impaired are offered braille signage on cabin doors and public rooms, large print format for the daily Carnival Fun Times (also available in an audio format), dining room menus and shore excursion information. A cabin visual/tactile alert system that notifies guests of a dock knock, a telephone call, an alarm clock or smoke-detection and the TTY (teletypewriter) in the cabin is linked directly to Guest Relations. Closed-captioned televisions also provide a safety briefing video available at all times throughout the cruise. Closed-captioning can also be requested from Guests Relations for the enjoyment of outdoor movies. Internet cafes provide screen-reader software on specific computers. For cruises starting and returning to an American port, sign language interpreters are on hand for the main production shows, port and shopping talks as well as other popular activities but must be requested a minimum of 60 days prior to your cruise.

Outside space is equally accessible and pool lifts, all with a 300-pound weight limit, are available on Carnival Horizon, Carnival Panorama, Carnival Radiance, Carnival Sunrise, Carnival Vista, and Mardi Gras.

Carnival is the first cruise line to be certified 'sensory inclusive' by KultureCity®, a leading non-profit organisation for individuals with sensory and invisible disabilities such as Autism, ADHD, Down Syndrome, and PTSD.

Carnival Cruise Line welcomes and encourages parents of special needs children to work with them so they can integrate the child into a program they will enjoy. KultureCity Sensory Bags are issued on a complimentary, first-come, first-served basis and contain items to help calm, relax and manage sensory overload. These can include comfortable noise-cancelling headphones, fidget tools, a visual feeling thermometer, and a KultureCity VIP lanyard to help staff quickly identify a guest. Youth staff have been specially trained to understand and assist guests with sensory and cognitive needs and with a number of resources at hand, such as weighted vests, sensory activities and conversation cards, they can help calm and entertain each child that is enrolled in the club.

Accessibility at ports of call vary hugely and ramped vehicles may not be available for shore excursions but

> **Don't Ask:**
> Who is driving the ship?
> (said to the Captain)

the cruise line does provide detailed information on which tours are accessible to wheelchairs and the anticipated physical activity for each shore excursion.

Half Moon Cay is Holland America's private retreat in the Bahamas that is also used by Carnival and Seabourn but there is no deepwater dock so visiting cruise lines have to anchor and tender their guests ashore. An accessible 25-passenger tram runs continuously between the Welcome Center and the Tropics Restaurant; for those that prefer to walk there is a barrier-free pathway that connects the tender landing with Fort San Salvador, the Welcome Center, the Straw Market, many food & beverage venues and accessible toilets. Complimentary beach wheelchairs are available on a first-come-first-served basis. The Rum Runners Bar and the Tropics Restaurant are listed as accessible, as is one of the cabanas, and Villas D and E are wheelchair-accessible throughout the first floor. (*carnival.co.uk*)

**Celebrity Cruises**
Every ship in the fleet, except for Xpedition-class, includes additional provisions for the mobility challenged passenger, including early boarding and wheelchair assistance during embarkation and disembarkation. Onboard conditions for wheelchair users are excellent with spacious corridors, step-free access and automatic doors to most decks, and there are a number of grab bars in high traffic areas. Theatres have dedicated seating areas, there is a lift or chair hoist for pool and jacuzzi access and the casino offers lowered tables.

Most accessible cabins come with automated doors that are wider than standard, with ramped thresholds and a generous turning radius of 5 ft (1.5 m) in bedrooms, bathrooms and sitting areas. Bathrooms feature roll-in showers, lipless entry and grab bars as standard - raised toilet seats, shower stools, commode chairs and bed blocks can be added to any standard cabin.

The vision and hearing impaired are catered for with closed-caption television, large print menus, qualified crew readers, tactile and braille signage and lift buttons (on some of their ships). They offer portable kits such as TTY/TTD and Alertmaster, and a strobe alarm can be requested. The TTY (teletypewriter) in the cabin is linked directly to Guest Relations, making contact with a member of the team effortless. The Alertmaster alarm clock has a vibrator that goes under either your pillow or mattress, and lights will alert guests to the doorbell, telephone or alarm being activated.

The outside space is equally generous with automatic doors to most decks, wheelchair-accessible toilets, plush sofas and lounge chairs. Celebrity have ensured that wheelchair users that enjoy the water can utilise the lifts for access to the pool and jacuzzi.

Celebrity Cruises put a real emphasis on accessible shore excursions for all and provide an efficient gangway docking service for easy port tendering. Celebrity's brand-new Edge Class ships offer their state-of-the-art Magic Carpet moving platform that has made industry-wide changes in tendering, especially for wheelchair users. An electric stairlift will take your chair down to the Magic Carpet, maximum weight is 225 kg (496 lbs), and from there it's plain sailing, though, as with all tendering, bad weather and rough seas can prevent safe boarding.

CocoCay, a private island found in the Bahamas, is leased exclusively for passengers sailing with Royal Caribbean and Celebrity. Wheelchair-friendly trams run along the pier and throughout the island. Oasis Lagoon freshwater pool, the wave pool in Thrill Waterpark and the infinity pool at Coco Beach Club all have pool lifts. The Beach Club is accessible and includes courtesy beach wheelchairs (cannot be operated solely by the end-user as it needs to be pushed), a low bar counter and ramps to the dining area. The new floating accessible cabanas are amazing and can accommodate eight people. Accessible toilets are placed conveniently all around the island. Unfortunately, not all the island is accessible, as the towers to the waterpark's slides and zipline are only accessible by steps, and the hot air balloon is also not suitable for guests in wheelchairs. (*celebritycruises.co.uk*)

## Disney Cruise Line

Disney Cruises feel that every family should be able to enjoy a cruise holiday to the fullest, regardless of their abilities, and most areas on their ships, including the theatres, restaurants, shops and public restrooms are wheelchair-accessible. Disney Dream has a dedicated youth program with specially trained

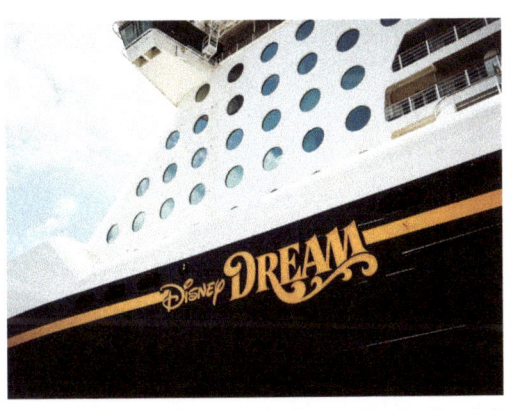

Credit: Christian Lamber, Unsplash

counsellors experienced in working with children with special needs. Cast Members cannot provide one-on-one assistance, but parents are encouraged to participate in the Open Houses program so they can enjoy the session with their child. Families with a disabled member are catered for with 24 accessible cabins that house open bed frames, bed boards, bed rails, ramped bathroom thresholds, portable or raised toilets, adjustable-height shower heads, shower stools and transfer benches on request. Accessible cabins also have auxiliary aids, stateroom communication kits with door knock and phone alerts, bed shaker notification, strobe light smoke detector, and TTY.

There are a number of services for guests with hearing disabilities, including scheduled American Sign Language (ASL) interpreters for a variety of onboard shows and entertainment - the schedule is aligned with the main (first) dinner seating and the second (late) performance in the Walt Disney Theatre. ASL interpreters are shared by all guests that request the service and must be confirmed with the Special Services Department at least 60 days prior to your sail date for US-based cruises and 120 days prior to your sail date for European cruises.

Located in the Bahamas, Disney's island, Castaway Cay, has its own dock, eliminating the need to tender and making it easily accessible for wheelchair users. There are wide and evenly paved pathways, as well as accessible toilets, throughout the island. Additionally, there is an accessible open-air tram service (first car) connecting the main areas and Serenity Bay (adults only). Cabana 1 is located on the family beach and is wheelchair-accessible, offering complimentary beach wheelchairs for those wanting to access the sand. (disneycruise.com)

**Holland America**
Holland America provides accessible experiences for all disabilities, starting with hydraulic lifts at most airports and cruise piers, and assistance during embarkation, all the way through to disembarkation and everything in between including a ship orientation tour. Most of their fleet have fully accessible cabins with ramps out onto the balconies, with larger numbers of cabins - up to 30 available on each of their Vista and Signature Class ships. The cabins also provide wide interior and exterior doors, wheelchair access to both sides of the bed and a roll-in shower with grab bars, shower seat, accessible shower controls and a handheld shower head. A raised toilet seat is available on request. Finally, pool lifts are available on the Amsterdam, Koningsdam, Volendam and Nieuw Statendam.

For the vision or hearing impaired there are optical and tactile alerts, closed-caption TVs, amplified telephones, assistive listening systems, visual alarms and large print or braille menus. Window-Eyes software, available throughout the ship, reads text for those that have impaired vision.

The whole fleet, with the exception of the Amsterdam, Veendam and Volendam, features an innovative scissor lift system which makes it possible for guests to roll *directly on and off tenders without leaving their wheelchair, however, heavy electric mobility devices are not permitted. Note, these lifts may not be available on all tenders in all ports.*

*As part of its Signature of Excellence program, Holland America has produced 'Access to Excellence', a 10-minute DVD that illustrates how their ships accommodate guests with a variety of special needs, including those requiring wheelchairs, scooters or service dogs, those who are sight or hearing impaired, and those using oxygen. More information can be found at:* http://book.hollandamerica.com/pdfs/guests/AccessToExcellence.pdf

*Half Moon Cay is Holland America's private retreat in the Bahamas that is also used by Carnival and Seabourn but there is no deepwater dock so visiting cruise lines have to anchor and tender their guests ashore. An accessible 25-passenger tram runs continuously between the Welcome Center and the Tropics Restaurant; for those that prefer to walk there is a barrier-free pathway that connects the tender landing with Fort San Salvador, the Welcome Center, the Straw Market, many food & beverage venues and accessible toilets. Complimentary beach wheelchairs are available on a first-come-first-served basis. The Rum Runners Bar and the Tropics Restaurant are listed as accessible, as is one of the cabanas. Villas D and E are wheelchair-accessible throughout the first floor. (*hollandamerica.com*)*

**Norwegian Cruise Line**
*Norwegian welcomes the disabled onboard its ships and takes the needs of individual passengers seriously. A dedicated Access Officer is available for disabled guests should any problems arise while aboard. Among its vessels, Norwegian Epic has 27 disabled-friendly staterooms, with extra-wide doors for ease of entry and bathrooms which feature grab bars, shower seats and alarm pull rods. Raised beds and adjustable hanging rails are also available in the cabins, and some of the fleet has alarm buttons beside the beds.*

*Public areas are wheelchair and disabled friendly, with clear signage, braille indicators and complimentary packs for those that are hard of hearing, including pagers for announcement alerts, hearing aids and cabled cabins with optical and tactile stimuli; some ships even provide sign language interpreters. The theatres provide special seating areas and the brand's newest liners have electric hoists for access to the pools and Jacuzzis.*

*Not only were they the first to offer a private island retreat to their passengers, but NCL now offers two. Great Stirrup Cay is located just 60 miles north of Nassau in the Bahamas. The Port Centre is akin to a modern cruise port with*

numerous restaurants, five bars and colourful stalls selling excellent souvenirs. A paved path takes you to the main facilities, but accessibility can be hard as the rest of the island has stretches that require walking through sand, however beach wheelchairs are available. The bar, dining and toilet facilities on the island are all wheelchair-accessible.

Harvest Caye is found at the southern end of Belize in the Caribbean. A wheelchair-accessible gangway is available at the pier where your ship will dock, and shuttles are provided for those with mobility limitations, though the island has good paved paths to some areas. If tendering, two of the tender boats are wheelchair-accessible, with roll-off capabilities at the Harvest Caye Marina as well. The Main Plaza is predominantly wheelchair-accessible, but a large proportion of the island is soft sandy beaches with unpaved paths which might prove difficult. Complimentary beach wheelchairs are available and there are two lifts for access to the pool. The pier is long (1200 ft) so mobility-impaired guests may have to make arrangements on the ship for wheelchair assistance if they do not have their own, or they can utilise the pier shuttles. There is a wheelchair-friendly tram available to guests signed up for a beach villa, one of which is fully ADA accessible, as are a few of the cabanas. The dining, bars, shopping venues, and toilet, are all accessible. For those that want to explore, Roam Belize has great accessible private tours for NCL guests, including visits to the ancient Mayan site of Nim Li Punit and boat safaris along Monkey River. (*ncl.com*)

## P&O

The line provides a dedicated section of their website for cruisers with special needs. All ships have wheelchair-accessible cabins with wide access doorways and ample space for freedom of movement in a wheelchair or mobility scooter, and the balconies have ramped access. Bathrooms are kitted out with roll-in showers, grab rails and pull-down shower seats. Ramps are available for all outside areas.

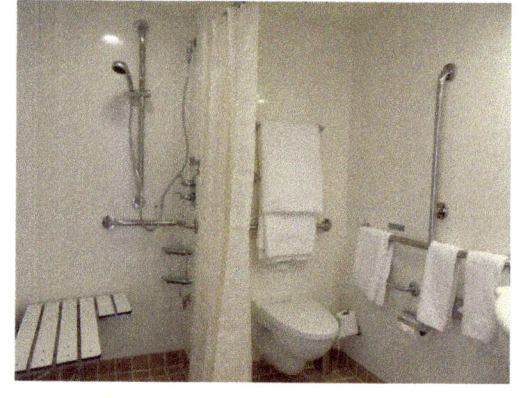

*Credit: P&O Azura - Cathie O'Dea, Flickr*

*Cabin numbers are given in braille, as are the lift buttons, across the entire fleet. The theatres provide a dedicated seating area and some show lounges provide infrared hearing support. Disabled public bathrooms are easy to find throughout the ship. All of the fleet: Arcadia, Oceania, Ventura, Azura, Aurora, Britannia and Iona have chair hoists available at the pools. Large print daily programs and menus can be arranged. Each ship has a few wheelchairs that can be borrowed, but they cannot be reserved in advance. The cruise line also offers accessible excursions and adapted vehicles in port, but you must inform the cruise line in advance of sailing if you wish to use these facilities.*

*P&O's newest additions, Britannia and Iona, provide wheelchair-accessible thermal suites. However, the pool does not have an ADA hoist, only steps into the pool. For those who purchase a spa package and are confined to a wheelchair, assistance is not provided onto the loungers in the Retreat but a caregiver will be granted free access, however they would not be able to obtain the benefits attached to the package. (pocruises.com)*

**Princess Cruises**
*Princess Cruises has long placed a high priority on making cruise holidays accessible for all guests, including those with special needs. The company initiated its award-winning 'Princess Access' program in 1992 to raise standards of cruise ship accessibility across its fleet. Accessible areas include spacious lifts, theatres, entertainment lounges, restaurants and spas, and shore excursions are available to all passengers, regardless of their special needs. Also, special gangway mechanisms on most Princess ships simplify embarkation and disembarkation for wheelchair users in many worldwide ports.*

*All ships provide a minimum of 31 accessible cabins with widened doorways, wheel-in showers, handheld showerheads and bath distress alarms. There are also lowered closet railings, sinks, handrails and ramped thresholds. Additional equipment, including toilet seat raisers, shower stools and bed boards, are available on request.*

*Braille panels, infrared listening assistance systems and tactile alarm systems are provided for the hard of sight or hearing, as well as telephone amplifiers, visual smoke detectors, door knock sensors, text telephones (TDD), audiobooks and close-captioned movies.*

*Exclusive to Princess Cruises, Princess Cays lies just 30 miles from Nassau in the Bahamas. Walkways and ramps offer an easy access link to all of Princess Cays' facilities, with disabled toilets located on both sides of the island. The island does however require a tender. (princess.com)*

## Royal Caribbean

*All of Royal Caribbean ships provide for the disabled and are packed with facilities that make moving around the ship effortless for less mobile passengers, including wheelchair-accessible gangways, automatic doors and pool and jacuzzi hoists. Accessible staterooms offer ample turning space and ramped bathroom thresholds, with roll-in showers, shower seating, handheld showerheads, grab bars and lowered sinks and dressing tables. There are even deck plans that show the accessible routes of travel throughout the ship. Quantum-class ships offer wheelchair access to tenders and its 360-degree vista observation capsule, The North Star.*

*The vision and hearing impaired are also well catered for, with assisted-listening devices, braille panels, visual and tactile signage, and alerts for door knocking, telephone ringing, alarm clocks and smoke detector activation. Closed-caption televisions and large print daily programs and menus can be arranged, and amplified telephones are provided in cabins and public areas of the ship. Dedicated sign language interpreters can be provided on request for guests travelling from America or Canada and use American Sign Language (ASL) as their primary means of communication.*

*Royal Caribbean offers an autism-friendly initiative for families living with autism, Down's syndrome and other developmental disabilities. This includes sensory-friendly films and toys, menu options for most dietary requirements, and specialist training for their Adventure Ocean staff.*

*Perfect Day at CocoCay, Royal Caribbean's private island in the Bahamas, is partly accessible, with docking facilities for two ships. Wheelchair-friendly trams run along the pier and throughout the island. Oasis Lagoon freshwater pool, the wave pool in Thrill Waterpark and the infinity pool at Coco Beach Club all have pool lifts and there are accessible toilets throughout the island. The Beach Club is accessible and includes courtesy beach wheelchairs (though they cannot be operated by the end-user as they need to be pushed), a pool lift, low bar counters and ramps to the dining area. The new accessible floating cabanas are fabulous and can accommodate eight people. Not all the island is accessible though, as the towers to the waterpark's slides and zipline are only accessible via steps, and the hot air balloon is also not appropriate for a wheelchair user.*

*Labadee in Haiti is another of Royal Caribbean's private retreats. Well paved pathways allow good access to select areas of the island, including the marketplace, where Haitian vendors compete with each other to sell you island memorabilia. An accessible tram that can accommodate up to two wheelchairs makes a continuous circuit of the island, with access via a ramp platform at the rear of the vehicle.*

Café Labadee, the Artisan Market, the Native market and the adjacent toilets are all barrier-free. The main bathroom facility has raised toilets and 36" doors. Complimentary beach wheelchairs are available on a first-come-first serve basis. There are three accessible Barefoot cabanas for hire, but they do not have private bathrooms. (*royalcaribbean.com*)

## Seabourn Cruises

Seabourn Cruises are an excellent choice for the disabled cruiser as they have had all their ships specially designed for those that are physically challenged. The Odyssey, Quest and Sojourn all offer wheelchair-accessible suites with wider entryways and roll-in showers with grab bars, seating and handheld showerheads. They have lowered the towel and wardrobe hanging rails, helping the mobility challenged be independent. Mobility scooters and electric wheelchairs are welcome onboard, but you will need to make your requirements known at the time of booking so the right cabin is allocated to you.

For travellers with visual difficulties, the cruise line has made the daily activities sheet, the daily news and the menus all downloadable, so those that have laptops with screen reader programs enabled can easily access all the information. For large print or braille menus, simply inform the company at least 45 days in advance of sailing.

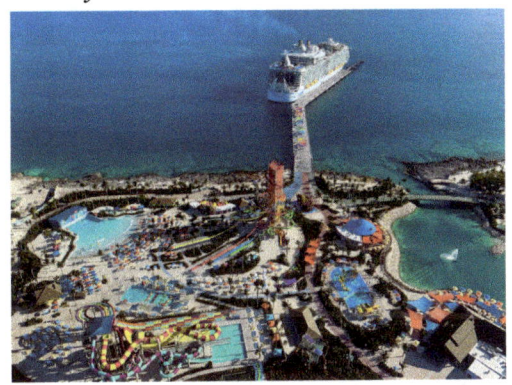

Credit: CocoCay - Fernando Jorge, Unsplash

For travellers with hearing disabilities, the provided suite kits include a visual and tactile alert for anyone knocking at the cabin door or ringing on the phone; the kit will also alert the guest if the ship's alarm is activated. Cabins are also equipped with close-captioned televisions, telephones with amplified sound, and Assistive Listening Systems with portable receivers in the showrooms. All disabled guests will be offered a familiarisation tour before sailing.

Half Moon Cay is Holland America's private retreat in the Bahamas that is also used by Carnival and Seabourn but there is no deepwater dock so visiting cruise lines have to anchor and tender their guests ashore. The island offers an accessible passenger tram that runs continuously between the Welcome Center and the Tropics Restaurant. A barrier-free pathway connects the tender landing with Fort San Salvador, the Welcome Center, the Straw market, many food & beverage venues and accessible toilets. Complimentary beach wheelchairs are available on a first-come-first-served basis. The Rum Runners Bar and the Tropics Restaurant are listed as accessible, as is one of the cabanas. Villas D and E are wheelchair-accessible throughout the first floor. (seabourn.com)

## Best for Seniors

### Cunard
As of 2019, Cunard is the only shipping line to offer scheduled classic transatlantic crossings between Europe and North America as well as annual world cruises on its distinctive red and black funnel fleet. Preferred by an older clientele who enjoy the trademarks of traditional cruising, with quiet spaces, few children and musical recitals. Onboard, passengers still dress up for formal dinners and enjoy ballroom dance parties, with social hosts on hand for unescorted ladies and gentlemen who want to don their dance shoes. Passengers love to indulge in the age-old traditional custom of a British afternoon tea, complete with delicate cucumber sandwiches, fresh scones, clotted cream and strawberry jam. All Cunard ships are fully accessible. (cunard.co.uk)

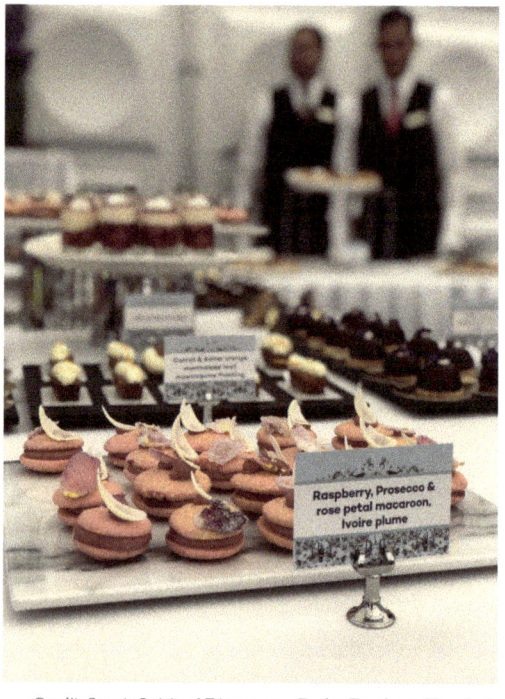

Credit: Saga's Spirit of Discovery - Becky Fantham, Unsplash

### Fred. Olsen Cruise Lines
Fred. Olsen has always been a favourite with pensioners and widowers, with the average age hovering around the 65 mark, rising slightly on world and out-of-season cruises. The company caters exclusively to the British Market and operates four

*small, understated ships with a focus on ensuring the key elements of your holiday are on point. Smaller ships mean less walking and a chance to meet more of your fellow passengers. Expect traditional dining and very few children, with tea dances complete with social hosts for unescorted ladies. Deck quoits, shuffleboard, lunchtime melodies and a late supper club means no one goes bored. There are a limited number of adapted cabins on all of Fred. Olson's ships. (fredolsencruises.com)*

**Docking Bonus:** *Fred. Olsen has announced that all cruises on the popular Braemar will now offer 'closer docking'. This is good news for the 929 guests that travel on each cruise as the company is guaranteeing that their guests will be within 1 km of the city centre upon docking. This new company initiative, which is capitalising on Braemar's small size, will enable each guest to fully utilise the amount of time they can spend ashore. Bigger is not always better.*

### Saga
*You can't get on Saga's three ships unless you're over 50 (although you can bring a guest as long as they are over 40), so you can expect like-minded passengers. The fleet is very traditional, with superb cuisine offering familiar menus, British afternoon teas, bridge, deck quoits, UK style pubs and 24-hour room service. The line will also ensure you find a companion for a day ashore and a dance partner to glide across the ballroom floor with. Saga cruises include travel insurance, delivery of foreign currency to your home, free chauffeured transport to and from your vessel and all tips for luggage porters, bellhops and waiters. Adapted cabins are available on each of Saga's ships. (sagacruises.com)*

## Best for Families with Children
Kids' clubs are extremely popular not just for the children but for parents who need to grab some alone time. If travelling with an infant and you are looking forward to enjoying some of the evening activities, choose a ship with a nursery and babysitting facilities. Likewise, if you want to pamper yourself in the spa while in port then check whether the children's club offers activities when the ship is not at sea or whether you can leave your child in the youth club if you want to go ashore. Royal Caribbean, Disney and Carnival offer this service, but P&O insist a parent or guardian stay onboard. Norwegian Cruise Line asks the same if the child has any special requirements. MSC stipulates that children cannot remain onboard if their parents or legal guardian go ashore unless you are booked on one of their shore excursions and then only if authorised by the youth staff one day beforehand.

Although not a legal requirement, Royal Caribbean International, Norwegian Cruise Lines and Disney Cruises are the only three cruise lines who have added trained lifeguards to the company payroll. In light of recent drownings, the guards are stationed at family pools on select ships during the pool's opening hours. Complimentary floatation vests are available on several other lines that offer family pools, including Carnival Cruise Lines and Celebrity Cruises. Other lines do employ lifeguard-certified attendants but don't advertise the fact, as they want to promote active parental supervision.

**Water Baby:** *Never leave your children unattended in any water, regardless of whether a lifeguard is on duty or not.*

### Carnival

*Children will be in their element onboard a Carnival cruise, with experienced counsellors ensuring everyone has a fantastic time with oodles of fun-filled, age-appropriate activities. Kids' menus offer firm favourites like mac & cheese, chicken nuggets and pizza. Seuss at Sea includes a parade and story hour with Dr Seuss characters, Build-a-Bear Workshops bring a stuffed friend to life and, to top the day off, there are Night Owls Parties (late-night babysitting).*

*Little ones can have a blast in their own clubs: Penguins (2-5 years), Stingrays (6-8 years) and Sharks (9-11 years), Circle C for tweens (12-14 years) and Club O2 for teens (15-17 years). Carnival even offers shore excursions just for 12-17 year-olds chaperoned by the youth staff. All the clubs have a full schedule of activities, including scavenger hunts, video gaming, dodgeball, T-shirt decorating and dance parties.*

*Outdoor facilities include movie screenings, ropes courses and mini-golf for all day fun while Carnival Vista offers the first IMAX at sea and a Skyride bike course. Carnival's newest addition Panorama incorporates two fun slides, a kids' spray park and the first trampoline park at sea*

*Carnival's onboard water park, WaterWorks offers fun for the whole family. Try the Twister Waterslide, one of the wettest and fastest rides at sea or the side-by-side racing slides that end with a massive splash in the pool below. Speedway Splash features hundreds of feet of racing action complete with lighting effects while the 300-gallon Power Drencher tipping bucket is not for the faint-hearted. The Dr Seuss WaterWorks has been a big hit with little ones with life-size statues of their favourite Dr Seuss character, the ever-popular tipping bucket and tons of water spray toys. (Horizon). Staying with the theme, Carnival Horizon will also feature Dr Seuss Bookville family reading and play area and the Seuss-a-palooza Parade and Story Time.*

Half Moon Cay, Carnival's private island resort is a hit for water-lovers with a two-mile expanse of pure white sandy beach and a lagoon aqua park. Pirate-themed it comes complete with its own water cannons, and climbable water toys. All Carnival ships are fully accessible. (carnival.com)

## Disney

Parents with tiny tots will appreciate the nursery that Disney offers for youngsters from six months to three years (fee payable). Disney's Oceaneer Club has pure Disney fantasy-character-driven performances, special storytelling sessions, larger-than-life playgrounds, dress-up opportunities and cool interactive activities that are sure to delight tiny tots and older kids alike. Toys and games, an open seating area for arts and crafts and ongoing Disney movies mean there's never a dull moment. Disney's Oceaneer Lab screens movies on a 103" plasma wall. Kids get to enjoy interacting with their favourite characters, immerse themselves in the workshops, the science laboratory, the Animator's Studio, Playmation and The Wheelhouse, a multiplayer computer room.

Tweens and teens have their own places to play and hang out, equipped with high-tech entertainment including flat-screen TVs, computers and video games. The interactive play space is very popular, as are the parties and karaoke sessions that are hosted by the entertainment team.

Several pools grace the Disney fleet each named after one of the brand's famous characters. Mickey's pool (Wonder, Dream, Fantasy) is a firm favourite among children, with its winding waterslide and shallow depth. Disney Dream and Disney Fantasy feature AquaDuck, a four-deck high water flume which sends the fearless two at a time through twists and turns, up, down and all around the ship on its 765-foot long track, including a transparent section that swings out 13 feet over the side of the vessel, 150 feet above the ocean. Guests step inside the AquaDunk's slide's capsule-like entrance and endure a nail-biting wait until the floor drops out beneath sending them plummeting straight down. The ride curves around over the side of the ship, before splashdown several decks below (Disney Magic).

A dedicated 1800 square-foot recreation space AquaLab, is a sprawling water playground that delights all members of the family, with leaky pipes, water jets, bubblers, geysers, pouring paint cans, raining showerheads and rotating wheels and levers. (Fantasy, Magic). The area also incorporates the Twist 'n' Spout Slide, a double looping water flume and Dory's Reef, an entertaining 400 square foot

**Don't Ask:**
Will the Captain let me drive the ship?

splash deck dedicated to infants and toddlers. Kids of all ages love that extra touch of Disney as the ship's horn plays an iconic Disney song at sailaways.

Castaway Cay, Disney's private island provides serious water fun with sprawling beaches, sparkling lagoons, snorkelling, stingray adventures, jet skis and splash-worthy water play areas including twisting water slides, a floating platform, dripping pipes, hissing misters and a giant 'bucket dump'. All ships are fully accessible. (*[disneycruise.com](disneycruise.com)*)

## MSC Cruises

As well as age appropriate clubs for 3-17 year olds, MSC are the only fleet to offer a Baby Club with dedicated facilities for 0-2 year olds. They even offer a dedicated overnight laundry service that washes infant and toddler clothes separately from anything else. Children have their own menus in the main restaurants and the specialty venues as well as a dedicated Kid's Corner in the buffet restaurant. Once every cruise there is a special Lego entertainment event onboard suitable for the whole family.

**Medical Essential:** *Infants below the age of 12 months will require a 'fit to travel' certificate.*

MSC Preziosa features a 390-foot-long Vertigo water slide that sits imposingly atop Deck 18, an elevation of 42 feet, taking its thrill-seekers, at speeds of up to 13 mph, downward through a series of twists and turns. The water slide becomes even more impressive when the ride takes you over the edge of the ship through a 30-foot transparent section that provides a glimpse of the sea below.

With a new ship popping up almost every year, the company has now given the MSC Seaside a sister ship named Seaview, home to two full-sized bowling alleys and a multi-storey waterpark at sea. The Forest Aquaventure features five different flumes, including two high-speed racing slides with clear loops extending over the side of the ship and a 367-foot water chute with lights and music. Thrill seekers can climb up to the top deck and experience the Adventure Trail, a ropes course with two of the longest aerial runways at sea (394 feet).

The Doremi Castle Kids Aqua Park perched atop Deck 16 also provides its younger guests with plenty of thrills with interactive sprays, water pistols, fountains and a tipping bucket guaranteed to drench those that dare stand under it. The younger tots will love the AquaPlay and AquaSpray Adventure Park complete with its own adventure trail, a ropes course that includes spray canons.

MSC's private Caribbean island offers water lovers over ten gorgeous beaches, a vast lagoon and an aquatic sports facility suitable for all the family. All ships are fully accessible. *(msccruises.co.uk)*

**Norwegian Cruise Line**
*Splash Academy is divided into four age groups: six months - to two years (one parent must remain with their children), 3-5 years, 6-9 years and 10-12 years old. Activities range from interactive dance mats, jungle gyms, Circus School, arts & crafts, Wii tournaments and movies in the surround sound cinema.*

*The Teen Club enjoys the 'freestyle' approach – no set dining times, no strict dress code and plenty of choice for entertainment and food. The club offers gaming, a video jukebox, table football and air hockey, and at night the space transforms into a teen disco.*

*Outside the club there are sports courts, a mini-golf course, a bungee trampoline, a ropes course, ziplining, glow parties (Breakaway class ships), bowling (Epic, Pearl) and rock-climbing (Breakaway class, Epic, Pearl, Gem).*

*Soak it all up at the Aqua Park with five multi-storey towering water slides, splash parks, two swimming pools and four hot tubs. Practice cannonballs or take the plunge on Free Fall and drop at the speed of 4Gs, the fastest drop slide at sea or feel the rush of The Whip, two racing side-by-side twister slides that are wet and wild on the Breakaway Class ships. Feel the exhilaration as you slide down the four storeys high, 200-foot long Epic Plunge, the most exhilarating of Norwegian Epic's three flumes. Youngsters who are into serious water play can splash the day away in the Kids' Aqua Park complete with water slides and water shooters*

*The giant Aqua Park on Norwegian Cruise Line's biggest ship Bliss features the Aqua Racer slide, where adults can twist and turn side by side in tandem on inner tubes. There's also the Free Fall, side-by-side slides with floors that open up, dropping riders into a thrilling loop and for the family-friendly, there's an open-flume body slide. Kids have their own aquatic area kitted out with a multistorey tower, rope bridge, lookout platform, spraying cannons and tipping buckets. All Norwegian ships are fully accessible. (ncl.com)*

**Royal Caribbean**
*Cruising with a small baby can be difficult, but the Royal Babies program takes tiny tots from 6-18 months and offers a babysitting service. Babies 2 Go allows parents to pre-order nappies, wipes, cream and organic baby food right to your stateroom so they are there for you on arrival and don't need to be packed, and you can also re-stock by ordering more throughout the cruise.*

# The Autonomous Cruiser

The award-winning Adventure Ocean youth program has three clubs catering for 3-5 years, 6-8 years and 9-11 years old. Tweens and teens also have their own age-specific programs and spaces. The DreamWorks Experience offers films in the 3D theatre and your stateroom, while life-size characters from Shrek, Madagascar and How to Train Your Dragon roam about the ship and are a big hit with pre-teens (Allure, Oasis, Liberty, Freedom, Quantum, Voyager and Mariner of the Seas).

Harmony, Oasis and Quantum-class ships each include rock climbing, ice skating, bumper cars and Scratch DJ Academies. Quantum-class ships have SeaPlex, a multi-purpose sports facility offering circus school, roller-skating, dance parties and SeaPods, a live gaming suite. Oasis of the Seas offers onboard ziplining and another first at sea, Ripcord by iFly, an amazing indoor skydiving experience (Quantum, Anthem). These ships also feature an H2O Zone Water Park and Splashaway Bay Aqua Park are both aimed at the pint-sized cruiser offering a lively, aquatic play area overflowing with fun, including interactive geysers, climbable sculptures, water cannons, pools and waterfalls.

With multiple pools and whirlpools, some cantilevered, extending 13 feet over the edge of the ship, Royal Caribbean has it all including the onboard 40 ft long surf simulator FlowRider, which has been such a hit that RC now features it on 13 of their ships. For the real thrill-seekers, check out Perfect Storm. Three storeys high, this water slide takes excitement off the chart. Race through twists, turns and transparent panels offering jaw-dropping views to the bottom. The ride encompasses a trio of terror although not necessarily the same three on each ship.

In all cases, two of the slides are Cyclone and Typhoon, both racers while the third varies depending on your chosen ship. On Harmony of the Seas, Perfect Storm is joined by Supercell, a champagne bowl slide that snakes down twists and turns, then swishes around a circular 'bowl' before depositing its rider into the plunge pool at the bottom. On Liberty of the Seas, the third option is Tidal Wave, the first boomerang style slide at sea. Plummet down a steep slope gaining speed until you are propelled up the side of an almost vertical wall, giving a sense of weightlessness before an exhilarating rebound down the other side into a splash pool. Harmony of the Seas' Ultimate Abyss is one of the tallest slides at sea, with a 100-foot drop and hair-raising twists and turns.

Labadee, Royal Caribbean's private island offers gorgeous beaches with kayaks, snorkelling, jet skis and a 300-foot long Dragon's Splash water slide that goes through ten twists and turns ending up in the splash area of Columbus Cove. The Arawak Aqua Park features trampolines, waterslides, rolling log, interactive water *activities and other floating inflatable aquatic toys. All Royal Caribbean ships are fully accessible. (royalcaribbean.com)*

## Best for Expedition & Adventure

### Aurora Expeditions
*Purpose-built for adventure, the Greg Mortimer, named after its co-founder, incorporates two unique viewing platforms that fold out hydraulically for unobstructed views of the stunning scenery. The four sea-level launching platforms enable the 15 Zodiacs to load easily and quickly, allowing more time to explore during the two or three daily landings in both Antarctica (Antarctic Peninsula, South Georgia and the Falkland Islands) and the Arctic (Svalbard, Franz Josef Land, East Greenland, Jan Mayen Island, Iceland and Norway). The Greg Mortimer has accessible cabins but you will need to negotiate a set of stairs to access the zodiacs or the Mudroom. (auroraexpeditions.com.au)*

### Hurtigruten
*Hurtigruten's skilled crew enable them to take you on fabulous itineraries, from the polar regions of the High Arctic, across to Europe and from the Americas, down to the end of the Earth, Antarctica. Explore Spitsbergen, the largest island of the Svalbard archipelago found midway between Norway and the North Pole, populated by Arctic foxes and mighty polar bears. Witness imposing icebergs, picturesque fjords and long-forgotten early whaling stations. All Hurtigruten ships, except for MS Nordstjernen and MS Lofoten, are wheelchair-friendly and have at least one accessible cabin onboard. Blind passengers need to travel with a seeing-eye companion, but deaf or hearing-impaired guests are permitted to travel alone. Several ports have accessible vehicles suitable for shore excursions. Explorer ships require a certain level of agility and are not suitable for less able guests as landings and some embarkations are by Zodiacs or tenders. (hurtigruten.co.uk)*

**Saving the Seas:** *Norwegian-based expedition cruise line Hurtigruten has taken a massive step in protecting the oceans by removing all unnecessary single-use plastic from their vessels. The cruise line offers its passengers the chance to participate in beach clean-up programs to help preserve several of the marine species already on the verge of extinction. Hopefully, others in the industry follow suit.*

## Seabourn

The Seabourn Venture is due to launch in December 2021, with its sister scheduled to launch in May 2022. Both ships will be purpose-built for diverse environments to PC6 Polar Class standards and will offer two bespoke submarines and a fleet of kayaks and 24 Zodiacs. The expedition vessels will feature scientists, historians, naturists and wilderness experts who will deliver a rich holistic travel experience to each guest. Seabourn is committed to providing accessible accommodations for all persons with disabilities. (*seabourn.com*)

## Scenic Luxury Cruises & Tours

Scenic's all-inclusive Eclipse is the world's first Discovery Yacht, allowing you to cruise to previously inaccessible destinations. The six-star vessel includes luxurious suites, six dining options, a dedicated onboard discovery team, a seven-seater submarine, helicopter and a fleet of Zodiacs. There is one suite with modified facilities onboard the Eclipse, with additional grab bars available on request. There are lifts on board, but they do not service the Marina platform, which is only accessible via approximately 12 steps. Guests must be able to step in and out of the zodiacs without a mobility aid and navigate stairs in the event of an emergency to reach the evacuation point which is located on Deck 3. (*scenic.co.uk*)

## Windstar Cruises

Gain access to hidden coves, bubbling brooks, tapered fjords and tiny hamlets in one of the 150 ports Windstar travel to. Witness spawning salmon in Alaska, the cloven-hoofed tree-climbing goats in Morocco, an incredible sunset over Santorini's turquoise-topped domes or a private concert set in the ruins of Ephesus. Windstar Star Breeze, Star Pride and Star Legend each have four accessible suites equipped for disabled guests. (*windstarcruises.com*)

## Best for Budget Cruises

## Carnival

Renowned for their emphasis on family fun and chilled onboard atmosphere, Carnival's 27 ships depart from every coast in the US, as well as from Europe, Canada, Mexico and firm favourite, the Caribbean. Specialising in low-cost cruising, Carnival offers frequent sales and early bird and last-minute deals on top of their already low prices. Cruises range from 2 to 16 nights, with some

# Where to Start?

*itineraries available for less than £100 per person per night. All Carnival ships are fully accessible. (carnival.com)*

## Costa Cruises

*Founded in 1854 and a member of the Carnival family, Costa Cruises is an Italian line based in Genoa. Costa is recommended for partygoers, families shopping for a deal and those with a disability. Costa offers lower rates and better last-minute deals on Mediterranean routes compared to its competition, resulting in their cruises having a good mix of European nationals taking advantage of the great prices. All Costa ships have a generous number of accessible cabins and lift access to most decks. (costacruises.co.uk)*

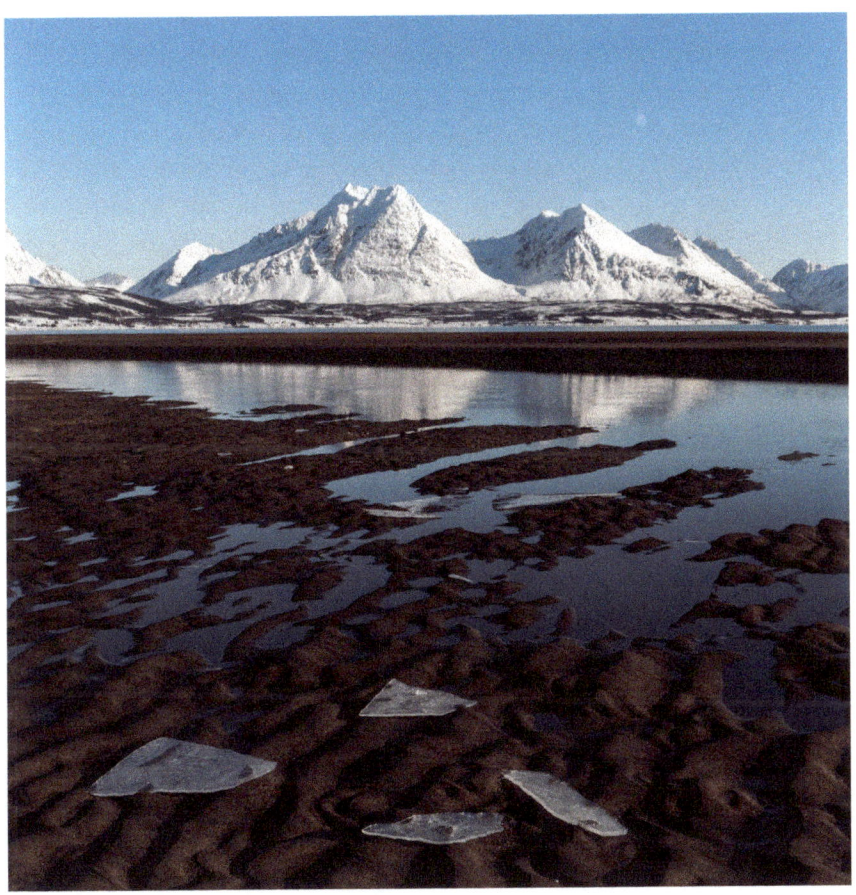

Credit: Norway - Tromsø Villmarkssenter

### Fred. Olsen

Another line that offers cruises primarily to the British market, Fred. Olsen offers a good choice of UK sailings from Dover, Liverpool, Newcastle, Edinburgh (Rosyth) and Southampton. Their four smaller-sized, classically-designed British vessels sail across Europe, the fjords of Norway and the Caribbean, visiting historical gems in a variety of jaw-dropping destinations. To take advantage of any deals on their already low prices, keep an eye out for their special offers, summer bargains on departures for June-December cruises, and any last-minute getaways. Fred. Olsen's ships offer adapted cabins. (fredolsencruises.com)

### MSC

Recommended for anyone looking for a deal on a cruise through the Mediterranean during the summer, MSC prides itself on its rich heritage and competitive pricing, with 'Early Booking' fares, 'Best Price Today', 'MSC Special', 'Last Minute' offers, 'Flight Included', 'Special Rates' for families and children, and they even offer deals on world cruises. A great bonus for families is that children under the age of 18 that stay in the same cabin as their parents cruise for free, paying only port taxes, registration costs, insurance, flights and transfers. MSC welcomes passengers of all disabilities. (msccruises.com)

## Best for Food & Wine Lovers

### Crystal Cruises

The Symphony and Serenity are the two Crystal ships that offer their bi-annual 'Ultimate Vintage Room' dinner feast - starting at $1000 a head, the experience offers the chance to sample some of the 230 vintages available from the ships' wine cellars, along with an eight-course gourmet French meal. Sushi fans will love Umi Uma & Sushi Bar, the Asian-fusion masterpiece of Chef Nobu Matsuhisa. The eatery offers an assortment of Nobu's inventive sushi and sashimi while Umi Uma features his renowned Japanese-Peruvian fusion dishes. During your voyage you can also enjoy the Italian inspired Prego restaurant, contemporary dishes at the Crystal Dining Room, informal buffet-style dining at the Marketplace, Brazilian fare at Churrascaria, Chinese comfort food at the Silk Kitchen & Bar, fast-food favourites at the Trident Bar & Grill, afternoon tea at Palm Court and fabulous dessert at the Ice Cream Bar. Designed to be accessible, both Serenity and Symphony are excellent for the physically challenged, with fully accessible cabins and bathrooms, and ramped access to most decks and public areas. (crystalcruises.com)

# Where to Start?

## Oceania

*Designed for gastronomes and travel connoisseurs, Oceania Cruises' most luxurious ship, Marina, offers guests multiple dining venues, six of which are surcharge-free, open-seating gourmet restaurants. Wine Spectator's La Reserve delivers educative seminars, tastings and gourmet food pairings, and master chefs give a range of classes at the onboard cookery school, The Culinary Center. Guests have a fabulous array of food choices, from the classic steakhouse Polo Grill, the French fare Bistro, Italian inspired Toscana, the Asian fusion of Red Ginger, the informal Terrace Café, and Waves Grill, serving gourmet burgers, tangy barbecue and delicious seafood. Modelled after a Parisian bistro, the eclectically-decorated Jacques is a gastronomic delight with an ambience that is distinctively French. Oceania's ships offer several staterooms that are accessible for travellers with special needs. (oceaniacruises.com)*

## P&O Cruises

*Hedonistic delights crafted by Marco Pierre White, wine selections from televisionHs grape expert Olly Smith, fabulous sweet treats created by master pâtissier Eric Lanlard, and Michelin-star chef Atul Kochhar's Sindhu Indian restaurant can all be found on P&O's newest additions to their fleet, Britannia and Iona. Celebrity chef James Martin's Cookery Club also gives you the option of creating your own culinary delights. Other options include The Horizon, Grab and Go, the Lido Grill, Java, The Market Cafe and for the ultimate experience, book a celebrity-hosted exclusive dinner on select 'Food Heroes' cruises.*

*If you love good food and wine, join Olly Smith for an intimate dinner and a choice of 38 handpicked wines from across the globe, in the stylish surroundings of The Glass House, on Aurora, Azura, Britannia, Ventura and the newest addition to the fleet, Iona (select cruises only). The British television personality, columnist, author and wine*

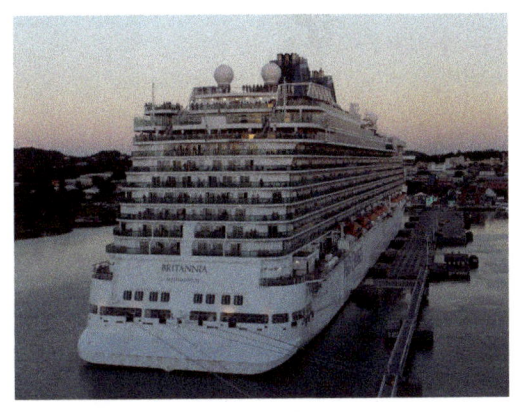

Credit: P&O's Britannia berthed in Antigua

*aficionado will share his expertise, top tips and trade secrets while walking you through the wine and food matching process.*

# The Autonomous Cruiser

Set to spend her summers in the Norwegian fjords, take a seat in The Epicurean for a lavish six-course Norwegian taster menu created exclusively for the Iona by Local Food Hero and award-winning chef, Kjartan Skjelde. The Glass House will feature tapas with locally sourced ingredients, traditional recipes and menus brimming with authentic flavours created by renowned Spanish chef José Pizarro when Iona moves to Spain, Portugal and the Canary Islands for the winter breaks. Taste 360, a new casual deck dining space which is exclusive to Iona, is home to street food dishes from across the globe. All P&O ships are fully accessible. (*pocruises.com*)

## Princess

Explore award-winning cuisine with a vast array of dining options, including delectable seafood bars and five-course tasting menus. Wine lovers can match their selections with fresh bites including sushi, tapas and artisan meats and cheese at Vines Wine Bar. As well as the two cafes, two pizzerias, a pastry shop, ice cream bar, grill room, Horizon Court, Planks BBQ and room service, food lovers have a choice of 9 specialty dining options, including an Italian restaurant, a steakhouse, crab shack, and Curtis Stone's first restaurant at sea, Share. Chocolate Journeys showcases decadent handcrafted sweet treats by world-renowned chocolatier Norman Love, and the Winemakers Dinner is a chance for guests to dine in a cellar-inspired private space and revel in a special menu designed with the help of respected winemakers.

Taking dining to another level, the Chef's Table is designed as a special treat for food aficionados and wine buffs - it offers the rare opportunity to be invited into the ship's galley to feast on memorable sights, tastes and conversation, and is hosted by the executive chef. This intimate private gathering, available for only ten guests at a time, offers a multi-course menu that might showcase local cuisine from a recent port. Each dish is served with a comprehensive explanation of its special features, and preparation methods. Specially selected wines accompany each course, chosen to complement the meal. All Princess ships are fully accessible. (*princess.com*)

## Seabourn

Seabourn is a member of Chaîne des Rôtisseurs, an international society of gastronomy devoted to the art of fine dining. Their consistent gourmandise is evident throughout the fleet, including its newest addition Seabourn Ovation - the ships have five distinct restaurants, each with its own menu with dishes crafted by expert chefs, including the three-time Michelin-starred American chef and restaurateur Thomas Keller. The gourmet maestro brings his highly-prized

French and American dishes to the cruise line, adding new flavours and finesse to Seabourn's already acclaimed cuisine.

Enjoy the refined dining of The Restaurant, embrace the view and an undisputedly perfect steak under the stars, savour inventive small-bite tasting menus at Restaurant 2 or sample classic dishes inspired by the American chophouse at The Grill. Sushi offers hot and cold bite-size dishes, and the Colonnade and Patio serve casual dining. The Ovation's new Artisan Gelato ice cream parlour tempts with unique flavours such as Blood Orange, Yuzu, Dulce De Leche and Cappuccino. All Seabourn ships have accessible staterooms, but features vary between vessels. (seabourn.com)

### Silversea

No matter which venue you choose to dine in, the influence of your cruise itinerary is undeniably evident in the vast assortment and freshness of your selections. Spaccanapoli, with its recently harvested ingredients, authentic dough and appreciation for the Italian lust for life, is a sublime eating experience, and Silver Note offers bite-sized tapas-style dishes. Indochine's stylish and delicate dishes, teeming with Asian essence, are sure to stir your culinary senses, while La Dame, inspired by the Eiffel Tower, features a bespoke menu by top chefs, and is a fabulous illustration of French dining excellence. Japanese restaurant Kaiseki's fine art of dining is ingrained in the country's culture and lies in its meticulous presentation of dishes while observing the 'Power of Five': the five methods of preparation – raw, simmered, fried, steamed and grilled - the prevalence of the five colours – white, black, red, green and yellow – all while immersing the five senses in a perfectly balanced menu respecting the equilibrium of yin and yang.

Launching with Silversea's newest addition, Silver Moon, the unique Sea and Land Taste program (SALT) offers travellers the richest epicurean experience by reflecting destinations through taste. Join market and vinery outings and tasting events, attend cooking demos with local chefs in the lab and enjoy special S.A.L.T dinners. Silversea has a limited number of accessible staterooms but welcomes all guests with special needs. (silversea.com)

## Best for Enrichment:

### Celebrity

Enrichment options are spread across 4 main categories: Taste, Learn, Play and Revive. Examples include wine tasting and appreciation classes, Molecular Mixology *workshops, interactive cooking demonstrations, Top Chef at Sea competitions and behind the scenes galley visits. Wellness activities feature fitness classes, nutrition tutorials, acupuncture, stress management and body-sculpting classes. Celebrity has partnered with several renowned companies, offering a plethora of educational opportunities to its guests. An alliance with Rosetta Stone grants access to learning 13 languages, Smithsonian Institution's educational travel program strengthens your knowledge on history, culture, art, and architecture, while Stargeezer's onboard program introduces guests to astronomy. The Beyond the Podium expert speaker series presents guest lectures on a range of topics, and cruisers can also enjoy craft lessons, photography instructions, destination education, technology tutorials, dance classes, art talks and the Celebrity iLounge, the sea's first authorised Apple specialist centre. All Celebrity ships, except for Xpedition-class, are fully accessible. (celebritycruises.co.uk)*

## Cunard

*You can experience the Cunard Insights speaker series across their entire fleet, offering regular talks on contemporary issues by well-known celebrities and personalities. The Cunard Book Club offers literary discussions and iStudy classes which take the mystery out of today's technology. Head over to the Planetarium for specially created shows courtesy of the Royal Astronomical Society during transatlantic crossings. Queen Mary 2 allows you to embrace your inner thespian with the Royal Academy of Dramatic Art's acting workshops, or you can try something completely new like fencing demonstrations, bridge lessons, craft tutorials, wine tastings or dance classes. All Cunard ships are fully accessible. (cunard.co.uk)*

## Fred. Olsen

*Fred. Olsen offers a varied daily program of activities across its fleet, including arts and craft lessons, quizzes, fitness classes and destination presentations so you can make the most of your time ashore. They present the award-winning Vistas enrichment series, offering talks and lectures hosted by experts in fields such as business, politics, gardening, antiques, and wine. Other enrichment opportunities range from singing lessons, theatre workshops, photography skills, watercolour tutorials, wine tastings, and ballroom dancing complete with dance hosts on every cruise. A limited number of adapted cabins are offered on all Fred. Olsen ships. (fredolsencruises.com)*

> **Don't Ask:**
> Can you ask the Captain to stop the sea? (said by a seasick passenger)

# Where to Start?

### P&O

P&O's Strictly Come Dancing themed cruises come complete with a special guest judge from the show and sequined, step-perfect professional dancers, who oblige with autograph sessions and intimate Q&A events. Get close to the costumes that dazzle you each show and meet the talent behind the show-stopping tailoring. If you are a fan of the popular BBC series, the whole cruise is packed with features from the show, including themed movies, book-signings, photograph sessions and fashion shows. Grab the chance to trip the light fantastic with private one-to-one lessons, or have dinner in a specialty restaurant with one of your favourite pro dancers as host. All P&O ships are disability-friendly. (*pocruises.com*)

## Best for After Dark

### Carnival

You would expect an extensive entertainment program onboard what's known as the party fleet of the seven seas, and you wouldn't be wrong. Choose from the piano bar, playlist productions, stage shows, live music, karaoke, late-night clubs, Dive-in Movies or Hollywood blockbusters at the IMAX theatre. Enjoy the adult-only Punchliner Comedy Club, take part in the Lip Synch Battle, play Hasbro the Game Show, immerse yourself in a multi-dimensional experience in the Thrill Theatre or take part in Clue: a murder mystery that unfolds as you cruise. Special 'Carnival Live' sailings present legendary headline acts – past shows have featured music legends Lionel Richie, Gladys Knight, and KC & The Sunshine Band. On the comedy front, they've hosted the hilarious Chris Tucker, Jay Leno and Jeff Foxworthy, while Carrie Underwood, Tim McGraw, and Trace Adkins have represented country music. All Carnival ships are fully accessible. (*carnival.com*)

### Celebrity

The newest additions to Celebrity's vast fleet, Celebrity Edge and Celebrity Apex, boast a total of 29 distinctive restaurants, cafes, bars and lounges to choose from, including the unique ice-topped Martini Bar with juggling bartenders serving more than 100 different varieties of vodka. Most ships showcase Las Vegas-style shows with guest aerialists, jaw-dropping circus shows, late-night comedy performances, open-deck parties, theme nights, karaoke and Rock City, a stadium-style concert. There's also the crowd-pleaser and great spectacle that is the Silent Disco. All Celebrity ships, except for Xpedition-class ships, are fully accessible. (*celebritycruises.co.uk*)

## Holland America

*Holland America presents the usual entertainment options such as nightclubs, disco, piano bar, live music and movies under the stars, but it also offers a whole lot more. Lincoln Center Stage showcases exceptional live chamber music performances, with world-class musicians performing multiple ensembles nightly. From rhythmic and brisk to soulful and fluid, you're sure to find live music you love - an eight-piece band performs in the legendary B.B. King's Blues Club, a five-piece play the best of four decades of rock and roll in the Rolling Stone Rock Room, and two pianists showcase their talent in Billboard Onboard. Following their highly acclaimed 'Frozen Planet in Concert', Holland America now presents 'Planet Earth II in Concert' on most ships in the fleet. Produced in partnership with BBC Earth, it combines live music with a backdrop of breath-taking footage from the award-winning BBC television series. All Holland America ships are fully accessible. (hollandamerica.com)*

## Royal Caribbean

*Ice escapade-style shows and acrobatic aqua-productions with high dives and hydraulic stage effects are just a glimpse of what Royal Caribbean has to offer across its vast fleet. Club 20 is the spot for dancing after dark, held under the Solarium Bar's retractable glass roof. If music isn't enough then the go-go dancers are sure to brighten*

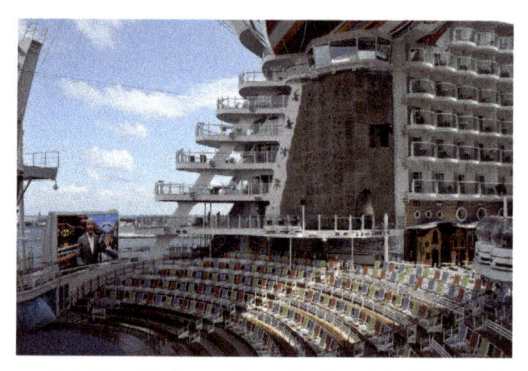

Credit: Royal Caribbean, Allure of the Seas - John Ostrom, Flickr

*the mood, bopping to the sounds of a Scratch DJ Academy-trained disc jockey. Guests are even given glow-in-the-dark light rings that flash to the beat of the music. There are high-tech productions, Latin American clubs, jazz clubs, comedy clubs, karaoke bars that allow you to create your own music in a private video booth, deck parties, indoor parades, and the classic British pleasure, a pub replete with guitar and vocals. All Royal Caribbean ships are fully accessible. (royalcaribbean.co.uk)*

# Where to Start?

## Best for Solo Travellers:

### Fred. Olsen Cruise Lines

Fred. Olsen beat off stiff competition to win 'Best for Solo Travellers' at the 2018 Wave Awards, where the industry experts believed that the company had excelled and gone above and beyond in the experience they offer their solo guests. The company provides 190 single cabins across its fleet of 4 ocean ships, Balmoral, Braemar, Bolette and Borealis, and their new river cruise, Brabant, with a reduced (or waived) single supplement on a number of cruises worldwide. Once onboard ship, solo travellers will find exclusive gatherings to enable them to get to know each other, with staff seating them together for dinner and arranging companions when going ashore if requested. There are also dance hosts onboard the ships to provide partners for solo guests. All Fred. Olsen ocean ships offer adapted cabins. (fredolsencruises.com)

### Norwegian Cruise Line

Norwegian Cruise Line (NCL) have repeatedly been voted Porthole Magazine's Best Cruise Line for Solo Travellers, and for good reason. The Epic, Breakaway and Getaway's snug studios are purpose-built for people cruising alone and come with no extra charges, and guests staying in them are given exclusive key-access to a double-height communal lounge to meet and mingle. There's a whiteboard to display messages for fellow guests, so it's easy to arrange a get-together or post a time for a shore excursion meet. Solo gatherings are available each day and provide a great way to get tablemates for dinners and shows. All NCL ships are fully accessible. (ncl.com)

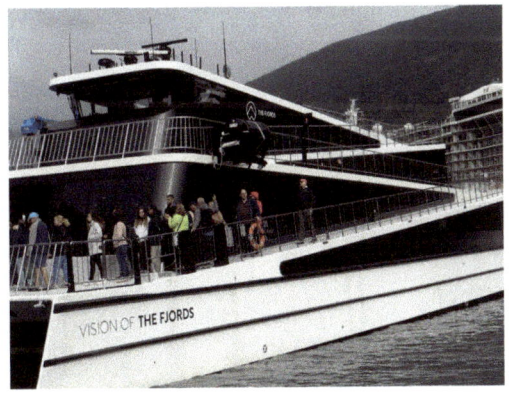

Credit: Visions of the Fjords, Flam, Norway

### Saga Cruises

More than a fifth of Saga's over-50 travellers prefer to travel alone and with more than 100 single cabins across the fleet they are well catered for. The 'Singles Mingle' drinks party and exclusive 'Singles Lunch' are an excellent opportunity to meet

# The Autonomous Cruiser

other solo travellers and organise meals or outings together. Cocktail parties are hosted for solo cruises and there are get-togethers before each port for those who'd like to go ashore with a companion, with dedicated Solo Hosts that will seat new friends together on shore excursions. All restaurants offer open seating so you can opt to share your meal with other single guests, reserve a table to share with new friends, or take pot luck and dine with different guests each night - the maître d' will be happy to arrange everything for you. The complimentary chauffeur service for passengers living within 250 miles of their departure port is especially attractive when travelling alone. Adapted cabins are available on all Saga ships. (saga.co.uk)

## Best Foreign Brands

### AIDA Cruises

Easy to spot with the familiar AIDA smile plastered across the bow of each of their ships, the company prides itself on offering a consistently excellent service with the highest international quality, environmental and safety standards. The epitome of casual cruising aimed at the German market, these are the perfect cruises for those wanting to adopt a wellness and fitness lifestyle with some of the largest spa and sports areas on the seven seas. Disabled cabins are available on all AIDA ships and almost all public areas are accessible to wheelchairs. (aida.de)

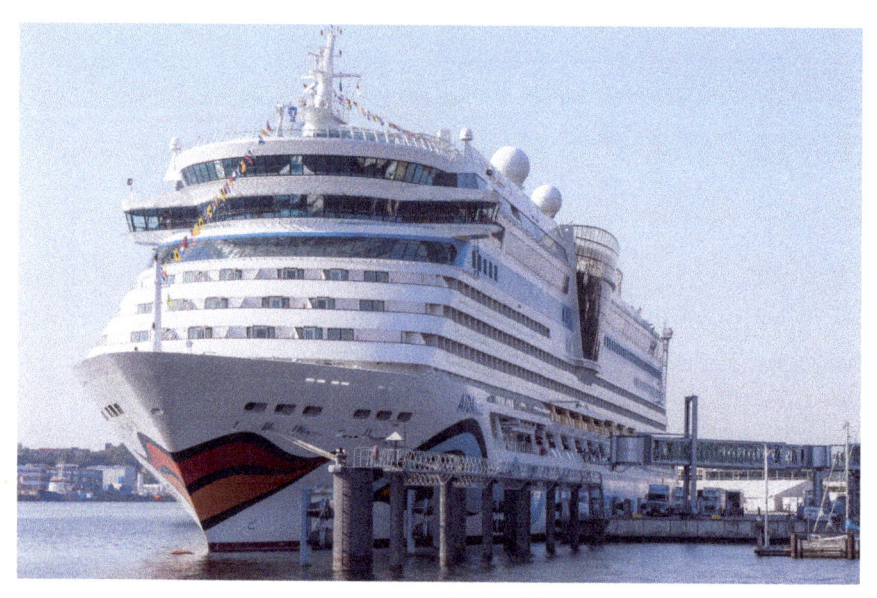

Credit: AIDA's famous smile - Bernd Schray, Pixabay

# Where to Start?

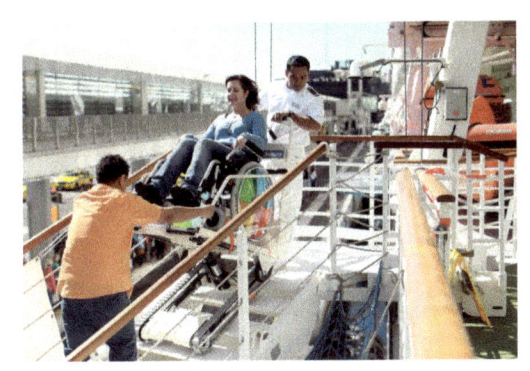

*Credit: Belted stair climber (Treppenraupe) - AIDA*

### American Queen Steamboat Company
*Climb aboard the iconic, richly-appointed steamboat American Queen, or the opulent paddle-wheeler American Duchess and experience a fragment of American history on an unforgettable Mississippi or Ohio River sailing. Travelling along American rivers means guests with special needs are provided for under the laws of the Americans with Disabilities Act. The accessible cabins are large with plenty of manoeuvrability and accessible balconies, and the bathrooms come with roll-in showers, shower seats and grab bars. All six decks are accessible via two sets of lifts. Enjoy complimentary pre-cruise hotel stays, wine and beer with dinner, shore excursions in each port, lectures from historians and culture specialists, and delicious regionally inspired cuisine. Most of the shore excursion buses have wheelchair lifts and the drivers are happy to assist. (americanqueensteamboatcompany.com)*

### Costa Cruises
*Geared mainly to Europeans, Costa embodies Italian style and hospitality and offers an all-inclusive experience to all its guests across its fleet of more than a dozen ships. Interactive stands with touchscreen screens are located throughout the ships that can interact with guests in six languages - they provide information about ship life, shore excursion sales, 4D cinema tickets, dinner reservations and you can access your onboard account from them. All Costa ships have a generous number of accessible cabins and most decks have lift access. (costacruises.co.uk)*

### Hapag-Lloyd Cruises
*You'd be forgiven for thinking this German company was just a cargo fleet, but Hapag-Lloyd offers international voyages on its beautiful ships, the Hanseatic*

# The Autonomous Cruiser

Inspiration and Europa 2. All documentation, menus, announcements, lectures, Zodiac instruction and the safety drill are provided in English. Europa 2 has one suite that can accommodate disabled guests while Hanseatic Inspiration has a fully accessible cabin and bathroom. All of the public areas and some of the outer decks can be accessed by lifts which are designed to accommodate wheelchairs. Guests with mobility problems must travel with a companion. MS Europa, Nature and Bremen also have accessible cabins but are German speaking cruises. (hl-cruises.com)

## Best European River Cruises

Below is a small selection of the major operators that provide European river cruises. Most are not suitable for wheelchair dependent travellers, but the newly renovated MS Viola and the Prins Willem Alexander are notable exceptions - they represent a first in the river cruising industry, both offering full accessibility throughout the ship. Tour agents Accessible Travel Netherlands and Enable Holidays have confirmed wheelchair users will be able to get off at every port.

### *MS Viola*

MS Viola is a luxury 61 cabin river cruise specially designed for people with physical challenges and special needs, with 34 fully adapted, spacious two-person cabins enjoying extra-wide thresholds, height-adjustable beds, wheelchair-accessible washbasins and a shared roll-in shower and toilet. The entire vessel is barrier-free, including the lounge, bar, reading room, restaurant, hairdresser and public toilet, with access to all four decks via several spacious lifts. Wheelchairs and scooters can be used at all times, and additional mobility equipment is available on the ship, including electric hoists and shower chairs.

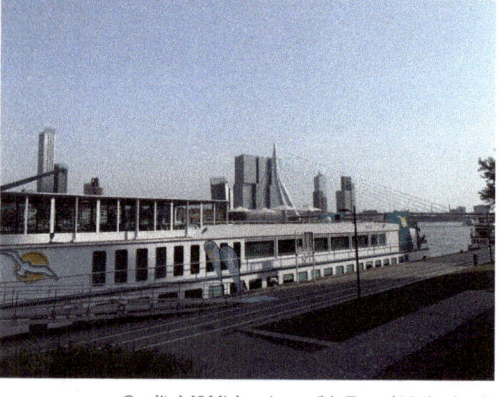

Credit: MS Viola - Accessible Travel Netherlands

The ship departs and ends in Bonn, Germany, where passengers can access the vessel via the wide ramp that makes it possible for guests to visit every port along its four routes through West Germany, the Netherlands, Belgium and France. At most destinations, a shore excursion is offered with an English-speaking guide who takes into account your accessibility requirements and provides a suitable step-free route to the town centre.

After a renovation costing more than €7.5 million, the MS Viola offers all the care options you might need, including onboard medical staff that are available 24/7, and kidney dialysis available in Germany. Nightly dialysis treatment is also possible as the ship is docked overnight at its ports.

Accessible Travel Netherlands and Enable Holidays are two of the agents taking bookings on this innovative river cruise. Accessible Travel Netherlands manages direct contact and bookings with the river cruise company in Germany and resells the cruises to travel companies, including Enable Holidays. (*accessibletravelnl.com*) (*enableholidays.com*)

## Prins Willem Alexander

The Prins Willem Alexander is a 48 cabin river cruise specially designed for people with physical challenges and special needs, with 25 fully adapted, spacious two-person cabins enjoying extra-wide thresholds, electric height-adjustable beds, and a wheelchair-accessible washbasin. Please note the cabins do not have en-suite bathrooms - instead, there is a generous oversized bathroom shared by three other cabins that includes a roll-in shower with a seat, grab bars, a handheld showerhead, lowered washbasin, and toilet with support rails on both sides. There are four additional accessible toilets on the main deck. Originally a hospital ship, the entire vessel is barrier-free, including wide spacious corridors and large lifts to all four decks. Wheelchairs and scooters can be used at all times and additional mobility equipment can be delivered to the ship, including electric hoists and commode chairs. Care assistance is available on the ship and is included in the price, but it must be requested at the time of booking.

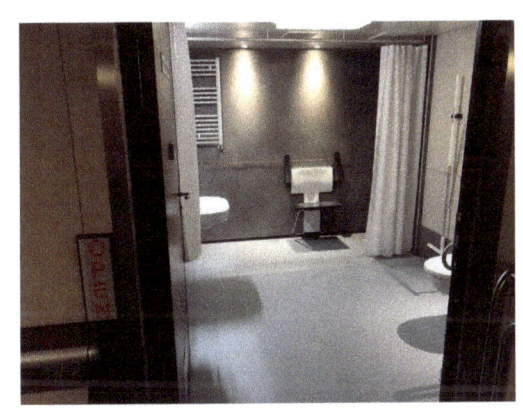

Credit: MS Prins Willem Alexander - Accessible Travel Netherlands

These select charter cruises are offered in spring and autumn, sailing along the Rhine and Holland's gorgeous waterways. Passengers can access the vessel via the wide ramp that makes it possible to visit every port along its various routes. A shore excursion is offered at most destinations, with an English-speaking guide who takes into account your accessibility requirements and provides a suitable step-free route to the town centre.

For an additional fee, wheelchair-friendly transfers to and from Amsterdam Airport and a pre-stay in a fully accessible hotel in Amsterdam can be offered before the start of the cruise.

The accessible river cruises that provide availability for international passengers are organised by Accessible Travel Netherlands in cooperation with a Dutch partner who hires the ship for four or five weeks a year. For the other weeks during the year, the river cruise ship is available for Dutch passengers only. So, if you'd love to enjoy a river cruise holiday with other English-speaking passengers, book well in advance and check the dates with Accessible Travel Netherlands or one of their trusted British agents, such as Enable Holidays. (accessibletravelnl.com) (enableholidays.com)

### Scenic Luxury Cruises & Tours

Unfortunately, it is not possible for wheelchair users to board Scenic river ships in their chair as the ramps used are not wide enough and are stepped with a steep incline. However, they do provide a limited number of accessible cabins situated near the reception desk on several of their ships that cruise the waterways of Europe. These feature wider doors to accommodate a standard manual wheelchair, a bathtub with grab bars and a wheel-in shower with a stool.

Scenic's ships operate a lift to the two main decks, giving full access to reception, the restaurants, the lounge, the bar and the shops. The lower Moselle Deck and the Wellness Centre (including the hairdresser) are inaccessible for wheelchair users, and guests will need to climb approximately 12 steps to reach the Sun Deck. Scenic's private butler service is available for each guest (except for Russian cruises) and the staff are excellent at lending a hand at the gangway and shoreside. (scenic.co.uk)

### Emerald Waterways

Emerald Waterways welcome disabled guests but point out that there are limitations which could exist onboard and during shore excursions. Emerald Sky and Emerald Star each have one disabled cabin, located next to reception so passengers have easy access to their cabins. Some of the bathrooms have been modified to allow wheelchair access, but all mobility aids taken onboard must be collapsible. Showers with grab bars are generally in a cubicle rather than over a bath, and there are a limited number of stools.

# Where to Start?

*Lifts serve two out of three decks on all their ships, but guests need to be able to climb approximately 12 steps to get to the Sun Deck. Unfortunately, a wheelchair user cannot embark the ships in a wheelchair as the ramps used are not wide enough as well as being stepped with a steep incline. The shore excursions offered sometimes provide for disabled guests, depending on their restrictions. (emeraldwaterways.co.uk)*

## Smoking Onboard

The issue of smoking on ships is still a divisive one, with cruise lines taking action to stamp it out but have yet to do so completely. The phasing out of smoking on balconies started in 2014, and gradually most cruise lines have jumped on the bandwagon, save Fred. Olsen, Costa Cruises, AIDA and Hapag-Lloyd. MSC's North American ship *Divina* and Oceania Cruises are probably the most restrictive, but aside from these, most lines still offer generous outside smoking areas. The premium lines also tend to offer their cigar-smoking guests a dedicated hideaway, typically decked out in dark panelled woods and plush leather seating, reminiscent of the private gentlemen's clubs from a bygone age.

**Smoking Penalties:** Most American cruise lines impose a minimum $250 cleaning fee for each violation of their smoking policy. If the policy is consistently ignored, the passenger may be asked to leave the ship.

Fire remains one of the major safety concerns at sea and so cruise lines have a strict policy on guests discarding cigarette ends or ash residue from cigars and pipes overboard, as they can easily be blown back on the ship and cause a fire. There are plenty of ashtrays in each designated smoking area, so use them to make sure whatever you've been smoking is completely extinguished before leaving the area. If smoking is allowed on your balcony, ask your steward for an ashtray if there isn't one already provided.

**Be Careful:** Smoking rules and regulations are subject to change at any time during your cruise as policies vary in different countries and will be dependent on the itinerary you are following.

E-cigarettes and vape pens are completely banned in certain countries, including but not limited to: Argentina, Brazil, India, Indonesia, Thailand and the United Arab Emirates. While some authorities will only confiscate the offending item if you're caught using one, some like Singapore can impose a fine of up to $5000, and according to the UK Foreign Office, an offender in Thailand could be fined or sent to prison for up to ten years.

The sale of e-cigarettes and vape pens, but not their possession, has been banned in some countries, as has the sale of nicotine-containing liquids, including Australia, Canada, Hong Kong, Norway and Japan. In February 2020, the *Washington Post* announced that the Trump administration had outlawed the sale of youth-friendly fruit, dessert and mint flavoured pods, though menthol and tobacco flavours have temporarily escaped the ban. Newspaper headlines about the legal status of e-cigarettes and vape pens are appearing daily, and it is likely that more countries will clamp down on the use of them sooner rather than later. Before you head on your next cruise, check the restrictions at the ports of call you might be visiting, as laws are evolving and a rising number of countries are banning them.

More information on the smoking policies of each cruise line can be found in the 'Smoking Facilities' section in the Directory.

## Religious Services

> **Don't Ask:**
> *Has this ship ever sunk?*

Cruise lines are under no obligation to provide religious services aboard their ships, but many do their best to accommodate their guests' beliefs and practices. The type and frequency of services vary enormously throughout the cruising industry and the information can be difficult to find. Below is a brief overview of which services are offered by each cruise line, and the religious holidays that are celebrated onboard.

**Azamara:** An interdenominational service is offered on Sundays, but only if the ship is at sea. A priest is provided for religious services over Easter and Christmas, and a rabbi is available for celebrating Pesach (Passover) and Hanukkah (Chanukah). Other holidays or festivals may be celebrated if a clergy or minister is onboard as a passenger and volunteers their services.

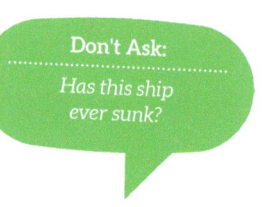

# Where to Start?

**Carnival**: There are no Sunday services unless a clergy or minister is onboard as a passenger and volunteers their services.

**Celebrity**: There are no Sunday services unless a clergy or minister is on board as a passenger and volunteers their services. There is often a self-led Shabbat service on a Friday.

**Costa Cruises**: All Costa ships have a chapel where passengers can go to pray. Mass is only celebrated on some cruises and only on the main Catholic feast days.

**Crystal**: An interdenominational service is offered on Sundays, but only if the ship is at sea, and there is often a self-led Shabbat service on Fridays. Jewish services are available during major holidays and Catholic services are offered on most cruises.

**Cunard**: Either the Captain or Staff Captain will hold an Ecumenical Service each Sunday and there is often a self-led Shabbat service on Fridays. A Catholic priest will now be sailing onboard all Queen Mary 2 cruises. There will also be Catholic and Protestant priests onboard Queen Victoria and Queen Elizabeth during key religious dates and festivals (e.g. Easter and Christmas), with services held accordingly. A rabbi is also offered to celebrate Yom Kippur, Rosh Hashanah, Sukkot and Pesach (Passover).

**Disney**: An interdenominational service is typically held on Sundays (except on sailings that depart on a Sunday) at approximately 9 am. Representatives of the clergy are brought onboard for special occasions (e.g. Christmas, Hanukkah (Chanukah), etc). There is sometimes a self-led Shabbat service on Fridays.

**Fred. Olsen**: The Cruise Director leads Sunday services on cruises which are shorter than 16 nights, and a chaplain is onboard for all cruises of 16 nights or more. There are also interdenominational services at Easter, Christmas, and on world cruises.

**Holland America**: A Catholic priest is onboard at all times and mass is held daily. Services are held on Sunday mornings and are led by the congregation when a minister is not present. Protestant ministers are on select sailings. Jewish rabbis sail on grand and legendary voyages.

**Hurtigruten**: No religious services are offered to passengers. If the ship is in port on Christmas Eve, passengers and crew are encouraged to visit a local church and join the service.

**MSC Cruises**: No religious services are offered to passengers.

**Marella Cruises**: An interdenominational service is offered on a Sunday and services are offered for most religious holidays.

**Norwegian Cruise Line**: No religious services are offered to passengers.

**Oceania**: A nondenominational service is given on Sundays and services are offered at Easter and Christmas. If a pastor, rabbi or other religious leader is on the ship as a passenger, they may conduct a service, otherwise one of the ship's officers will lead prayers.

**P&O Cruises**: Either the captain or staff captain provides an ecumenical service on Sundays and there is often a self-led Shabbat service on Fridays. A chaplain is on board all ships to hold services for the major Christian holidays. A rabbi is also offered to celebrate the four main holidays in the Jewish calendar: Pesach (*Passover*), Rosh Hashanah, Yom Kippur, and Hanukkah (*Chanukah*).

**Princess Cruises**: The Cruise Director provides interdenominational services on Sundays and there is often a self-led Shabbat service on Fridays. There is a Catholic mass service on Christmas cruises and a Seder service is held during Pesach (*including Passover meal*). For cruises during Hanukkah (*Chanukah*), services are available and will be guest-led with wine, challah bread, prayers and an electric menorah provided by Princess.

**Regent**: A nondenominational service is offered when possible.

**Royal Caribbean**: Interdenominational services are held onboard each week and during religious holidays. Guests of all faiths are able to host their own spiritual fellowship or group gathering by inquiring with the Guest Relation's desk onboard.

**Seabourn**: A nondenominational Christian service is typically held on Sundays while the ship is at sea. Ecumenical clergy will be aboard to conduct services on cruises that coincide with certain religious holidays.

**SeaDream Yacht Club**: No religious services are offered to passengers.

**Silversea**: A nondenominational service is offered on Sundays. Catholic, Protestant and Jewish clergy will be onboard during select holidays when possible.

**Star Clipper**: No religious services are offered to passengers.

**Virgin Voyages**: No religious services are offered to passengers.

**Windstar**: No religious services are offered to passengers.

## Where to Sleep?

Once you've decided when and where to go, your next decision is where to sleep. Choosing a cabin isn't easy, especially because there are hundreds to choose from, all with different prices and locations on the ship. There are several different types of cabin: crew, balcony, single, family, spa and accessible. There is no 'best cabin' - it remains a choice based on what is most important to you.

### Accessible Cabins
Most ships have a limited number of wheelchair-accessible, adapted or modified staterooms that are suited to guests with special needs so if your party requires one you should book well in advance as the need usually outstrips demand. Make sure to check exactly what each cruise line offers and that it is suitable for your group. Different cruise lines use slightly different terminology, but accessible rooms can be broken down into three main categories:

- **Fully accessible wheelchair cabins** are designed for guests with highly limited mobility who rely on the permanent use of a wheelchair, scooter or other similar assistive devices. They typically have wider doorways into the cabin and bathroom, ramped thresholds, and accessible routes with sufficient floor space for manoeuvrability. The bathrooms are usually equipped with roll-in showers, shower seats, grab bars, lowered sinks and alarm alerts. If you have booked a balcony grade cabin there will be step-free access out onto the patio.
- **Fully accessible wheelchair cabins** - single side approach cabins are also designed for guests who rely on the permanent use of a wheelchair, scooter or other similar assistive devices. They offer the same facilities as regular fully accessible wheelchair cabins (as above), while providing an accessible route and clear floor space on just one side of the bed in cabins configured to offer only one bed, or between beds in cabins providing two beds.
- **Ambulatory accessible cabins** (adapted/modified cabins) are standard cabins that provide accessible elements that would aid a person able to ambulate, as defined by an agreement between the Americans with Disabilities Act and the Carnival Corporation. These rooms are not purpose-built but instead modified from their original specifications, and consequently can cause difficulties to a permanent wheelchair user but are often ideal for guests who only use a cane or walker and who may benefit from certain accessible features like grab bars to help with balance. They may not have a sufficient turning radius for wheelchairs and there may be lipped access to the bathroom, shower and balcony.

Accessible cabins are specially designed to meet the needs of all passengers with mobility challenges and are usually available in all cabin grades. You might also find lowered closet rods, portable ADA kits for guests with hearing and visual impairments and closed-captioned televisions. Most modern cruise liners provide access to all decks by lift, including the sundecks, and most provide accessible bars and dining and entertainment venues.

If a wheelchair or motorised mobility device is needed for permanent use onboard the ship, you will need to book an accessible cabin and let your line know in advance that you require a wheelchair - some lines won't allow mobility equipment onboard without prior notice. If you have reduced mobility but don't use a wheelchair or scooter, you are not required to book an accessible cabin; there are a number of different options available, so it's best to speak with a cruise advisor about the specific features you need.

If you require an accessible or adapted stateroom but they are fully booked on your preferred cruise ship, it's wise not to book a standard cabin as there will be several limitations that could adversely impact your manoeuvrability, especially with bathroom access. Additionally, standard cabin doors and hallways may be too narrow for a wheelchair or scooter to access. For safety reasons, all wheelchairs, mobility scooters and walking frames must be charged and stored in your cabin, so fire doors, corridors and lift lobbies are kept clear in case of emergency. Most ships have one of either 110- or 220-volt outlets, depending on the vessel's nationality, however some of the newer builds offer both. You should ensure your equipment is compatible with your ship's electrical supply and bring any relevant adaptors for your device.

Do not book an accessible cabin unless you have a genuine need for one. Cruise ships have a limited number of staterooms equipped with features designed to help guests with impaired mobility and other disabilities, who may find a non-accessible stateroom restrictive. There have been offenders who have booked an accessible cabin just to gain the extra square footage that the room and bathroom afford, but cruise lines have grown wise and will now reassign guests to a standard stateroom when they have no genuine medical need for an accessible room, or even cancel the booking altogether.

Most cruise line operators have specially trained staff to assist guests with special needs. They are there to answer your queries before and during your voyage, including helping you to select the right cabin for your needs.

***Medical Essential:*** *Some cruise lines require 90 days' notice to implement a special request so make your wishes known as early as possible.*

The Disabled Cruise Club (*disabledcruiseclub.co.uk*) has details on the individual facilities (some with photographs) in disabled cabins on many of the most popular cruise lines. Likewise, Special Needs at Sea (*specialneedsatsea.com*) has a comprehensive list of all accessible features across every cruise line.

## Cabin Grade

The seemingly endless list of options you might find on a cruise line's website might seem overwhelming, but in reality, cabins generally fall into just four different types and each one will have a number of categories based on its size, location, features and view:

- **Inside cabins** are among the smallest on the ship and have no window, however, Disney, Royal Caribbean and NCL offer virtual or projected ocean views and balconies.
- **Outside and ocean view cabins** are as the name suggests, rooms with a porthole or window (*don't open*).
- **Balcony rooms** have floor to ceiling windows and a door to a veranda affording you the luxury of going outside without visiting a public deck.
- **Suites** are generally the largest and most luxurious cabins onboard, offering private balconies and larger living spaces that are often separate from the sleeping area.

Within these four types, all ocean cruise cabins have:

- Single, twin (convertible to queen- or king-sized) or bunk beds.
- A cabin steward who cleans your room and turns down the beds.
- Private bathrooms with showers, towels, soap, shampoo.
- A wardrobe stocked with hangers, a chest of drawers.
- A television, a small minibar or fridge (most ships) and one or two power sockets.
- A small safe (most ships), a wall-mounted mirror, a thermostat and a hairdryer.
- A phone featuring a wake-up call service.
- Lifejackets.
- Room service.
- Suites come with additional perks and extras, such as a fruit basket, flowers, iced champagne on arrival, afternoon canapés, preferential boarding and priority tender service.

CruiseMapper (*cruisemapper.com*) provides extensive information on all cabin grades of every ship on the market.

## Butlers

Premium category cabins or concierge class staterooms can have access to a private lounge and/or a private dining room and include the personalised service of a butler who is there to make your holiday as enjoyable as possible. They are assigned on a shared basis but will look after all of your needs, from unpacking your cases to stocking your minibar, serving canapes, handling your laundry needs or making any reservations you might want. On certain lines the butler will also book airport transfers, print boarding passes and facilitate priority disembarkation on port days and the last day of the cruise. They can offer advice about ports, problem-solve, and even organise an in-suite cocktail party. They won't, however, act as a personal companion, caregiver or babysitter.

## Cabin Size

One of the main distinctions between cabin types is their size. Basic interior and exterior cabins, regardless of their category, are referred to as a 'standard' and are generally the same size. Balcony cabins may also offer the same square footage except with the added bonus of outdoor space. While inside cabins are ideal for the budget-conscious, they are among the smallest on a ship, offer no daylight, and are not a great choice for passengers prone to motion sickness. If you need a generous amount of living space or need natural daylight, these cabins are not for you.

Most cruise ships incorporate a shower rather than a bath to save on space. Check the cruise ship deck plan if a bath is important to you, as they are clearly marked.

## Balconies

Some travellers spend all their time enjoying the public areas of the ship, so a balcony might not be a good investment, especially on a cold winter cruise. However, others like to avoid crowded areas and prefer their own private space where they can lap up the fresh air, enjoy room service and whale watch - for those types, a balcony would be ideal. They are by far the most popular cabin grade and with the huge demand for new ships over the last decade, shipbuilders have complied with the cruise line's requests to increase the volume of balconies, with the result that they account for around 75% of rooms.

Not all balconies offer the same view, nor do they all allow the same level of privacy. Depending on the ship's design you may find that you can see all your neighbours and they can see you, or that the balconies above yours look straight down into your 'private' space. Also, balcony dividers usually don't extend down to the floor and can be paltry thin, making it easy to overhear your neighbours' conversations and catch glimpses of their movements.

Just remember that not all balconies face out to sea, some face into the ship and have a view of a promenade deck or the passengers in the balcony cabins opposite. Royal Caribbean's Oasis-class ships have a great view of the Boardwalk and Central Park from the balconies, an area adorned with tropical plants and trees and the street-lined restaurants.

There are a lot of porthole and ocean-view cabins, as well as balconies, that offer views which are fully or partially obstructed by lifeboats, metal railings, bulkheads, beams, machinery or window cleaning gondolas (suspended platforms), and some, such as those on a promenade deck, are located so that nearby public deck space offers passengers a clear view of your balcony. These issues could be a deal breaker for some would-be travellers, but if, on the other hand, an obstructed view won't irritate you, then you will probably benefit from a better price deal as the downsides are reflected in the cruise fare.

Sometimes it's the structural design of the ship, rather than the nearby safety equipment, that obstructs the view from a balcony, like, for example, the aft cabins on P&O's *Ventura* which are affected by a slanted beam in front of the veranda. Several of these cabins are also near the ship's vents, so it isn't unusual to experience strange smells or a thin layer of black soot rain down on you. This problem doesn't just apply to P&O, any cruise line offering aft cabins located near a vent, will experience the same problem. Some of the cabins also experience vibrations from the ships' thrusters when manoeuvring in and out of ports and they are a long way from the lifts, so they are not suitable for everyone with

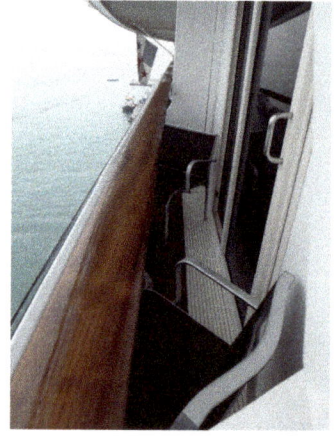

*Credit: MSC Divinia - cruisedeckplans.com*

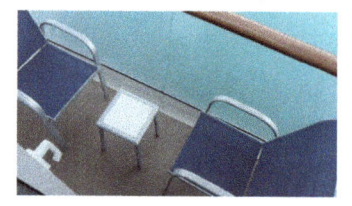

*Credit: Norwegian Breakaway - cruisedeckplans.com*

a mobility problem. On the flipside, there will be far less foot traffic outside your cabin, and the balconies are usually much larger and will comfortably fit a wheelchair.

If you're a lover of the Princess brand, then you'll be aware of the *Royal* and *Regal*'s innovative SeaWalk. This incredible piece of engineering sees a 60 ft glass-floored walkway cantilevered over the ocean 128 ft below. As fantastic as it is, it doesn't offer any privacy to the mid-ship odd-numbered cabins underneath the structure, especially M411-M423 on the Marina deck or the equivalent cabins on Riviera deck.

If you are looking to book a balcony cabin it is worth researching which side of the ship will afford the best views for your chosen itinerary. Take the time to study the route map, and in doing so, determine which side will be facing land more frequently. To be fair, each side will offer a similar experience, and on scenic cruises such as those to Geiranger in Norway or Glacier Bay in Alaska, the captain will typically execute a 360-degree turn of the ship so everyone gets a fabulous view. If sailing along a river, both sides of the ship will afford a great view, or if you find your balcony is on the wrong side whilst coming into a port then you can always pop up to the top deck to get great views from either side. If something special comes into view, like dolphins following the wake of the ship or the Northern Lights, the captain or Cruise Director will make an announcement as to what side to look from.

**Routing Tip:** *Getting the sun or shade requires knowing the direction the ship is heading in relation to the sun.*

It's also worth noting that not all balconies offer the same amount of space. Certain balcony cabins on Carnival, Princess and NCL ships have such a small outdoor space that even the furniture is pared down, sometimes with just two chairs that face each other rather than the view out to sea. As another example, the

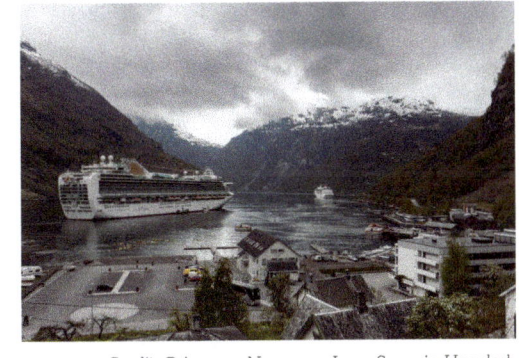

Credit: Geiranger, Norway - Jorge Segovia, Unsplash

MSC *Divinia* hasn't got so much as a balcony but rather a lip; more commonly known as a French balcony, they typically have sliding glass doors that open to a railing - if any deck exists it is a tiny strip. Finally, Disney's *Dream* and *Fantasy* charge the same for cabins 5188 and 5688 as standard balconies, but they are oddly shaped and so the outdoor space is much smaller.

Hump or bump cabins are located midship and jut out further from the side of the vessel than the balconies on either side giving you great views of the ship. Some are known to have much larger balconies than a standard cabin and because of the depth of the design they also have the added privacy of not being seen from other balconies. Celebrity *Solstice* has more than 50 cabins with triple the amount of balcony space, most of which are on the hump.

**Classified:** *The 8-forward-most balcony cabins on Deck 6 of Celebrity M-class ships are twice the size of other balconies on those vessels.*

**Balcony Essential:** *Check whether balcony doors are a push/pull or are sliding doors before you book - permanent wheelchair users travelling alone will find it difficult getting outside on their own if the door doesn't slide.*

**Balcony Essential:** *If you are a non-smoker, remember that AIDA, Costa, Fred. Olsen and Hapag Lloyd still allow smoking on their balconies, so it's possible you might see or smell other passengers smoking nearby.*

## P.O.S.H

*Although unconfirmed,* **P**ort **O**ut **S**tarboard **H**ome, *later shortened to 'P.O.S.H.', seems to have originated in 1935 when a letter was received by the editor of the London* Times Literary Supplement, *identifying port out starboard home as "an American shipping term describing the best cabins."*

*Merriam-Webster writes that the most elaborate version of the story associates the practice with the Peninsular and Oriental Steam Navigation Company, which from 1842 to 1970 was the primary steamship carrier of passengers and mail between England and India. The cabins on the port side on the way to India got the morning sun and had the rest of the day to cool off, while starboard cabins got the afternoon sun and were still quite hot at bedtime. On the return trip, the opposite was true. The cooler cabins were the more desirable and were reserved for the most important and wealthiest of society.*

## Suites

Choosing a suite or premium category cabin boils down to how much room you need and how much you're looking to spend. They often sell out very quickly, so you need to determine whether one is worth the investment early on in the booking process. Most suites are generous in size; some offer a king-sized bedroom, deluxe bathroom with a spa bath, and walk-in closets, while some of the 'super' suites have split-level living, several bedrooms, a balcony jacuzzi and a grand piano. Most upscale cruise lines provide a personal butler with your suite who will be available 24 hours a day and perform a lengthy checklist of duties designed to make your cruise stress-free. Assigned on a shared basis, the butler will also assist with packing and unpacking, offer a pillow menu, serve you afternoon tea and bring you your preferred newspaper daily. If you decide on in-suite dining, your butler will serve your meal course by course, either inside your suite or on your balcony. They will handle laundry and dry-cleaning requests, mix cocktails and deliver cappuccinos and espressos, draw bubble baths, and even organise in-suite parties.

Some suites provide a concierge service instead of a butler. Like their hotel counterparts, they can make reservations in the spa or your favourite restaurant, and secure a port tours on your behalf. Their desk is typically located in a restricted-access concierge lounge such as Celebrity's Michael's Club, MSC's Top Sail Lounge and Royal Caribbean's Concierge Club Lounge, which are exclusive to loyalty-club members or those who book a top-tier suite and provides a quiet space to relax or have hors d'oeuvres and pre-dinner cocktails.

## Family Cabins

Family cabins are offered across all category types, the only difference is that they are configured to house more people. Some have bunk beds attached to the walls that the steward will pull down during their evening service, while others have sofas which convert to an additional twin bed. To accommodate families more easily, Disney offers more space than you will find in most other cruise ships' cabins of the same grade - their standard inside rooms all feature a 'magical porthole', providing guests with a real-time view of the ship's exterior. If you are lucky, you might catch one of your family's best-loved characters or a pirate ship fly by. Another option for families is booking two (or more) adjoining cabins, offering much more space without separating you completely and without having to spend more on a cabin upgrade.

## Single Cabins

One of the banes of the single traveller is that very few ships have dedicated space for solo cruisers and those that do sell out quickly. Even just a few years ago, trying to secure a single cabin was a fruitless quest, but some cruise lines have now increased their range of cabin categories for those that want to cruise alone. With more solo cabins across its fleet than any other line, Norwegian Cruise Lines have ditched the single supplement and provide dedicated 'Studio Suites' - although small, these cabins do provide everything a solo traveller needs to cruise comfortably, with the added bonus that every guest in the room category has access to an exclusive private lounge. Another great choice for solo travellers is Royal Caribbean, whose *Anthem of the Seas* has studio staterooms (with space to sleep two people) available to solo guests. Their *Quantum*-class ships' inside studio cabins offer floor to ceiling virtual balconies providing real-time projections of the sea and ports of call, or you can opt for a balcony studio cabin with private outside space to chill out on. Either cabin type will give you access to staff-hosted meet and mingle events for solo travellers to get to know each other. Newcomer Virgin's *Scarlet Lady* has incorporated 46 of its cabins for solo travellers, and early indications look as if these will be a big hit.

The downside to having your own space on a ship, that either doesn't have any single cabins or are sold out, is that you will have to pay a hefty single supplement, the penalty charge of not having two people in the cabin, which can be as much as double the standard fare. The savings on food might be minimal but the money made from bars, tour sales, spa treatments, photography etc. are halved for single occupancy cabins, so the cruise line adds a premium to make up the shortfall. It's worth asking the price of a twin room for sole occupancy. Yes, there is a difference.

**Heads Up:** *At the time of going to print there are no cruise lines offering single accessible cabins. You can use a twin cabin for sole use but you'd have to pay the single supplement but remember you are only able to sail alone if you are fully self-sufficient in all your needs.*

## Spa Cabins

A new addition to contemporary cruise ships, this category of cabin is sometimes offered with direct access to the spa via a staircase or lift, otherwise your cabin will typically be located on the same deck as the wellness centre.

Enhanced perks could feature unlimited access to the spa's thermal suite, plush bathrobes, a rainfall shower, or an in-room supply of premium water. Although more costly, these living spaces offer health-conscious guests a more rewarding holiday experience.

## Cabin Location

Cabins of the same category are generally all very similar in terms of size and layout, but their location on the ship will massively affect your experience and also their price. For example, a cabin just one deck up from an identical one will cost slightly more, as do midship cabins compared to those at the front or back of the ship. Depending on your personal needs and preferences, there may be certain cabin positions to try to avoid when booking your holiday.

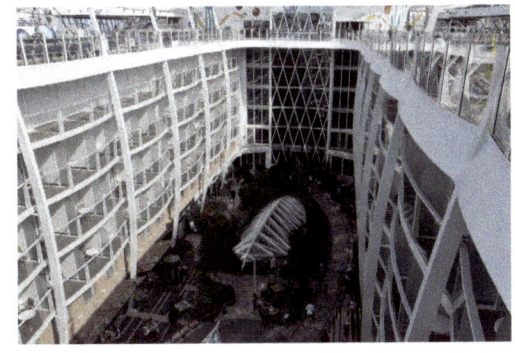

*Credit: Royal Caribbean Allure of the Seas inward facing balconies - John Ostrom, Flickr*

The first of these areas that might be worth avoiding is directly under the deck which houses the pools and/or buffet area (often called the Lido deck) - both these facilities are open extended hours and are a constant source of activity. You will most certainly hear furniture being moved about, especially during deck and pool parties. When the noise does start to abate after midnight, you'll only have a few hours of grace before the kitchen staff turn up to prepare for the morning shift at around 4 am. The ovens are fired up and the vacuum cleaners will be out in force preparing the restaurant for the onset of breakfast, and you may find it hard to sleep through this if you're directly below the noise. Getting back to sleep during breakfast hours may also be out of the questions, as the dishwashers hum in a constant struggle to keep up with the nonstop flow of diners.

***Cruise Tip:*** *Never book a cabin under the Royal Caribbean s Windjammer Café or Windjammer Marketplace, at least not if you ever want to sleep again!*

The noise coming from the casino isn't just affected by the people in them but also by dozens of slot machines with volumes off the Richter scale as they endeavour to tempt the customer away from their hard-earned cash, and then of course there's the resonating bell that indicates a big winner - all of these things can definitely disturb a good night's sleep. On a similar note, don't book a cabin under one of the nightclubs unless the sound of throbbing bass will lull you to sleep, or underneath the sports deck as the constant bouncing and thumping balls are sure to irk even the most tolerant of people.

The 'white space' on a deck plan indicate areas that are off-limits to passengers and tend to house crew only lifts, housekeeping closets and laundry rooms; industrial sized washers and dryers are not quiet and constantly run in order to supply fresh bed linen, towels, bathmats, tablecloths, napkins and crew uniform. Unlike passengers, the crew work around the clock, so these areas will be in almost constant use and could disturb your sleep if your cabin is nearby. This is the same for cabins located on the lower decks that are near the entrances to the 'I-95' or 'M1', the main corridor of the crew area, as the constant footfall and slamming doors day and night might be too much to bear.

Another problem area is directly above the bow of the ship, where passengers are often awakened at the crack of dawn on port days by construction-like noises and vibrations as the anchor is dropped, not the ideal alarm clock for most people. It's also worth trying to avoid lower-deck cabins at the rear of the ship, as they are likely to be near the ship's engine room and are thus victim to the constant hum spawning from the diesel generators.

> **Don't Ask:**
> Do the crew sleep onboard?

Whether or not you want to be near the passenger lifts completely depends on your circumstances. If you are a light sleeper or have small children, request a cabin away from congested passenger areas or lifts as they'll be in constant use as holiday makers make their way to restaurants, shows or the pool. On the other hand, if you have a mobility challenge, you might be best off choosing a cabin close to the lifts, otherwise it can involve sizable walks and deplete your energy before you've even started. Going one step further, it might be worth looking at the deck plan of your preferred ship and requesting a cabin near the set of lifts which will give you easiest access to the facilities you'll use the most. For example, several lines have designated 'spa staterooms', and on some of the luxury brands there are those with direct spa access, cutting down on the time you are traversing the decks in your robe and slippers.

If it's important to you that your cabin be a tranquil place, try choosing a cabin surrounded by other cabins as most of your neighbours will want peace and quiet themselves. Having said that, while adjoining cabins are great for large families, they might be best to avoid if you're not booking both of them - the extra door that connects the two rooms is not nearly as soundproof as a cabin wall and it'll be easy to overhear loud neighbours.

If a room with a view is high on your list of priorities, then the exterior cabins at the front or the back of the ship are your best bet. Forward facing cabins are usually suites and offer fabulous windows to the sea and to your ports of call, while the rear cabins offer fantastic unobstructed views of the ocean stretching out in an endless picture of blue. Your choice of cabins that run across the width of the ship will be limited, but they do offer larger balconies, and if you opt for a corner unit, you might even have the luxury of a wraparound veranda.

If you suffer badly from seasickness all is not lost, it is possible to choose your cabin to minimise the effect the ocean will have on your stomach. The saying "the more you pay, the more you sway" is usually quite true, as the higher up cabins that often cost a little more are also the cabins that experience the most exaggerated rolling motion. After this, the worst position is at the front of the vessel as the waves hit there first. The back of the vessel gives a slightly better ride, but if the sea is rough, the movement will still be felt. The general rule of thumb is the lower and more central your cabin is on the ship, the less motion you will feel. As such, your best bet will be a midship cabin on one of the lower decks close to the waterline. If your budget allows for it, opt for a balcony cabin where you can suck up all the fresh air you need at any time of day or night.

There are two great websites, *cruisedeckplans.com* and *comparethatcruise.com*, that allow you to check the placement of each cabin on most cruise lines. It is especially useful in that it explains what is directly above or below a specific cabin and provides photographs for some cabin types.

## Upgrades

If a free upgrade does sound appealing, there are a few things you can do to help put you near the top of the list. First of all, of course, is simply checking online if your preferred cruise line is offering any deals which include a free upgrade - they're a lot more common than you think.

The last thing to consider when it comes to booking your room is whether or not to opt for a 'guarantee' cabin - doing so means you're only reserving a particular category as opposed to a specific room. The benefit is that you're more likely to be upgraded as the cruise line releases cheaper cabins that will sell more easily; the downside is that you'll have no choice in the location of your cabin and you may not know which room you've been allocated until the day before you travel.

*Cruise Tip:* *What your cruise line sees as an upgraded cabin may not necessarily be an opinion you will share, as the room could be in a less favourable position on the ship or may have a restricted view. If you have sweated buckets to ensure you are happy with the cabin you've chosen, it might be best to decline any offers of an upgrade when you make your booking. If you or your cruise agent tick the 'free upgrade' box, you are giving up all control of where your cabin will be located.*

Being among the first to book any of the more affordable cabins can sometimes result in an upgrade. The demand for these cabins is only second to suites, so cruise lines may offer you an upgrade to a less in-demand mid-tier room so they can 'resell' the more sought-after cabin grade.

Many cruise lines have started to offer generous onboard credits as an extra incentive to book with them. Regrettably, you cannot use that same credit to apply for an upgrade before you sail, but once the ship has left its embarkation port, the rules change somewhat. If there is availability, and because the ship has already sailed, upgrades usually come at a reduced cost so you could apply your onboard credit towards it.

Whilst on board, your ship's daily planner will be full of future cruise deals to tempt you into booking another holiday before the one you're on is even finished, and you might like to take advantage of the added perks that the cruise line won't be offering elsewhere. For example, you might benefit from discounted cruise fares, that elusive cabin upgrades, a low booking deposit, free parking, onboard credit, and free Wi-Fi. Some cruise lines like Celebrity and Norwegian even entice future cruisers with a free drink's package on your next sailing, but take note you may be charged gratuities. All ships have their own future cruise specialist who will be happy to go through all the options available to you. They'll have the latest itineraries and sailing dates, and if you usually use a travel agent, they will ensure the booking is credited to them. Celebrity even allows you to change the sailing date or ship once you're back home without penalty and the benefits will be transferred automatically.

## When to Book?

When booking your cruise, the time of year, and even the day of the week, can make a sizable difference to what's available, the deals you might be offered and the level of service you might receive. With so much competition in the modern-day cruise market, some lines offer deals throughout the entire year, with a wide range of items designed to tempt you, like an all-inclusive drinks package, the inclusion of tips, free internet, cabin credit, free parking or door-to-door pick-up. However, if you're looking to secure a particular sailing or discount, like those often applied to seniors, military personnel, regional fares or families (at certain times of the year children might travel for free), it might have a bearing on what time of year you book your cruise.

The general rule to securing a specific sailing is to book as far in advance as possible, particularly if:

- you want a specific cabin or one of the limited high-end suites.
- you want a family cabin, especially over school breaks or seasonal dates like Christmas and Easter. Look at going in the last week of August, as most countries outside the UK are back at school - the lower demand might be reflected in the price.
- you are booking for a large party and hope to secure multiple nearby cabins or adjoining rooms.
- you dream of taking a maiden voyage, but remember there may be negatives to being among the first to sail on a new ship in the way of glitches and hiccups.
- your preferred destination has a short shelf life. For example, the Alaskan cruise season runs from late May to early September, and the majority will want to book mid-season when the weather is better and the wildlife sightings more abundant, meaning the best deals can be found at the start or end of the season.
- you want to book an expedition cruise to the Galapagos or Amazon River, as space is extremely limited.
- you wouldn't dream of sailing the seven seas without man's best friend. Cunard's *Queen Mary 2* has just 22 kennels, so the saying first-come-first-served certainly comes into play.

Another, albeit risky, method of securing a specific cruise at a good price is to check the date the holiday balance will be due (typically 90 days prior to departure, but this varies per cruise line) and hope that would-be travellers pull out, leaving cruise lines with a few cabins available that they'll want to shift quickly. Unsold tickets aren't just about the loss of one passenger's fare, but all the extra spending that a passenger would do. The real revenue loss comes from fewer drink packages, tour excursions, spa treatments, photography bundles and specialty dining, so cruise lines often sell these newly available cabins at a reduced rate to ensure their cabins are filled. If you are hoping for a cancellation, you can improve your chances by registering your interest with the cruise line so that you receive email alerts about any last-minute deals and ask your cruise agent to put you on a watch list. Sometimes you can get lucky.

When it comes to the age-old aim of grabbing a bargain, your two main options are booking early and booking last minute. There are certainly opportunities to secure fantastic early-bird prices, but they are usually only in place for a limited period. Also, on top of saving you money, being among the first to book gives you a free choice of cabin category and its location on the ship. Loyalty passengers are generally offered special fares even before the brochure hits the high street.

At the other end of the scale, waiting until the last-minute in the hope that a cruise line will offer its unsold cabins at basement price is risky but can be rewarding. Your preferred itinerary, travel dates, cabin placement and dining times will most likely be unavailable, but if you're flexible and spontaneous, this won't matter too much and you may find an excellent deal. Also, larger travel agents often reserve blocks of cabins to sell to potential passengers and offer significant discounts in order to offload the last few cabins on their books when the sailing date gets close.

Finally, when you're looking to make first contact with a cruise line or agent, it might be best to avoid calling on a Monday or Tuesday, as they are often playing catch-up on a backlog of weekend enquiries. Calling midweek is probably optimal as the agents will be at their least busy and will spend more time on your enquiry.

# Where to Start?

## How to Book?

Technology has made it so that nearly anybody can research every single detail of their holiday on their own, but once you have made all your decisions about when and where to go and who to go with, you will finally have to decide how to book. Booking online is an option, but unless you're an experienced cruiser, it's not highly recommended. The whole experience is a lot less personal, with nobody to answer your questions, submit any special requests or execute a complicated booking. The discounted fares offered online are there to attract your attention, but they tend to have limited validity, surcharges and even hidden fees that end up offering a far less competitive deal than you might find elsewhere. In general, you should probably only consider three methods of booking: cruise line agents, independent cruise specialists or accessible travel agents.

### Cruise Line Agents

The main reason you may want to book directly through a cruise line with one of their agents is if a flight is involved, otherwise, you're probably better off with an independent cruise specialist or accessible travel agent. The cruise agent can take away all the frustration of trawling through websites, looking for the right connections at the exact times to marry up with your ship's departure. Instead, they will handle your booking for you, but bear in mind, you will have no guarantee of a direct flight, your arrival time, and the airfare may be higher than other options. Having said that, most of the major cruise lines have 'bulk fares' which could even save you money compared to booking independently - for example, Royal Caribbean guarantees you the lowest possible airfare, otherwise you will receive a 110% refund of the difference in onboard credit. Other advantages of booking directly through the cruise line is that you don't have to pay for your flight until the cruise line sends out your final invoice, and they can organise ground transportation and pre- or post-cruise hotel stays on your behalf. Plus, if there is a flight delay or cancellation and you miss your cruise embarkation, the cruise line will work with the airline to get you to the next port of call and cover any extra costs incurred.

Another bonus of booking directly is, in the unlikely event the ship is delayed getting back to its home port through bad weather, the cruise line

> **Don't Ask:**
> Why is my microwave not working? (referring to the cabin safe)

will automatically rebook a suitable connection and put you up in a hotel if required. If you book your flight independently, through a cruise specialist or through an accessible travel agent, you'll have the onus of ringing them yourself to organise your trip home. It's also worth noting that budget airlines tend to only offer one flight a day to a given destination, giving you less choice if you experience a delay.

*Travel Agent Request:* *If you would prefer to book directly through a cruise line, you can do so and still transfer your booking to a travel agent, if requested within 30 days, and gain their perks as well.*

## Independent Cruise Specialists & Accessible Travel Agents

A growing trend over the last few years has seen more and more travellers seek advice from independent cruise specialists and accessible travel agents - aficionados whose experience, contacts and knowledge of the cruise market cannot be matched with any amount of internet searching. Unlike high-street travel agents who deal with all aspects of the travel industry, most of these experts are also seasoned cruisers themselves, meaning they'll be answering your questions and addressing your needs through first-hand experience. Accessible travel agents, especially those that are disabled or mobility challenged themselves have typically travelled and overcome those same obstacles that you might have to face, and have a level of expertise that is hard to match when it comes to getting the best deal. Any travel arrangements they make on your behalf will be guaranteed and not just requested.

The big bonus of booking through a specialist is that they are there to look after your interests, not those of a cruise line - simply knowing this can alleviate a lot of the stress and anxiety for a first-time cruiser. Your specialist will hunt out the best deals and can offer you special perks that are generally not offered if you book directly through the cruise line, including onboard spending money, cabin upgrades, free Wi-Fi, free port parking or a bottle of bubbly on ice in your cabin. Cruise lines depend on these specialists to sell their sailings, so they usually won't undercut the agencies they work with. Another advantage is that your cruise specialist will act as a point of contact, almost like a personal concierge, and can add accessible excursions, a rental car or a hotel for you. Also, if you have a genuine complaint on your return, you won't be left to your own devices to deal with the corporate complaints department, but instead you'll have someone to help you fight your battle.

Contrary to what a lot of people believe, these booking experts do not charge any more than a high-street travel agent. Travel industry personnel are usually rewarded via commission generated when booking a hotel room, cruise or tickets to an attraction. If your trip involves complex crossovers that require a lot of research, legwork and phone time, you may be charged a small planning fee, but it will often be offset by the fact that the agent's expertise and connections will have saved you money. The leading providers of these specialised services are listed in the Directory.

## The Fine Print

Having made all of the big decisions about your holiday, the hardest part is certainly done; however, your trip can easily be ruined if you forget to consider just a few more things, namely the small details contained within the fine print of your booking. We have all done it - just ticked the 'I've read the terms and conditions' checkbox without actually taking the time to read them, and it's exactly the same thing with the 'Booking Conditions' printed in the back of every cruise lines' brochure, posted on their website and printed on your confirmation documents. They're always the same, - technical jargon in incredibly small print, filling reams of pages, but the reason it is there, and the reason you should read it, is that it forms part of the contract you agree to when you book your cruise.

There's no doubt the terms and conditions are boring to read, but you really should know what you're actually agreeing to. For example, it is your responsibility to make sure everyone in your party has valid travel documents, including your mandatory visas and vaccinations; if you cannot provide the correct evidence, you might find that you are prevented from boarding. This might seem obvious to some, but it wasn't to the lady that turned up for her Amazon cruise without getting her yellow fever jab…… the ship left without her.

At the time of booking every passenger is obliged to inform the cruise line of any condition, including but not limited to reduced mobility or any disability of any guest travelling in the booking, which may require special arrangements, medical equipment, supplies, care or assistance. This also applies if you are travelling with a service dog, or if you are pregnant. The cruise line has the right to ask a guest to produce evidence of their fitness to travel. If you turn up at your embarkation port without informing your cruise line, you will probably never see the gangway.

***Medical Essential:*** *Pre-notifying your cruise line of any special needs you have is essential because without doing so you have no legal guarantee that you'll get the assistance you need on your journey. ABTA (abta.com) recommend you download their 'Checklist for Disabled and Less Mobile Passengers' and give it to your travel agent or cruise operator at the time of booking.*

One final thing to note, though there's nothing much that can be done about it, is that the fine print will always state that the cruise line has the right to change, omit or substitute the itinerary for whatever reason they see fit. So, if you had your heart set on visiting Bermuda and the port is bypassed because of bad weather, a guest emergency, mechanical or technical problems, or because of assistance to another vessel...... tough luck.

## Price Promise

Some cruise lines offer a price promise, with which you'll have up to 24 hours after booking to find a cheaper quote for the same cruise. Doing so will see your cruise line effect a reduction on the balance payable for your cruise. If you have already paid for your holiday in full, you can either apply for a refund or have the amount applied as credit to your onboard account.

**Hidden Costs**

The most frustrating part of the fine print is often the hidden costs, and while not knowing about them in advance won't ruin your holiday as such, having to fork out a lot more than you expected can put a damper on things. First off, make sure you understand exactly what is and what isn't included in your cruise fare. For example, people are often stung when booking an 'all-inclusive' and are surprised to find that the small print stipulates extra charges for specialty restaurants, coffee cards, drinks packages, excursions, Wi-Fi, photographs, spa treatments, gym classes, money exchange and tips.

***Onboard Account:*** *You can request a copy of your statement at any time from Guest Relations, and most cruise lines have the facility for you to check your account through your cabin television.*

# Where to Start?

Crew tips are expected on most ships in some form - a few lines include them as part of your cruise fare, while others will charge you between £6 and £9 per person per day, directly to your onboard account. In most cases, you can go to Guest Relations and ask that these charges be removed from your account, but some companies have grown wise to this and are making it more difficult. For example, NCL are now making you pay tips upfront, and you have to apply for a refund once you return from your cruise if you want the money back. It is not that passengers necessarily want to avoid tipping, it's just some like to pay cash to those crew members that have served them particularly well, especially to the steward that delivers the luggage or room service, who might not get a cut of the daily fee. Tips can be a big bone of contention with some travellers, so much so that some cruise companies have taken to scrapping the tradition altogether, instead adding a 15% service charge onto all beverages and spa services. Finally, while room service used to be free, some lines now charge a service fee for each order you place. Among the lines that offer free room service, there are still some menu items that carry a premium.

Expensive adverts placed in newspapers might advertise a seven-night Caribbean cruise for under $500, but the advertised fare rarely includes the flight to Miami or Barbados where you will board the ship. Cruise lines will be happy to secure your flights on your behalf and often offer a ground transfer from the airport to the cruise terminal, but both will come at a price. If there are several of you travelling it might be cheaper to share a cab to the port.

> **Don't Ask:**
> What's the combination for the safe?

Visas will always come at your own expense. You will be informed which ones you personally need to apply for prior to your departure, and others will be handled directly by the cruise line upon arrival in port. In the latter case, costs will be charged to your onboard account (at the conversion rate on that day). Note, you will be charged for a visa regardless of whether or not you wish to disembark at a port. The visas needed for a world cruise can add a hefty chunk on top of your initial cruise fare, especially those for China and India. There are even some ports that no longer require a visitor's visa, but your cruise ship could still add a processing fee to facilitate your temporary passage in that country.

***Child Watch:*** *There are fantastic facilities for your little ones during the day, but babysitting in the evening will typically incur hourly rates.*

Thousands of cruise passengers descend upon ports of call and stay for less than eight hours, behaviour which is generally seen as not contributing to the local economy. We all know of those that sneak back to the ship for their 'free' lunch, and on average a passenger might only buy a cup of coffee or a small souvenir while in port. In retaliation, as of 1st January 2019, Amsterdam levied a controversial tourist tax aimed specifically at cruise ships staying 24 hours or less, charging lines an €8 per person flat fee which is passed onto passengers. Cruise lines calculate their budgets two or three years in advance of a port visit and, with the late introduction of this tourist fee, some lines are not prepared to absorb the cost themselves. MSC has fought back and replaced or axed the waterfront city for the near future. Venice is also due to impose day tax from the 1st July 2020, but it gave cruise operators more than a year's notice, unlike the two months provided by Amsterdam. It remains to be seen if any other countries follow suit, or if cruise operators will be happy to carry on visiting the destination despite the tax.

There are a few other miscellaneous charges that you might find listed in the small print. Cruise lines reserve the right to reintroduce a fuel supplement surcharge if the price of oil tops a predetermined amount. It hasn't happened in several years, but you won't be able to avoid the fee if it is applied. Excursions are rarely included in your cruise fare as tour sales account for a considerable portion of a cruise lines' profits. Also, despite being complimentary for many years, shuttle buses laid on from the ship to a town centre now often incur relatively hefty price tags. There are plenty of free onboard activities included in your cruise fare, but there might be supplementary costs for certain exercise classes or speciality activities. Lastly, it's rare that an internet package is included in your cruise fare and buying one could add a significant amount to your onboard account. It is often better, if possible, to wait until you can get free Wi-Fi in port.

***Water Sting:*** *Beware of the bottle of mineral water waiting to greet you in your cabin when you embark. Ships charge as much as $5 for this tipple and, to add insult to injury, another 15% service charge may also be applied.*

# Where to Start?

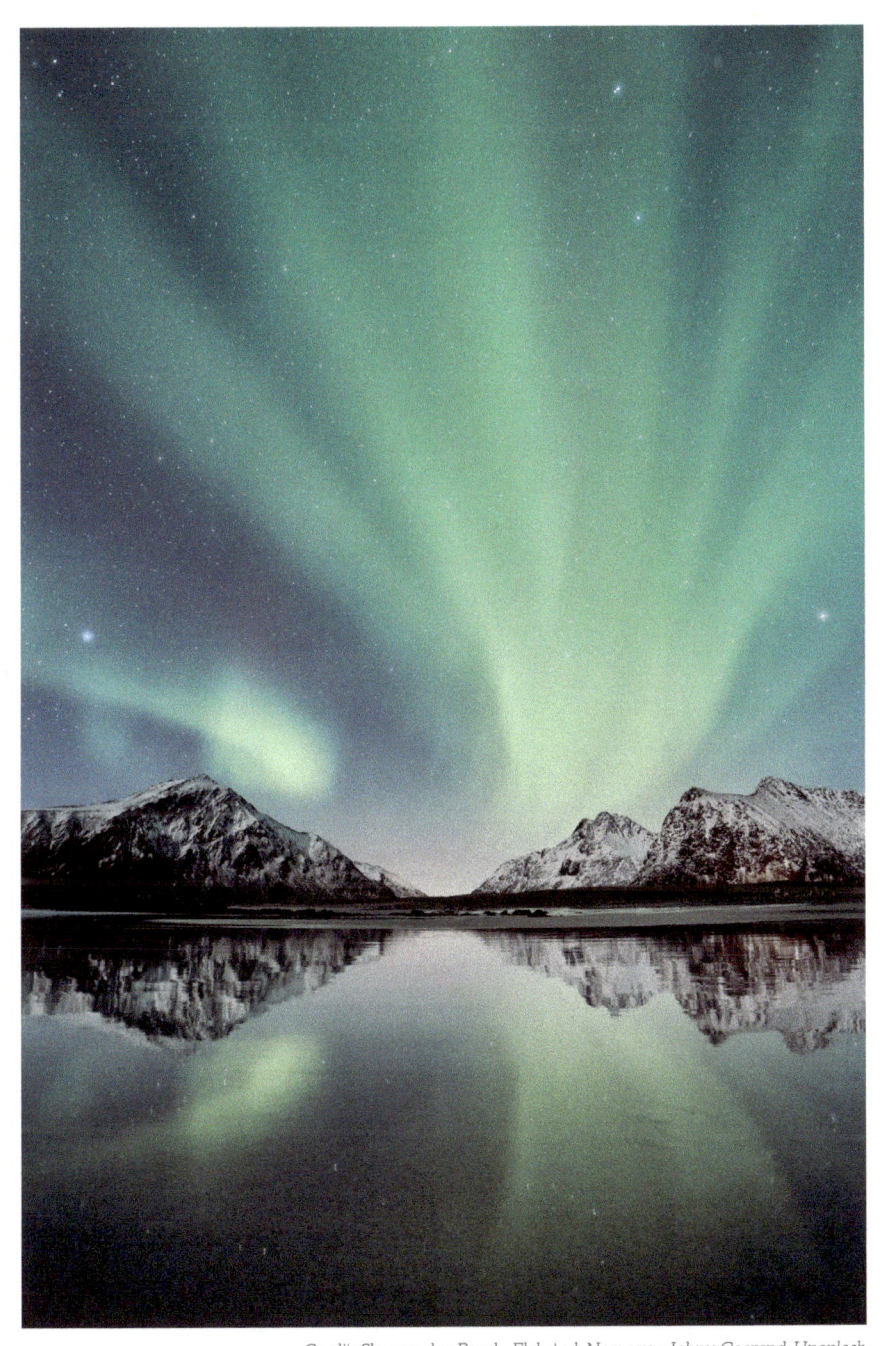

*Credit: Skagsanden Beach, Flakstad, Norway - Johny Goerend, Unsplash*

## Booking Confirmation

Before you pick up the phone to actually make your booking, make sure you have considered all your special needs at every stage of your cruise, including departure, while onboard, when visiting ports of call, through shore excursions and at your final destination. Prepare a list of any questions you might have for your booking agent.

You will be asked for your preferred dining time and table size at the time of booking. There are usually two different options when it comes to the time of your sit-down dinner, the more popular early sitting (typically 6 pm) and the late sitting (typically 8.30 pm), with table sizes usually ranging from two to ten people; tables for two, however, are extremely scarce as they use the space in the dining room least efficiently. You should choose early dining if you prefer to eat before catching the main show, are travelling with children or like to retire to bed early, though do bear in mind that the crew will need to ready the dining room for the late sitting, so your meal may feel rushed. Late dining is generally the better option if you prefer a more relaxed and quieter experience in the restaurant. Ships tend to stay in port until late afternoon, so the late sitting is also best if you don't want to rush back and want to spend each sailaway on deck.

***Dining Tip:*** *On popular cruises your preferred dining time or table size might not be available at the time of booking but you can always try and get it moved on embarkation day.*

Some ships offer alternatives to traditional cruise dining. Flexible, freedom or anytime dining gives you the option of eating when and where you want - you simply turn up at the restaurant when you are ready to eat; for some, not being locked into a specific time for the entire cruise is sheer bliss. The main difference is that you will have different table companions each night, offering a chance to meet new people or to avoid those you don't fancy eating with again. The downside of this option is that you might have to wait for a table.

To recap, when booking a cruise:

- Ensure the destination is right for you and that if there are any tender ports on the itinerary they are accessible.
- Ensure the ship and your cabin meet your special needs.

## Where to Start?

- Inform the cruise line if you have special needs and if assistance is needed at the terminal.
- Fill out the special needs/medical form if it applies to you.
- Inform the cruise line if you are bringing a wheelchair, scooter or any medical equipment.
- Inform the cruise line in writing if you are pregnant and submit a letter from your doctor stating your due date and fitness to travel.
- Confirm which dinner sitting you require and any special dietary requests you want noted.
- Inform the cruise line if you are travelling with a service dog, check that you can both get off at ports of call and that you have all the documentation required for your animal.
- Check on accessible excursions with the cruise line.
- Ask for written confirmation that your requests have been noted.

If you have booked a fly-cruise, on top of the above, you also need to consider your special needs when going through security, through departures, whilst onboard the plane, during stopovers, and with port transfers, and at your final destination.

To recap, when booking a flight:

- Notify the airline of your special needs and request airport assistance if needed.
- Inform the airline if you are bringing a wheelchair, scooter or any medical equipment.
- Consider pre-booking your aircraft seat.
- Confirm any special dietary requests you require.
- Check that the flight is on a DEFRA approved route and inform the airline if you are travelling with a service dog and that you have all the documentation required for your animal.
- Inform the airline if you need instructions in braille.
- Check that airport transfers are wheelchair-accessible.
- Ask for written confirmation that your requests have been noted.

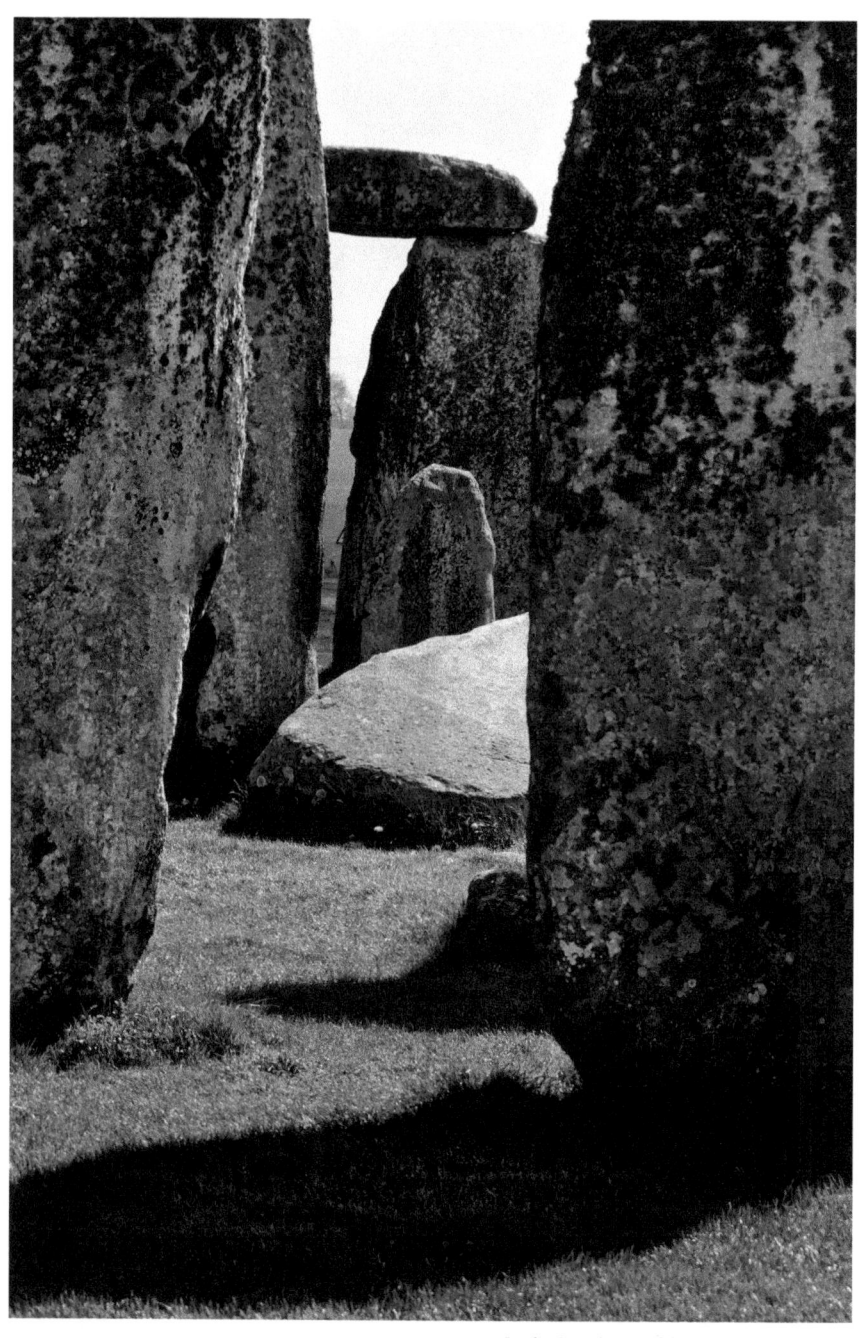

Credit: Stonehenge, Edward Dalmulder, Flickr

# Before You Go

Whether you book your holiday a year or just a few weeks in advance, there are certain things that you need to have in place or act on before you step foot on your chosen ship. This section of the book will walk you through everything you need to consider or implement before leaving for your holiday, from guidance to the documents you need to have ready and completed, to advice on the options that can be pre-booked.

## Holiday Admin/The Bureaucratic Stuff

There is always a fair amount of paperwork when it comes to planning any holiday, and while frustrating and sometimes overwhelming, getting it all in place early will massively reduce your stress levels whilst you're away. The following information aims to cut through the red tape and provide concise practical information on all of the paperwork and administration you need to consider before leaving for your holiday.

## Passports & Visas

Passengers are personally responsible for obtaining any travel documents required by their airline or cruise line, including in-date passports, any necessary visas and wedding documents. If you can't present all the papers needed upon embarkation, your cruise line may prevent you from boarding and will not offer a refund.

British passengers are required to carry a full passport that is valid for at least six months after the date of disembarkation. If you need to replace a passport or apply for a new one, allow plenty of time - leaving it until the last minute can be needlessly stressful and costly. Also, as a disabled passenger, it's particularly important to make sure the emergency contact details in the back of your passport are up-to-date.

**Passport Essential**: If you're thinking about renewing your passport anytime soon you should be aware of changes the UK Government recently made to the process as part of post-Brexit decisions. These changes have not been widely advertised. Until recently, when you applied for a renewal, any time left on your existing passport would carry over to your new one, up to a maximum of nine months. This is no longer the case: validity is no longer being carried forward from one passport to the next.

**Driver's License:** Not everyone is happy about taking their passport off the ship in a port of call. If you feel the same way, take your driver's license instead, as it is an acceptable form of ID in most situations (as long as your picture is visible). Your daily cruise ship planner will advise you the night before docking as to whether a port demands that you take your passport off the ship with you.

British passport holders can visit over 170 countries without the need for a visa, but there are exceptions; most reputable cruise companies will supply a list of visa and health requirements for your chosen itinerary, but it may still be worth doing your own research - check on *gov.uk/foreign-travel-advice* or with the relevant embassy, high commission or consulate for each of the ports on your itinerary. Note, you might still need a visa even if you don't want to get off the ship.

**Cruise Tip:** In case of loss or theft, take pictures or make photocopies of your passport, driver's license, travel documents and credit cards, and make a note of the 'lost or stolen' notification phone numbers.

For the countries that do require a visitor's visa, such as Egypt, Turkey, and Vietnam, your cruise ship may obtain a blanket visa for all passengers on short visits, though you will still be charged for this through your onboard account. Most cruise lines use the company CIBT to supply visas to passengers, and whilst it is convenient to let an agent do the work, it may be more cost-effective to source them yourself. If you choose to do it yourself, be sure to do your research to avoid falling victim to the websites who are charging up to 18 times the official price for certain visas. For example, British tourists wanting to visit the US must obtain an electronic system for travel authorisation, available directly from the US Government site for £12, however some sites are charging unsuspecting globetrotters up to £65. Another common scam to keep an eye out for, British tourists travelling to Turkey were forced to pay for a real visa on the spot when it was revealed that their pre-purchased e-visas were fake.

**Visa Facts:**
Australian visas are free – *border.gov.au*
US visas cost under $15 – *esta.cbp.dhs.gov*
Indian visas cost $25 – *indianvisaonline.gov.in*
Turkish visas cost $20 – *evisa.gov.tr/en*
Canadian visas cost $7 – *cic.gc.ca*

Please note, prices can increase without notice, and if you do want an agency to do the legwork for you, there will often be an additional administration fee. Visit the Foreign Office website (*gov.uk/foreign-travel-advice*) for links to alternative official visa sites. Acquiring a visa can be time-consuming, so allow at least two months for the whole process.

### How will Brexit affect my holiday?

The UK's transition period ended on 31 December 2020, after which UK tourists are still allowed entry to EU countries, Iceland, Liechtenstein, Norway and Switzerland without a visa for up to 90 out of every 180 days. This will remain the case as long as the same courtesy is extended to EU citizens wanting to visit the UK.

The European Commission confirmed that UK holidaymakers would not need a visa post-Brexit, however, Brits will need to apply for a visa waiver to travel to member states. The European Travel Information and Authorisation System, is now in effect, cost €7, and is valid for three years. Passports are only valid for travel if they are less than ten years old and still have at least 6 months validity.

## Vaccinations

Some countries will recommend certain vaccines, like hepatitis or malaria shots, but they are typically non-compulsory, and the decision to have them is up to each individual traveller. The main exception is the yellow fever vaccine, which is compulsory on certain cruises. On a particular voyage to the Amazon, a cruise line threatened to refuse boarding if proof of vaccination wasn't presented at check-in. The NHS 'Fit for Travel' website (*fitfortravel.nhs.uk*) has vaccination information for every country in the world.

*Vaccination Essential:* Some vaccinations are administered in several doses spread over a couple of weeks or months, and some have to be given in advance to give your body time to develop immunity, so allow enough time to get them done. It is advisable to make an appointment to see your doctor or travel health clinic a minimum of eight weeks before your travel date.

## Prescriptions & Medication

Countless medical conditions require a regular drug regime, and in every instance, you will need to carry a doctor or specialist's letter explaining any relevant to your condition, such as whether you have any implants, if you're susceptible to seizures, your dialysis treatment records, any clinical notes, your most recent EKG or kidney function test results, copies of scans, or confirmation that you are fit to travel.

*Generic Essential:* Ask your prescriber for a letter listing your medications with their generic names as this could prove useful during border control checks, if medicines need to be replaced or medical treatment is required.

If you are flying, you will need a letter from your doctor to show security for all your medication, particularly for liquid prescription or intravenous medicines that fall outside the 100 ml allowable limit, including lubricants for catheterising, liquid nutritional supplements, or immunoglobulin and infusion supplies that are required while in flight. The name on each prescription must match the passenger's ticket and be kept in its original packaging. The letter must also cover sharp medical items that could be seen as a security risk, such as syringes and hypodermic needles. Most surgeries will charge for this service and it can sometimes take some time to process, so make sure to contact your doctor long before your cruise. Medication that may be required during the journey, or soon after arrival, should be carried in your hand luggage.

*Diabetes Essential:* Carry extra insulin, blood testing equipment or any other prescription medicines you take so you don't get caught short.

All medicines, prescribed or otherwise, should be correctly labelled and kept in their original packaging, and it is advisable to carry a copy of your prescriptions in case your medication is lost, additional supplies are needed or security checks require proof of purpose; if your issuing chemist retains the original prescription, ask for an attested copy. That being said, not all your prescription medication will be available abroad, so you should make sure to pack ample supplies to meet your needs, allowing for delays in returning home or lost luggage. Please note, while the name and physical appearance of your UK prescribed medicine may look the same in other countries, the dosage and active ingredients may be different, and it may be out of date or fake. If you need contact details of an overseas medical practitioner, contact the International Association for Medical Assistance to Travellers (*iamat.org*).

When travelling across multiple time zones, it can be easy to lose track of when your medication is due. If you take time-dependent medicines, it may be sensible to keep a watch or mobile phone on 'home time' and continue to take your medication accordingly. Talk to your doctor to clarify any changes you may have to make if you are travelling to a time zone with more than a two or three hour difference. Also, if you have diabetes and require medication or have a dietary restriction, you and your doctor should work out an individual schedule for mealtimes, taking into account the length of your journey and any change in time zones.

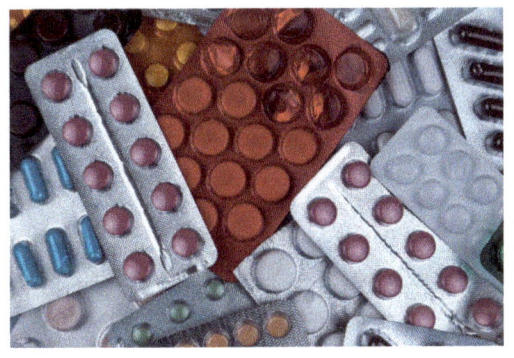

*Credit: Volodymyr Hryshchenko on Unsplash*

Travellers need to be aware that the legal status of their medication may differ outside the UK and result in delays, disruption or medicines being confiscated at border control if the correct paperwork and permissions are not in place. On rare occasions, travellers who have been found to have drugs that are illegal at the destination or transit country, including tramadol and codeine, have been deported or even imprisoned.

The United Arab Emirates (UAE), for example, has a rigid, zero-tolerance anti-drugs policy. Possession of even the smallest amounts of medications which are illegal in the UAE can incur a minimum prison sentence of four years. Some drugs and medicines that can be purchased over the counter in some countries are classified as controlled substances in the UAE and are illegal to possess in any quantity, including some cold and cough remedies, sleeping pills, antidepressants, hormone replacement drugs, Viagra and medicines containing codeine or similar narcotic-like ingredients. Codeine is also classed as an illegal drug in Greece, which will lead to severe ramifications even if found in your bloodstream, which constitutes an offence of trafficking. To get more information on carrying medication abroad, check out Travel Health Pro (*travelhealthpro.org.uk/factsheet/43/medicines-abroad*), a useful website set up by the Department of Health.

**Drug Restrictions:** *Before you travel, check with the appropriate Embassy or High Commission of the country you are visiting that your medications are deemed acceptable.*

If you are flying with controlled drugs such as diamorphine, diazepam or morphine, you may be required to obtain an export license if you have supplies for more than three months - an application is available from the *gov.uk* website and should be submitted by email to the Home Office Drugs & Firearms Licensing Unit at least ten working days before you travel.

**Brexit Essential**: *Post-Brexit, the rules for taking medicines containing controlled drugs to Europe has not changed.*

My Medicine List (*safemedication.com*) can help you keep track of everything you take to keep you healthy, including pills, vitamins and herbs. Having a list of all your medications in one place also helps your doctor, pharmacist, hospital or other health care worker take better care of you. Download a PDF copy of the list and fill it in electronically so that you can print out a copy to take with you when you travel. If you are unable to fill it in electronically, simply print it out and fill it in by hand.

## Travel Money

It's a good idea to have some local currency for each port on your itinerary for when you go ashore, even if you've prepaid for everything you plan to do - you never know when you might want to go exploring on your own and you might find yourself needing cash for taxis, snacks, souvenirs, tickets or tips. Changing money at the airport, cruise terminal or on the ship is expensive, and it's entirely possible that these places may not even carry the currency you want. As such, it's usually best to change your money in advance. You can check exchange rates from multiple providers online with *compareholidaymoney.com* or *travelmoneymax.com* and choose the best deal. If you prefer, you can order up to 80 foreign currencies from the Post Office (*postoffice.co.uk/foreign-currency*), all without commission, and collect from your nearest branch or get it delivered to your home the next day.

**Money Tip:** *Cruise ships charge high rates for foreign exchange, and you'll be charged again if you want to change it back.*

Prepaid currency cards are a safe alternative to cash. For example, the Post Office has its own Travel Money Card which is accepted in 36 million locations in over 200 countries and is able to store 13 currencies. The downside is that almost all of the 35+ prepaid cards currently on the market either have monthly fees, reload fees and/or transaction fees, and unlike a credit card, they offer no protection against loss or faulty items. Caxton FX offer a service which waives ATM fees and doesn't apply any overseas charges if used outside of the UK, but a lack of internet access or security concerns might make it difficult if you need to top up the card during your trip. It can also take three days to load money onto the card, possibly leaving you without funds when you need them.

Paying by credit or debit card is often the most convenient and safest way to spend money abroad, but a lot of debit cards charge a flat rate of up to £1.50 on every sale, plus extra fees for using an ATM to withdraw cash. Having said that, an ATM is generally the easiest and cheapest way to get your cash overseas and their rate is often much better than using a money exchange bureau. There is usually a fee applied every time you withdraw cash, it's more cost effective to take out a larger amount as opposed to several small ones. Check with your provider beforehand as to their policies, and consider opening a debit card with no fees when used abroad.

**ATM Essential:** *Most ATMs only accept a personal identification number (PIN) as a security measure. If your card uses letters, change to a numeric code before travelling.*

Credit cards are a safe bet for international use as their rates can be competitive and purchases over £100 are protected under section 75 of the Consumer Credit Act, but it's important to shop around for a good deal as some cards have hidden charges and squeeze you every time you withdraw cash from an ATM. The Halifax Clarity card, the MBNA Horizon card and the Post Office Platinum card are all free and don't charge for foreign purchases, though they will all charge interest from day one if you use them at a cash point. The bonus of the MBNA card in particular is that you earn 0.5% cashback on purchases at home or abroad which is automatically credited to your account every January.

The Barclaycard Rewards Card has no fees on purchases or cash withdrawals, and you'll get 0.25% cashback on whatever you spend at home or abroad. If you pay off the balance in full each month, you will not be charged interest on overseas cash withdrawals, unlike most other cards who charge daily interest until it is paid off.

***Did You Know:*** *The back of your card will indicate what networks your credit card is associated with. Make sure your card is linked to the Cirrus (Mastercard), Maestro (Mastercard) or PLUS (Visa) network as these are accepted in hundreds of countries, with each system offering compatibility with a million ATMs.*

When using your card abroad, whether to pay for something or withdraw cash from an ATM, always opt for the transaction to be paid for in local currency and not sterling; in the latter case, it's the local bank which sets the conversion rate and it will almost certainly work out more expensive. This is because you'll be hit by Dynamic Currency Conversion that is notorious for offering poor rates, and the merchants often apply additional fees, sometimes costing up to 10% more on every bill or ATM transaction. By law, all vendors have to give you the option of paying in the local currency, if they don't demand it.

***Credit Card Essential:*** *You are less likely to have a protective hold enforced on your debit or credit cards if the company is aware of your travel plans. Call your credit card company before leaving home and give them the dates you'll be away and where you're going.*

Make sure to keep a spare credit card or extra cash in your cabin's safe to protect you in the unlikely event your card is lost, stolen or eaten by an ATM. It is always safer to have a back-up plan.

***Credit Card Essential:*** *Check the expiry dates on all your credit and bank cards you plan on taking away with you, and if they are about to lapse, ring the bank and ask them to issue a new one.*

## Staying in Touch

As of 1 January 2021, the guarantee of free mobile phone roaming throughout the EU, Iceland, Liechtenstein and Norway ended. You will need to check with your mobile phone provider about any additional roaming charges that will apply to your phone plan although a new law will mean that you will be protected from charges over £45 being applied to your account without your knowledge. If you want to continue to use the internet while you are away, after you reach the £45 threshold, you will need to 'opt in' to spend more. You will need to check with your mobile phone provider on how to do this.

## Cruise Booking Confirmation

When you originally made your cruise booking you will have been sent a confirmation from your chosen booking agent, verifying your exact cruise booking and any pre-booked flights, hotels or transfers. Typically, 90 days before departure you will be able to manage your booking online using the 'cruise personaliser' service. The benefits afforded by your online account vary across the industry, but often include the ability to reserve a table at a specialty restaurant, book tour excursions, secure spa treatments or order a champagne breakfast for a special anniversary. You'll receive exclusive email updates, deals and insider tips, and it's a handy way of accessing your itinerary, cruise history and Loyalty Club information.

### Cruise Personaliser

You can manage your booking by logging into your cruise personaliser (different lines have different names) sometimes as soon as 24 hours after your booking is confirmed - simply log in with your first and last name, date of birth and booking reference number. If an error message pops up, check you have not entered any spaces in your telephone number, and if travelling on an American cruise line, your date of birth must be entered as month, date, year. If you have booked through a travel agent, make sure you enter your cruise line's reference number and not the travel agent's reference. If you continue to encounter problems, ring the cruise line directly.

## Flight Booking Confirmation

Once your fly-cruise booking has been confirmed, you'll be required to fill in the Advance Passenger Information to comply with security regulations. You will be required to give your full legal name, passport and insurance details, and the destination address. Do this as soon as possible as it is one less thing to worry about later.

## Tickets & Boarding Passes

Long gone are the days when cruise lines sent out plush travel wallets, leather luggage tags and spiral booklets. In fact, the mass market mega-ships don't even put a stamp on an envelope for their clients anymore - this service is now reserved for the privileged few who book with the more elite companies, such as Silversea and Regent Seven Seas. The cruise line and/or airline you have booked with will have a bearing on when your documents will be issued, anywhere from 24 hours in advance to 30 days beforehand, and how you will receive them, more frequently online nowadays, but still sometimes by post.

## Online Check-In

While online check-in is still optional on a few cruise lines, most companies insist you complete their online registration before arriving at the port. It is usually available 90 days before departure and must be completed by no later than three days before sailing. It only takes a few minutes to log in and create an account, and the form simply requests your contact details, passport information and health insurance particulars. Even if the service is optional, it can save you a lot of time and senseless queuing at the terminal. Once logged in, you will have access to your e-ticket and travel documents which you should print, as well as luggage labels that you need to affix to your luggage before arriving at the terminal.

***Luggage Tip:*** *Cover luggage tags with clear tape to prevent them from being torn off easily or by accident.*

Most airlines also offer the opportunity to complete their check-in process online, anywhere from 60 days to two hours before departure. You will need to visit your airline's website and sign in using your last name and your booking or confirmation number. You will normally have the opportunity to choose your seat, pay for any checked luggage, and sometimes even upgrade to premium economy or first-class. The earlier you check-in, the greater the choice of available seats. You'll be given the option of printing your boarding card at home, or you may print it at one of the airport's self-serve kiosks on the day of your flight. You should be careful if choosing the latter option as the cut-off times vary by airline and destination, and there may be queues. Download your airline's app to your mobile phone as some companies will accept (and often prefer) electronically-stored boarding cards that will be scanned in the same way a physical ticket would.

***Online Check-in Tip:*** *Some airlines, such as EasyJet, Ryanair and Wizz Air, have made it mandatory to check-in online and impose a fee if you check-in at the airport or have not pre-printed your boarding pass. Check your airline's website to check what services are open to you.*

***Accessible Check-in:*** *You won't have the option of online check-in if you need special assistance at the airport. Wheelchair users and those travelling with a service dog will need to check-in at the airline's counter so that the ground staff can allocate the best seating to suit your special needs and direct any medical equipment to the aircraft's hold.*

***Boarding Pass Tip:*** *EasyJet will not accept your boarding pass as a PDF file, but recommends that you store it on their EasyJet Mobile app, which is available offline. If you prefer, you can print your boarding pass out before going to the airport or have EasyJet print it out at the airport for you.*

The Autonomous Cruiser

## Boarding Documents

Once at the check-in desk in the terminal, you will be required to show your passport, any applicable visas, booking confirmation, and boarding card. You'll also need to fill out a health questionnaire with a few questions about your current wellbeing, a simple safeguard against you spreading germs that could adversely affect other passengers. A few cruise lines have taken to adding the health questionnaire to the online check-in to save time at embarkation. Single parents travelling with children might need a letter of permission from the absent parent. You'll also need to set up a cashless onboard account by filling in a credit card authorisation form. Lastly, your photograph will be taken and added to your digital profile and your cruise card will be issued.

## Baggage Allowance

> **Don't Ask:**
> Why can I only see the car park when I booked a seaview? (said while docked in Southampton)

If you don't need to catch a flight to join your cruise, there will be no restriction on the amount of luggage that you can bring aboard, though cruise lines encourage passengers to limit their packing to two suitcases and a carry-on. If you have booked a fly-cruise, or are flying to a UK embarkation port, the amount of accompanying baggage will be limited by your airline's baggage allowance. As there are no separate storage facilities on ships, all bags must be kept in your cabin; the space under the beds is usually ample for storing suitcases which don't exceed 9" (23 cm) depth. If you bring several bags or holdalls with you, store the smaller ones in the larger cases to save space.

### Locked Luggage

*Although it is not obligatory, most passengers prefer to lock their luggage before leaving it at the baggage drop-off point. The Transportation Security Administration (TSA) has authority over the security of the travelling public in the United States. One of their specific duties includes screening bags for prohibited and dangerous objects and materials. As such, they can open and search any of your belongings at any time without informing you in advance. For this reason, if travelling to or from the US to meet your ship, use a TSA approved lock to avoid them cutting it off to gain entry if your bag is chosen to be searched at random. A Notice of Inspection should be placed in the bag if it has been inspected and, although the screening shouldn't damage your suitcase, if your lock had to be cut off your bag will remain unlocked until it reaches its destination.*

## Travel Insurance

Doctor's fees, hospital bills and repatriation flights can be extremely costly if your holiday gets cut short because of illness, with most medical facilities requiring cash up front. Insurance will be your only protection should you need to cancel your travel plans or require medical care while abroad, so make sure you're fully covered. Among other things, your policy should include cover for: medical and repatriation expenses, cancellations or delays, lost luggage and mobility equipment such as wheelchairs, personal injury, personal liability to others and legal costs.

**Insurance Essential:** *Take your policy out the same day you book your cruise, otherwise you won't be covered if you need to cancel your trip before your travel date.*

It's a good idea to book through an independent company and not through your cruise line so that you're insured from the moment you book until the day you come back. The exception is Saga, who have one of the best cruise insurance policies on the market for the over 50s and have recently announced that treatment abroad for Covid-19 and repatriation to the UK if a guest contracts the virus, will be included as standard on their travel policies as of 1 June 2020.

If you simply want to compare travel insurance quotes, then Medical Travel Compared (*medicaltravelcompared.co.uk*) will search through over 40 specialist providers, so you do not pay a penny more than you have to. Designed especially for people with pre-existing medical conditions and their travelling companions, they offer a free independent service to help you find the right travel insurance solutions for you.

You can often organise a 'free' travel insurance policy through your home insurance policy or your bank account; if you choose to do so, be sure to read the small print as most only offer basic protection and do not cover pre-existing conditions. Medical bills or repairs to damaged mobility equipment can soon add up, and you don't want to get home to find your insurance company won't pay out. If your bank doesn't offer comprehensive cover, it might be better to look elsewhere.

When you declare a pre-existing medical condition, you will generally have to undergo a medical screening; for instance, you might have to call a medical helpline to give details of your health, or ask your doctor to complete a questionnaire or declaration of your fitness to travel. Alternatively, you may have to sign something stating that you are not travelling against doctor's orders, you have not received in-patient treatment in the last six months, you are not awaiting or travelling to obtain treatment and you do not have a terminal prognosis.

**Checklist:** *Download the 'Checklist for Disabled and Less Mobile Passengers', compiled by the Association of British Travel Agents.*

If you use a comparison site to buy your insurance, it may be best not to opt for one simply because it is the cheapest option, as it could mean you wont have enough cover (if at all) in the areas you need. Do your research and make sure to cover yourself for what you need. For example, £1500 of cover against cancellation is almost useless if your cruise cost £3,000. Whatts more, breaking an ankle in Tenerife could set you back £7,000, and an air ambulance in the US is a heart-stopping £50,000 - healthcare costs abroad can really add up, so don't skimp on medical cover.

**Health Alert:** *A UK Global Healthcare Insurance card (GHIC) is free (ghic-healthcarecard.co.uk), but remember, it only covers you for 'NHS type' treatment in European hospitals. It will not offer the full range of insurance cover you'll need for a cruise, including care in the ship's medical centre. You should buy travel insurance just as you would if visiting a non-EU country to ensure you get any healthcare treatment you might need.*

**Coronavirus Update:** *The spread of COVID-19 has resulted in considerable disruption to travel plans. Subsequently, some insurers have made changes to policies bought or renewed on or after 12 March 2020 and may not offer cover for coronavirus-related claims.*

The recent and unexpected demise of Monarch Airlines, Flybe, Thomas Cook, Cruise & Maritime and Pullmantur Cruises are prime examples of the importance of cover against missed departures and repatriation, due to the losses one can incur if your cruise is cancelled or you are stranded abroad due to the collapse of a travel company. Similarly, unforeseen costs can arise if you miss your departure due to a delay in public transport or a serious traffic incident, but with the right cover, you will be protected.

Another less known type of cover you'll want is for cabin confinement due to inclement seas or illness. In the event you are struck with norovirus (or similar), your cruise line will enforce a three-day cabin confinement to safeguard the health of other passengers - not only will you lose valuable holiday time, but it may mean missing out on expensive prepaid shore excursions.

On purchasing insurance, thousands of travellers assume they have insured all aspects of their trip and are horrified to later find out that it isn't the case and their policy is full of exclusions, the most common of which are:

- Flights purchased with miles or points
- Claims due to pre-existing health conditions, particularly when undeclared
- Dental care
- Psychiatric disorders
- Planned overseas medical procedures
- Pregnancy and childbirth
- Extreme sports accidents
- Business equipment
- Acts of God - defined as an accident or event not influenced by man but by nature, such as hurricanes, floods, tsunamis, earthquakes and tornadoes
- Acts of War - generally defined as an act of invasion, insurrection, revolution, military coup or terrorism

A lot of policies limit the amount you can claim in damages or losses on individual possessions. When you add up the replacement costs of items such as laptops, mobile phones, cameras, hearing aids, false teeth, passports and cash, you'll quickly find that most policies would leave you at a sizable loss - make sure your policy will cover your most expensive items comfortably.

***Insurance Essential:*** *Whichever cover you choose, you must reveal any pre-existing medical conditions to your insurer, otherwise you will void the policy. If you have trouble finding the right cover, you can always get a free broker from the British Insurance Brokers' Association (biba.org.uk) to help you. It might feel redundant to declare an illness from years ago, but if that condition recurs while you are away, the insurance company could very well refuse the cost of the treatment. While there are* some companies that will not insure you at all if you have a pre-existing condition, there are plenty that will; they will assess the risk and alter your premium accordingly.

The over-70s often have a hard time getting cover as they are deemed to be more at risk than a younger traveller, but there are several companies who will be happy to insure you. Insure and Go (*insureandgo.com*), and Saga (*saga.co.uk*) will both cover the over 70s, and Good to Go (*goodtogoinsurance.com*) and All Clear Travel (*allcleartravel.co.uk*) offer policies with no age limit and provide specialist cover for pre-existing medical conditions, including diabetes, angina, cancer, heart conditions, epilepsy and strokes.

**Excess Policy:** Some companies (like Saga) will not charge you for the excess on your policy if you can use the UK Global Health Insurance Card to reduce the cost of treatment.

It may sound obvious, but make sure your policy protects the entire length of your cruise, especially if you're planning a longer or even a round-the-world trip, as the average policy covers just a 31-day period. PJ Hayman (*pjhayman.com*) offers single trips of up to 186 days, has no upper age limit and, for an additional premium, will consider a traveller with a pre-existing medical condition. Just Travel (*justtravelcover.com*) provides single-trip cover for up to 365 days for people up to 70 years old, and will protect all pre-existing medical conditions, including terminal prognosis. Avanti Travel Insurance (*avantitravelinsurance.co.uk*) safeguards single trips of up to 550 days with no upper age limit and with protection against pre-existing conditions.

Several companies will cover pre-existing conditions to some extent, but you need to shop around to ensure your policy covers every aspect of your condition. For example, there are four types of multiple sclerosis (MS), an illness that is expensive to treat and hard to find cover for, but there are specialist policies that are tailored to protect you from all MS-related costs throughout your cruise. Boots Travel Insurance (*bootstravelinsurance.com*) have single-trip policies with no upper age limit and that cover any medical condition, including all types of MS (e.g. benign, relapse remitting, primary progressive and secondary progressive).

Free Spirit (*freespirittravelinsurance.com*) is one of the UK's largest specialist travel insurance providers and aspire to be different by offering to help people of any age who have been declined travel insurance cover elsewhere due to pre-existing conditions.

Travel insurance companies will provide cover for mobility aids but the value might be insufficient to cover the costs of replacing a state-of-the-art wheelchair, oxygen or dialysis machine so you should consider taking out specialist equipment travel insurance.

*Insurance Essential:* If you need to make a claim, keep every receipt and all paperwork, however innocuous it might seem. Your insurance company might not pay out without a full paper trail.

*Insurance Tip:* Check the 'Travel Planning Disability Resources' section in the Directory for a comprehensive list of companies who provide specialised travel insurance.

# Special Needs

If you did not liaise with your cruise line in regards to your special needs (anything from special dietary requirements to mobility issues) at the time of booking, now is the time to contact them to make sure you receive the support required. Requests need to be made as soon as possible as some lines require a 90-day notice period to implement special meal requirements. Several cruise lines provide refrigerators (as opposed to minibars) in their staterooms, which are suitable for storing certain medicines.

*Dietary Tip:* It is unlikely that any kosher or halal meal you requested at the time of booking will be loaded onto the ship until late afternoon so you will need to make alternative arrangements for embarkation day.

### Travelling with Compromised Immune Systems

The risk of acquiring an infection whilst abroad among immunocompromised travellers may be higher due to deficits in the immune system, especially for those with HIV, multiple sclerosis, and people receiving steroid, stem cell or chemotherapy treatment. First off, carry a doctor's letter detailing your medical problem, treatment and medication, and wear an identity bracelet for specific medication, such as steroids.

It is important to plan early and visit your doctor for advice on immunisation, vaccines or malaria tablets, which might require treatment starting several weeks before your travel date. Some vaccines, such as those made from live viruses (e.g. yellow fever), may not be suitable for people whose immune systems are weak, so you will need to ask your doctor for a medical waiver instead and discuss other protective options.

Extreme temperatures at either end of the spectrum are a common trigger for people with multiple sclerosis, meaning some destinations may present more of a challenge than others; however, there are a few things you can do to counteract these problems if you've already booked a potentially problematic itinerary. Hot weather can be combated in several ways, perhaps the most effective of which is by wearing a cooling garment, such as those that contain specialised gels or ice packs. Also, regular use of a water mister or portable fan on your face and wrists can make a big difference, as can simply staying hydrated.

Radiotherapy, stem cell transplants and certain cancer drug treatments can make the skin more sensitive to the sun for several years, so take particular care to wear clothing that covers your skin and head and avoid the sun during the hottest times of the day. Also, be sure to use a sun cream with a high sun protection factor (preferably at least 50).

Spasms and muscle stiffness occur more often in cold weather and can severely impact your mobility if you are susceptible to them, so keeping warm is an absolute must: layer your clothing, wear hats that offer ear and neck protection, and invest in heat packs that you can activate as needed. If you are a wheelchair user, cover yourself with a fleece blanket when going outside. Hot drinks and food will fuel the body and generate internal heat.

Bladder weakness or an overactive bladder is a common problem especially for people with multiple sclerosis, and while it is not a big issue whilst aboard an aircraft or ship as the toilets are generally nearby and always perfectly clean, some countries definitely won't offer the same level of facilities. If you are planning on going ashore in any capacity, but especially if you plan to enjoy an excursion, it might be wise to wear an absorbent pad and carry wet wipes and toilet paper. Make sure to maximise each coach stop so you don't get caught short, and if travelling in a non-English speaking country, try to learn the phrase for 'where is the toilet'. The web site *sitorsquat.com* can help you locate public bathrooms around the world.

Immunosuppressed travellers are often prone to diarrhoea, so pay particular attention to what you drink and eat and avoid tap water, fountain drinks, unpasteurised dairy products, ice, unpeeled fruits, and raw foods. Also, use the ship's sanitising stations and wash your hands with soap frequently.

Some countries, including Saudi Arabia, Brunei and Jordan, have travel restrictions in place for those with HIV, even for short-term stays, though these restrictions are not always enforced. The HIV Global Database (*hivtravel.org*) has details on each country's travel restrictions.

## Travelling with Epilepsy

To avoid any security concerns, carry a letter from your doctor explaining your epilepsy and the medication you take to control seizures. Because epilepsy is one of the 'invisible' disabilities, it is also wise to wear a medical bracelet or carry an epilepsy ID card so that people can be made aware of your condition and existing treatment should you experience a seizure in public. Epilepsy Action (*epilepsy.org.uk*) offers an epilepsy ID card free of charge, which you can get from their online shop or by phone on 0113 210 8800.

## Travelling with Diabetes

If you have diabetes it is advisable to wear a medical ID bracelet that details your condition and, as with other special needs, carry your prescription with you. Ask your endocrinologist or doctor for a letter stating that you have diabetes (specifically type 1 or type 2) and that you require insulin, pumps, syringes and needles with you at all times. Carry double the required amount of medication, blood testing equipment, test strips, and insulin with you, including spare batteries for your blood glucose monitor and insulin pump. Discuss a back-up plan with your doctor about what dose of insulin to take if your insulin pump breaks. If you do run out of insulin and want to try and source it locally, you need to take into consideration that the strength can vary as some countries still use U-40 or U-80 instead of the UK's U-100 strength.

***Don't Forget:*** *The UK Civil Aviation Authority (CAA) and Airport Operators Association (AOA) have sponsored the new Medical Device Awareness Card, which covers insulin pumps and continuous glucose monitoring systems for those with type 1 diabetes, which the CAA offers as a free PDF download (caa.co.uk). Regulations allow passengers with these medical devices to ask for an alternative security screening process.*

Passengers should never be asked to remove a medical device from their body for screening, though they can stop working if taken through an x-ray machine; instead, notify security staff in the cruise terminal that you are wearing an insulin pump or continuous glucose monitor and opt for an alternative screening method, such as a pat down. If you are carrying a spare device in your carry-on luggage, remove it, as it should not be screened by an airport scanner but instead an alternate security screening process such as a hand search. Also, be sure to advise one of the security officers if your sugar is dropping during the screening process or if you need medical assistance at any point.

Carry a bag with you to hold your insulin, glucose or dextrose tablets, and snacks like cereal bars, biscuits, fruit, raw vegetables and nuts to prevent episodes of hypoglycaemia, especially when venturing ashore. On any outing, take a spare pair of socks to help keep your feet dry and be disciplined in checking your feet for chafing and blisters, which can lead to ulcers. Diabetes can reduce blood circulation and cause damage to the nerves in your feet which in extreme cases can lead to gangrene.

**Diabetes Passport:** *The credit card sized Insulin Passport is used to keep an up-to-date record of the type of insulin, syringes and pens that you use. It also contains emergency information on what to do if you become ill or found unconscious, and can be obtained from your doctor, diabetic practice nurse or chemist.*

If your travel plans include time zone changes, keep detailed notes of exactly when your insulin is due - the National Diabetes Education Program suggests keeping your watch on your home time zone until the morning after arriving at your destination. It is also a good idea to set the alarm on your phone for an alert so you don't miss an insulin dose. Another thing to keep in mind is that travelling east means shorter days so less insulin may be required, whereas travelling west means longer days so more insulin may be required. Because of changes in time zones, levels of activity and alterations to your diet, check your bloods more frequently than if you were at home in case the variations have an impact on your blood glucose levels.

**Research is Key:** *Contact your insulin supplier and verify that your insulin is available in the countries you are docking in and if it is sold under the same name. Before you go, plan where you can get supplies during your itinerary, as in an emergency, your prescription can be faxed or emailed to the destination.*

Most of the major cruise lines have fridges in their cabins that can store medicines, but those that don't will provide a unit for your insulin with 24-

hour access, either through reception or room service. They will also provide a sharps container for the safe disposal of needles.

**Diabetes Essential:** *Some cabin minibars might not be designed to reach the necessary temperature that your drugs need to be kept at. Some of the newer cruise ships can provide Medi coolers on a first-come-first-served basis, but if not, the medical centre will be happy to store your medication at the correct temperature.*

If travelling to a hot climate, your biggest threat is the sun, so make sure you keep covered, pack a high factor sunscreen and wear UV sunglasses to protect your eyes. If you suffer from neuropathy, protect your hands and feet by wearing gloves or thick socks and cover any exposed areas with sunscreen as you may not be aware your skin is burning. Likewise, take extra precautions in cold climates to prevent frostbite if you suffer from poor blood circulation or have neuropathy, as the numbness in your feet might mean you are unaware of how the extreme temperatures are actually affecting you.

### Travelling with Heart Disease

You will need to carry a letter from your cardiologist or doctor outlining your condition and if you have an implantable device. You'll also need to carry copies of your medical history, repeat prescriptions, any clinical notes, most recent EKG results, scans, or anything else you might need to produce, including confirmation that you are fit to travel. Carry extra prescription medication with you to allow for any travel delays, and make a list of the brand and generic names of any medicines you take regularly.

Heart devices such as a stent or pacemaker are able to pass through the screening detectors safely without setting off the alarms or damaging your equipment. However, don't allow a handheld detector to be passed directly over your device as they do not always react well. If you have any concerns, ask for a physical search. If you are travelling with a cardioverter defibrillator (ICD), pacemaker or insertable cardiac monitor, carry your device identification card with you and brief the security team that you have a device inserted. Identification cards can be downloaded for free at *www.heart.org* and are available on Amazon.

## Travelling with Dementia

Make sure you go over all the travel plans several times with the person under your care and ensure they wear a wristband, lanyard or ID badge around their neck at all times - it should be clearly printed with their name, your mobile phone number, and your ship's name and your cabin number. Dementia is often an invisible disability, and confusion, anxiety or fear can sometimes be perceived by strangers as rude or aggressive behaviour. A simple identifier might prevent unnecessary problems with ship security or with people unaware that the person has a special need.

***Photo Alert:*** *Carry a current photo of your loved one for identification purposes.*

Make sure you go through shipboard security behind your companion, as doing so means you'll be able to assist them if they encounter a problem during the procedure. However, if you have gone through the screening process first, you will not be allowed to return.

***Tile Alert:*** *A Bluetooth 'Tile' tracker can attach to a piece of clothing or placed in a pocket so you can keep tabs on a loved one.*

Disorientation can lead to wandering, a common and serious concern for many loved ones. It is easy to get lost on a large ship but using GPS tracking enables a guest to be found quickly. The Guardian Pro by GPS Trackershop (*trackershop-uk.com*) attaches to your loved one's clothing and can only be removed by the guardian. It offers all-day monitoring, real-time mapping and sends an immediate alert if the person under care has ventured out of a pre-set location or safety zone. There is even an SOS button on the device that will send a text alert to three emergency mobile numbers. There is no range limitation for the service as long as you have an internet connection.

***Location Alert:*** *Some people find that dressing their loved one in bright or distinctive clothing makes it easier to find them if they get separated in a crowd. Take a photo on your mobile each time a new outfit is donned so that if your ward gets lost, it will be easier for the crew to spot them.*

***Luggage Delivery:*** *Take snacks, noise-cancelling headphones or downloaded YouTube videos in hand luggage that can be used as distractions as your suitcases might not be delivered to your cabin until late afternoon.*

## Travelling with Cognitive, Intellectual & Developmental Disabilities

Cruise lines welcome all guests with cognitive, intellectual and developmental disabilities, such as autism, cerebral palsy, Down's syndrome and Alzheimer's, and at the time of booking you should have discussed any special requirements needed during your cruise. It may be a good idea to reconfirm that assistance will be available if you need it, especially for embarkation.

Make sure you have a doctor's letter confirming your party's fitness to travel and giving permission to take their medication or equipment aboard the ship. Also, for passengers with autism spectrum disorder (ASD), it might be wise to carry an 'ASD Attention Card' so that staff can discreetly be made aware of the passenger's needs. The Wallet Card Project is a communication tool for people with autism or intellectual and developmental disabilities used to disclose a special need when interacting with first responders - the card is available worldwide and is designed by Just Dig It (*justdigit.org/wallet-card-project*).

You might consider boarding the ship later rather than earlier as the lines through the terminal will usually be much shorter. Waiting for a wheelchair can be a long process so if you don't need any special assistance after check-in, you can go straight to security. Make sure security staff are aware of medications or medical accessories the person in your care has with them. The screening process can be daunting for all parties involved, including companions or caregivers travelling with someone prone to exhibiting physiognomies of anxiety and meltdowns in unfamiliar situations. However, you will need to keep as calm as possible so that your angst doesn't transfer to the person you are travelling with and perhaps make the situation more difficult.

*Motion Sickness Tip: As people with autism may be more prone to seasickness than neurotypical travellers, nausea relief wristbands may help.*

Preparing the passenger for change can, hopefully, reduce their fears and resulting negative behaviours. Use visual aids such as photos, videos or similar tools to help a traveller become more familiar with a new means of transport, and help in areas they may struggle with, such as the security screening, dining in unfamiliar eateries and sleeping in a strange room. Make a plan together and explain each part of your day so your companion knows what to expect.

Most people with autism find travelling abroad a little easier if they're able to maintain some of their normal lifestyle and daily routine. As such, it is best to plan mealtimes similar to those at home and bring with you anything that provides them with comfort; for example, if they have a favourite television show, download a few episodes to a handheld device before leaving home. Comfort aids such as sensory headphones and textures, fidget spinners and weighted blankets can also help reduce the stress of being on a ship.

If the traveller suffers from auditory sensitivity, use noise-cancelling headphones or ear defenders when sailing as the noise of the ship's engines could frighten them. They can also be useful in public restrooms because of sensory input overload - flushing toilets, automatic hand-dryers and strange smells can all cause problems. If the headphones are not effective, it might be useful to use your cabin's bathroom where there is less foot traffic and fewer unexpected noises.

**Travelling with a Breathing Disorder**

First off, you should carry a doctor's letter describing your medical history and including a notation of all prescription medications you are taking, specifying your hours of oxygen use and associated flow rate. On top of this, some cruise lines will insist that your doctor fill in a medical form approving you for travel.

As well as travelling with an adequate supply of metered-dose inhalers and spacers, it is best to bring an extra cannula hose for your oxygen tank, as they are known to malfunction on occasion and it's better to be safe than sorry. Always have an oximeter on you and check your oxygen levels regularly. You should also research the names of local doctors, clinics or hospitals in the destination ports you'll be visiting in case you need extra supplies.

Anyone with a breathing-related mobility restriction is entitled to help from the wheelchair assistance team at the cruise terminal with taking you through security, check-in and onto the vessel. Even if you're not a permanent wheelchair user, it can be a long walk from the terminal to the ship, with long waits at security and check-in; riding instead of walking will save you time, your energy, reduce your stress levels and conserve your batteries if you use a portable oxygen concentrator (POC). If you didn't make the request for assistance at the time of booking, do it as soon as possible.

Pack enough fully-charged batteries to power a POC, plus extras to cover for potential delays, and be sure you have the correct power adaptors with you. Whenever possible, plug your device into an electrical outlet to recharge your batteries, making it much less likely that you run out of power at an untimely moment. Always have an oximeter on you and check your oxygen levels regularly.

Medical centres onboard most ships are not equipped to provide guests with oxygen other than on an emergency basis. If you're receiving oxygen therapy at home, you are solely responsible for ensuring you have all the equipment and supplies you need. This may mean bringing your own, however you will need to make arrangements for your necessary supplies to be delivered to the ship on embarkation day, a service which is offered almost everywhere in the world. You will also be responsible for off-loading the equipment at the end of the cruise. Note, while certain lines will allow guests to bring their own oxygen equipment onboard with them or use any company for equipment hire, some lines have designated suppliers and will only allow those appointed vendors to deliver to the ship, primarily for security and safety reasons. For example, Norwegian Cruise Lines have designated Scootaround (*scootaround.com*) as the only outside vendor that they will permit to deliver oxygen supplies to their ships while P&O will only accept the hire of an oxygen concentrator or a gaseous or liquid system from their approved supplier, Omega Advanced Aeromedical (*omegaoxygen.com*). Their team will deliver your order directly to your cabin and set everything up ready for your arrival. Take note that most lines will not permit liquid oxygen onboard their vessels. If you wish to use an independent supplier, please refer to 'Travel Planning Disability Resources' in the Directory.

***Oxygen Machine Essential:*** *If you choose to travel with your own personal oxygen machine (BiPAP, CPAP, Concentrator, Nebulizer, etc.), it must be carried in your hand luggage. Packing oxygen cylinders and/or tanks in your checked baggage and putting them through a security x-ray machine is strictly prohibited as they are highly flammable.*

### *Sleep Apnoea*

You will need to inform the cruise line if you intend to bring a continuous positive airway pressure (CPAP) machine on the cruise with you, and they are usually accommodating if they have been given advance notice. It is also important that your doctor provide a letter of medical necessity for you to use the machine during travel. Your doctor will also need to provide a prescription for CPAP and any other necessary equipment (heated humidifier, mask, filters and tubing).

Some cruise lines do not permit CPAP machines being packed into checked bags; regardless, you definitely don't want to risk damaging or losing your equipment, so it's always best to take it onto the ship in your carry-on luggage whenever possible. Also, though a costly investment, it is worth carrying a backup battery for your machine, just in case of an emergency. British cruise ships will have standard three-pin plug sockets onboard, but European and American ships probably won't; be sure to check with your cruise line as to what type of outlets, including their operating voltage, are available for use. Alternatively, you could rent a machine for the length of your cruise. Speak to the Online Sleep Clinic (*onlinesleepclinic.co.uk*) for more information, but bear in mind you cannot get a CPAP machine unless a doctor prescribes one.

Check with your cruise agent as to whether your ship can provide distilled water for the unit, and whether or not you will be charged for it. In cases where you would have to pay, you can avoid the fee by carrying your own water with you in your luggage. Most cabins do not have an electrical outlet by the bed, so pack a 12-15 ft. (4-5 m) extension cord to ensure the machine can be plugged in and kept near enough to you while you sleep. Extension cords aren't usually permitted on board, but those to be used with medical devices are an exception to the rule, though you should clarify this with your cruise line; alternatively, you can ask the cruise line to provide one for you.

**CPAP Tip:** *Bring a spare mask in case of a fault or damage to your primary unit. A working unit is worthless without a mask.*

### Travelling with Kidney Disease

Passengers will need to bring with them all related medical documents, including a full medical history, dialysis treatment records, recent kidney function test results, and your current dialysis prescription. Your doctor will usually need to fill in a medical health form and approve you for travel.

> **Don't Ask:**
> *Does the lift go to the front of the ship?*

Patients are now able to take a peritoneal dialysis machine onboard and administer their own treatment; if you choose to do so, make sure you pack extra supplies, including gauze sponges, antiseptic, disinfectants and surgical gloves, to cover any eventuality. Even if you plan to self-administer your treatment, it is important to make a note of the dialysis centres who offer transient dialysis treatment in the ports you'll be visiting during your cruise, as they will make every effort to accommodate a patient in the event of an emergency.

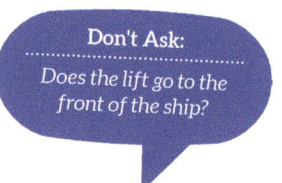

It is relatively easy to stick to a kidney-friendly diet when on a cruise ship, with copious amounts of salads and fresh vegetables and fruits available in the buffet. Advise the maître d' if you require a low sodium diet but you'll find most cruise lines offer healthy options on their menus and are willing to prepare dishes to suit special diets.

Your kidney function can deteriorate quickly if you become dehydrated, so increase your fluid intake whilst away, especially if travelling to a hot climate or if you experience vomiting or diarrhoea at all. Pack some oral rehydration salts to compensate for any fluid loss you might face.

## Travelling with a Visual Impairment

If you requested assistance through the cruise terminal at the time of booking, it is a good idea to doublecheck the request has been logged at least 48 hours before travelling; if you are yet to request any assistance but feel you may need it, do so as long before your cruise as possible. You will be met at the entrance to the terminal, escorted through security and check-in, and taken onboard the ship.

*Travel Tip:* Tactile bump dots (made of plastic with a self-adhesive backing) or markers can be used to help you easily identify a variety of things whilst onboard, including your luggage, your cabin door, buttons on a remote control, or hot tap.

*Travel Tip:* The cabin bathroom usually has wall-mounted shower products, an easy way to distinguish between certain items is to use elastic bands as identifiers, e.g. one band around the shampoo bottle, two around the conditioner.

*Travel Tip:* Use a cane whilst onboard as it can help you navigate uneven surfaces and steps around the ship, and they alert others that you are blind or have low vision.

## Travelling with a Hearing Impairment

As with all special needs, you will need to inform the cruise line of your travel plans at least 48 hours (but preferably a lot longer) before your departure date, especially if you require assistance through security and onto the ship. Some of the ports' terminals have public address systems that include induction loop facilities, but you can also request that someone informs you personally as soon as the ship is ready to board passengers.

When passing through security, you are not required to remove your hearing aids, but the TSA recommends that you advise a security officer that you are wearing them before the screening process begins. Disability notification cards offer a discreet way of informing people of your hearing loss and any other health conditions. Visit the TSA website to find a printable card and fill it out before arriving at the cruise port.

Security scanners won't harm hearing aids, but it may be a good idea to lower its volume as you go through as the scanners can occasionally cause them to make excess noise. If you're travelling with a service dog, ask for your screening to be done by a hand-operated detector so that you're not separated from your companion and also because your dog's harness, leash and collar may be made of stainless steel and could activate the metal detector.

Before leaving home, pay a visit to your audiologist and make sure your hearing aids are as ready for the trip as you are. Discuss the latest assistive listening devices designed to complement your hearing aid prescription and augment what it can do - Bluetooth wireless technology is one of the most cutting-edge consumer electronics, offering connectivity between your hearing aids and telephones, televisions, radios, FM systems, and more.

While hearing aids are available from the NHS as a free long-term loan, private ones can cost hundreds if not thousands of pounds. As such, talk to your audiologist or your insurance company about purchasing comprehensive cover for your hearing aids. Underwritten by Lloyds of London, Asset Sure (*assetsure.com*) protects against loss or damage to analogue or digital hearing devices, including unexplained disappearance cover as standard, and includes unlimited trips abroad of up to 60 days each trip.

If you have a spare hearing aid, take it with you in case of loss or damage. Also, remember that hearing aid batteries and tubing might not be easy to buy in the countries you are visiting, so take extras and pack them in your carry-on luggage along with a converter if they are rechargeable. Your hearing aid is vulnerable to damage from moisture and condensation, so if you are visiting hot and humid or very cold climates, bring a hearing aid dryer kit or dehumidifier and run it overnight in your cabin so it is moisture-free in the morning. Lastly, pack a protective waterproof case and cleaning kit.

## Rental Equipment

Transporting your personal special needs equipment across an ocean or around the world can be bothersome and not always trouble-free. Inept baggage handlers or awkward cobblestone streets can easily damage mobility aids, and should the worst happen, trying to source spare parts is not easy in a foreign port. A better option that might give you peace of mind is to lease any equipment you need from a specialised independent provider. A full list of independent suppliers is in 'Travel Planning Disability Resources' in the Directory.

***Mobility Tip:*** *Even if you don't usually use a mobility aid at home, you might want to consider hiring one for your holiday as cruises can involve a lot of walking, with long corridors to navigate and tiring days ashore. Once at a port, a lengthy trek might be required just to reach the terminal, so you could be worn out before you start.*

***Medical Essential:*** *For security reasons, Norwegian Cruise Line will only accept medical equipment from the supplier: Special Needs at Sea.*

## Equipment Insurance

Wheelchairs can come under tremendous abuse while travelling, and with the exorbitant costs of mobility aids, the last thing you would want to face is the financial consequences of having to replace your chair, aside from the complications of being without it. Several companies will insure your special needs equipment - see the 'Travel Planning Disability Resources' in the Directory for a list of some stand-out providers.

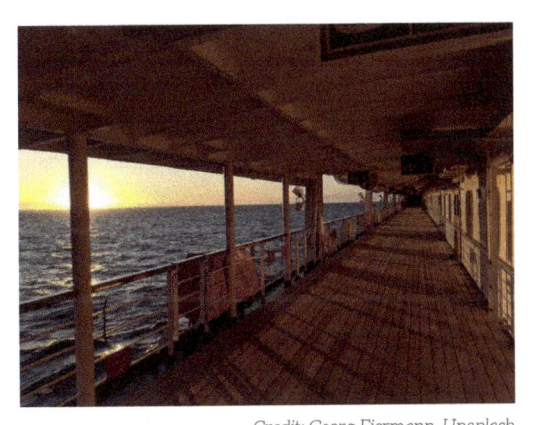

*Credit: Georg Eiermann, Unsplash*

***Wheelchair Essential:*** *Always carry a small tool kit and spare parts for emergency repairs. It could prove invaluable if your tyre suffers a puncture or your seat comes loose.*

## Pregnancy

If once you have booked your holiday, but before your departure date, you find out that you are pregnant, you will need to inform your booking agent immediately. A doctor's letter or medical certificate is required stating the estimated due date, that mother and baby are both in good physical health and fit to travel, and that the pregnancy is not high-risk. Most cruise lines will not accept guests who will have entered their 24th week of pregnancy by the time their cruise concludes. If you discover that this will be the case, you should receive a refund for your cruise, but a doctor's letter will be needed and must be supplied on stamped, practice-headed paper.

Don't forget to contact your travel insurance company and inform them of your change of circumstances and confirm that their policy covers both you and your unborn child in case of any complications or a premature delivery.

Your pregnancy might make your skin hypersensitive to the heat and sun, so avoid direct exposure, especially at the hottest times of day. Be careful when choosing your sunscreen or insect repellent as some are not safe for expectant mothers, and keep especially hydrated. Completely harmless but itchy and uncomfortable, atopic eruption of pregnancy causes itchy bumps on the skin which looks similar to eczema. Some people have invested in a rash guard which protects the wearer against rashes caused from extended sun exposure.

## Pre-planning

With your cruise fully booked there are a number of things that can and should be pre-booked, especially if missing out on a specific experience would ruin your trip - first-time cruisers are often disappointed on embarkation to find that something they wanted to secure has limited availability or is sold out. The other benefit of pre-planning is that certain items are offered at a pre-board rate. For example, pre-booking a dining package on Royal Caribbean offers a substantial saving, sometimes up to 45%, and includes gratuities and service charges.

### Children's Clubs

Children's clubs are extremely popular and most are limited in how many children they can accommodate on each sailing, so if having use of them is important to you, register your children with the club(s) as soon as possible so they are not excluded from the program. Similarly any special children's events, like character meet and greet opportunities, get booked out fast despite their additional cost, so secure your place early.

Most cruise lines offer online registration which can be accessed through your cruise personaliser, typically within 90 days of sailing. You will need to fill in a form for each child so that they can participate in the club designed for their age group. Let the youth team know if your child has a special need, a food intolerance or an allergy. If your chosen cruise line doesn't offer an online service, you can register your child either at a dedicated desk in the terminal on embarkation day or once aboard the ship.

## Gifts

If you are celebrating a special occasion, your family and friends may wish to treat you with a thoughtful gift like a 'Bon Voyage', 'Welcome Onboard', or 'Ultimate Celebration' package. Other choices include onboard credits, spa certificates, romance packages, wine, flowers and gourmet treats. You might even want to spoil yourself with a champagne breakfast in bed. Most cruise lines allow you to pre-order a wide range of gifts before you travel.

## Dining

There are usually two different options when it comes to the time of your sit-down dinner, the more popular early sitting (typically 6 pm) and the late sitting (typically 8.30 pm). If you didn't select an option at the time of booking, do it as soon as possible. Some people prefer flexible, freedom or anytime dining, (available on select ships) which gives you the option of eating when and where you want - you simply turn up at the restaurant when you are ready to eat.

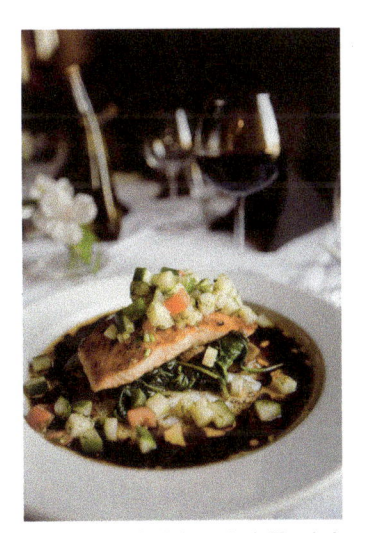

*Credit: Deleece Cook, Unsplash*

## Specialty Dining

Larger cruise ships offer several alternatives to dinner in the main dining room - some have multiple specialty restaurants that offer select menus for a cover charge. You can make your reservations before sailing online, through your cruise ship app or with your booking agent.

## Drinks Packages

If a drinks package was not included in your cruise fare, you may consider buying one before your holiday starts, though they are rarely worth it unless you really like a tipple. For instance, with some packages you may find yourself having to drink several bottles of wine every day just to break even. If you don't want to pre-book a drinks package before leaving home, there will still be plenty of opportunities to purchase one, namely in the terminal after you check-in and at any bar on embarkation day.

If you decide to purchase a drinks package, which do you pick? The problem is there are just so many on

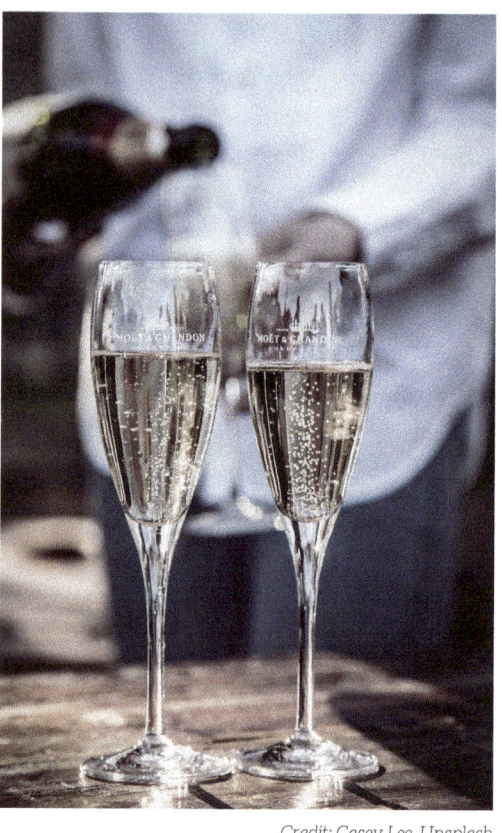

Credit: Casey Lee, Unsplash

offer and most have restrictions: some cruise lines charge extra for premium brands, some require purchase before your sail date, some put restrictions on the number of drinks you can order a day, some lines don't include drinks from your cabin's mini bar or room service, some packages are only valid during certain times of the day, and some do not include gratuities - an extra 15-20% on every drink can soon add up. It is best to try and calculate what, where and how much you might want to drink while on your cruise, and pick the cheapest package that covers it all, bearing in mind that on port days you will spend less time onboard. You could find there isn't much difference between a drinks package and what you might spend if buying drinks individually at the bars onboard.

Beware of the sharing clause - most cruise lines have made it compulsory for everyone over the age of 18 (21 on American lines) in a given cabin to purchase a package. Celebrity and Princess don't impose this same rule, but they in turn will only allow you to 'buy' one drink at a time. If there is a medical reason as to why one person in a cabin cannot drink, take a letter from your doctor to Guest Relations and ask if they would remove the drinks package charge for that passenger, but remember if you are caught flouting the rules, you might well lose your package altogether.

You can still save money on drinks without a package by taking advantage of the ship's happy hour deals, drink promotions, drink tasting events, beer buckets, casino offers and by going on shore excursions that include drinks, like brewery visits or booze cruises. Free champagne and drinks are usually offered at the Captain's Welcome Aboard party, art auctions and member's loyalty lunches. Holland America, Princess and Oceania offer a bottle service in your cabin. Ordering a bottle of gin and six mixers will let you indulge in a drink before dinner whilst saving money, as buying the equivalent at one of the onboard bars will cost a lot more.

## Swimming Pools

Most modern cruise ships launched after 2012 have been built to include swimming pool lifts for the disabled, and some of the older vessels have retrofitted them. On some ships, the equipment is a permanent feature, but on others, such as Disney's fleet and Holland America's *Koningsdam, Niew Statendam* and *Ryndam*, the equipment is only brought out and installed by request. If the latter is true of your cruise line, make sure you request the equipment in advance from the respective special services department.

## Spa Treatments

If you want to enjoy a morning full of pampering or a series of treatments on days that suit your schedule, check if your cruise ship gives you the option of pre-booking spa treatments to make sure you get appointments on the days and at the times you want.

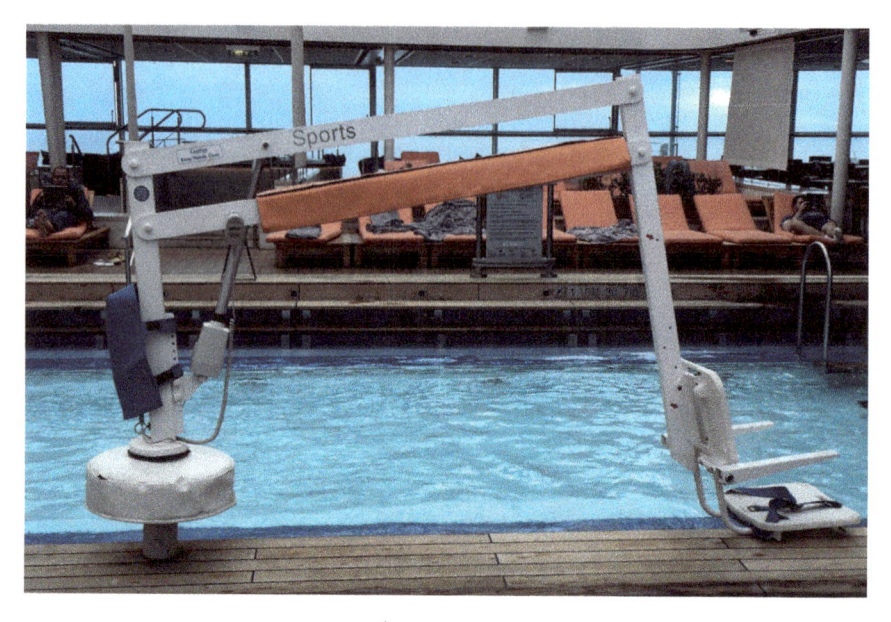

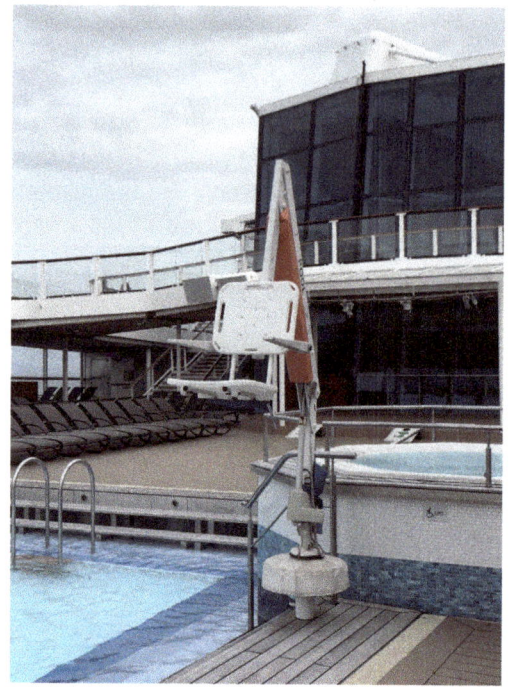

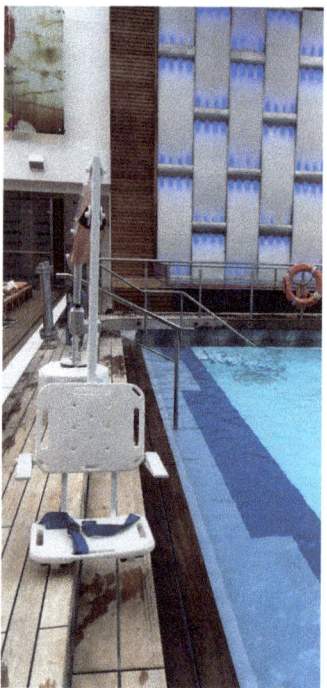

*Credit: Celebrity Silhouette pool hoist*

## Ports and Shore Excursions

One of the big selling points of any cruise itinerary is its excursion program, but finding accessible tours can often be difficult. Certain destinations and ports throughout the world simply don't have accessible vehicles, making it hard (or even impossible) to explore anywhere that isn't immediately next to the port. Some cruise lines do their best to secure accessible vehicles for their passengers, but unfortunately it's not always enough; for example, Holland America will endeavour to book a sedan vehicle, but a wheelchair user will still need to transfer from their chair to the car. Even when accessible vehicles are available, most do not have the capability of carrying scooters safely.

*USA Tours:* *Because of the Americans with Disabilities Act, the rights of people with disabilities to access public and private transportation are guaranteed under federal law. It also ensures access to restaurants, retail stores, museums, parks, attractions and tours.*

However you choose to explore a port, do not take expensive jewellery or large amounts of cash with you ashore. Theft happens in every town and city throughout the world, with tourists a very common target, so no matter where you are visiting, it's always best to only take the things you need ashore. Most staterooms feature an electronic safe, so you can store your valuables and cash securely while you are ashore.

*Cruise Essential:* *Your watch and phone should always be set to ship time when exploring ports. Most people that miss their ship do so because they forget to adjust their timepiece.*

In most places in the world there is little or no reason to take your passport ashore, but there are certain destinations, including Hamilton in Bermuda and St Petersburg in Russia, where port security or immigration will insist on seeing your passport. Ships will advise their passengers whether a passport is required in the visiting port. If it isn't needed, it might be prudent to carry a form of photo ID anyway, just in case you wish to make a credit card purchase.

# The Autonomous Cruiser

***Cruise Tip:*** *Always take the ship's daily planner ashore with you so you have your cruise line's details handy. In the event of a medical emergency, vehicle accident or unexpected delay, contact the port agent immediately so that they can advise the captain.*

Whilst in port, especially if you have a tour booked, comfort is key - there's nothing worse than being hot, sweaty and suffering from blisters. Unless your plans dictate otherwise, you're probably best off simply wearing shorts and a t-shirt, or a sundress over your bikini. Throw on flip-flops for a day at the beach, or don a comfortable pair of shoes if you intend to do a lot of walking.

When it comes to exploring the ports and booking excursions, you have four main options, each with their own set of advantages and pitfalls: you can book tours through your cruise line, book through an independent tour company, hire a private guide, or you can go it alone.

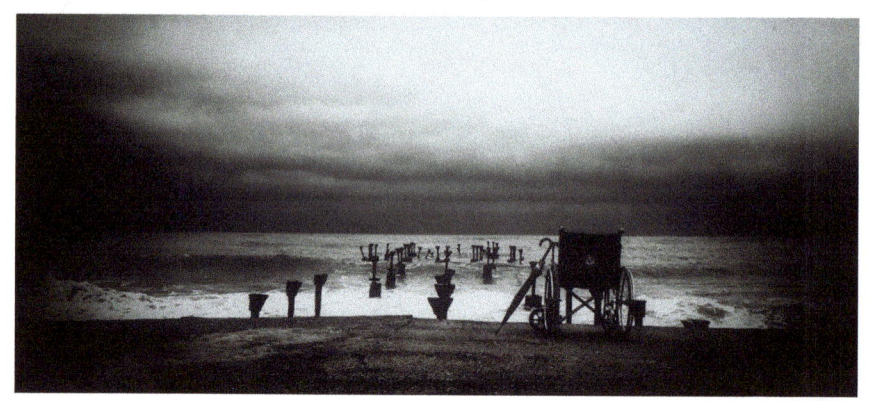

*Credit: Sabeel Ahammed, Pexels*

## Cruise Line Bookings

Your cruise line will issue a shore excursion booking form around eight weeks before embarkation, outlining the selection of tours on offer, along with their mobility restrictions and price. Most cruise lines give, at the very least, information on the physical ability required for each outing, while some, including Princess Cruises, provide a detailed explanation of the embarking and disembarking difficulties for those with limited mobility, in case that impacts on a tour a guest wants to do.

To avoid disappointment, it is strongly suggested that you take the time to go through the tour options and take advantage of booking any 'must-do' shore excursions in advance, as popular tours tend to sell out fast. You might think that you'll be fine waiting to book, but there could be three or four ships in the same port as you and they will most likely all be using the same tour operators as each other. That being said any spaces that don't get booked in advance will be available on embarkation day onboard the ship. If the tour manager offers to place you on a waitlist because an excursion has sold out, don't be too disheartened, as sometimes the excursion office will be able to increase the capacity of a tour because of demand, and passengers pull out at the last minute quite regularly. Talk your plans through with the excursion team, and they will do their best to accommodate your choices. Tours can be cancelled online before a pre-sail cut off period, after which you will need to visit the shore excursion office onboard the ship. Refunds will be given as per the terms and conditions of your cruise line.

**Booking Alternative:** *If a specific cruise ship tour is already sold out by the time you enquire, or you would have preferred it at a different time, then look for the same experience online. Chances are an independent tour operator will have the same or a similar excursion, and it may even be cheaper.*

Cruise ship tour departure times are arranged to maximise their bookings, and sadly the guest's convenience is sacrificed in the process. For all those who have wondered why a tour leaves as early as 7.30am when the ship is in port until early evening, it's because the tour company can utilise the same tour vehicles and schedule an additional afternoon departure, thus capitalising on their revenue.

**Ship Tour Essential:** *One key benefit of booking an excursion through your cruise line is that your ship is more likely to wait for you if your tour is delayed for any reason. Only in extreme circumstances will the captain decide to leave, but in such cases they will usually arrange passenger transportation to the next port of call.*

Booking an excursion through the ship is not necessarily a time-efficient way of spending your day ashore. People don't account for having to meet in the theatre half-an-hour beforehand, then wait for the signal to be herded out to the terminal's parking bays; by the time the coach is loaded, you've waited for latecomers and a final body count is made, you could well have wasted more than an hour of your day. In fact, every rest stop or attraction you visit will involve a reasonable amount of time-wasting, and it's very possible that booking with your cruise line will actually make your day less efficient.

***Take Note:*** *If a shore excursion is operated by minibus, there will usually be no storage space for mobility scooters or wheelchairs.*

Several cruise lines have recently added fully accessible excursions to their brochures, a start to what is hopefully a growing trend. For example, Disney's Port Adventures offers a good selection of fully accessible tours in 26 countries. They have comfortable vehicles equipped with wheelchair lifts or ramps and they provide step-free routes, accessible bathrooms and a professional tour guide familiar with serving disabled guests. Other cruise lines, including NCL and Fred. Olsen, will try to accommodate disabled guests on their tours, but they are limited by whether or not they can secure accessible transport. Azamara also offers shore excursions in select ports with accessible vehicles that are lift or ramp equipped for full-time wheelchair users and guests who are unable to walk or negotiate coach steps.

***Mobility Essential:*** *Wheelchair users have booked tours in the past, only to find that they were expected to be able to climb the steps into the tour bus unaided. If a tour does require you to access a vehicle yourself, you or your caregiver are responsible for collapsing your wheelchair or scooter and placing it on the bus.*

Another major benefit to booking directly with your cruise line is that some offer exclusive outings that you can't book elsewhere. For instance, Azamara and Celebrity Cruises offer the chance to go shopping around bustling markets for fresh ingredients with their chefs, and Hurtigruten let you join their 'Clean up Svalbard' team to take part in a beach clean-up activity during one of their landings in the area.

***Missed Port:*** *Shore excursion offices are generally loath to give your money back, but weather, medical emergencies, or mechanical issues can all cause a port to be missed, and in these circumstances, the ship's excursion team will automatically issue a refund.*

## Independent Tour Operators

If you booked your cruise through a specialised travel agent, they will be able to recommend local accessible tour companies in each port. Booking excursions through these companies often incur additional costs, but they will have knowledge that your cruise line and most 'normal' tour operators lack, meaning they can usually offer more appropriate sightseeing options and experiences, and more flexibility.

**Shore Excursion Tip:** *Even if you don't know which cruise terminal you will be docked at on the day of your arrival in port, independent tour operators will, and they will be standing by the terminal ready to greet you.*

There are a number of specialist companies that are owned and run by people with disabilities who have spent years evaluating the accessibility of each port and know the problems a passenger can face first hand. One of the best is Sage Travelling (*sagetravelling.com*), set up by full-time wheelchair user John Sage after sustaining a T-4 incomplete spinal cord injury. The company sells complete cruise packages as well as custom accessible tours for people with special needs, including wheelchair, scooter, cane and walker users, and senior travellers, in both Europe and the Caribbean. Sage Traveling offers reasonable prices, a pre-trip consultation, an accessibility guide for the port of call and emergency support during your trip. Check out the 'Travel Planning Disability Resources' in the Directory for alternative travel specialists.

Health and safety laws have tightened over the years and as a result a lot of cruise lines tend to only offer more sedentary experiences, like a city or island bus tour. The more thrilling experiences, such as zip-wiring, Segway rides, and quad biking, have all but disappeared from their offerings. This means you'll often have to go directly to independent tour operators in order to secure some of the more adrenaline-inducing activities a port has to offer, but you'll usually have plenty of choice. If your ship does offer something a little more adventurous, it could be cancelled at the last minute due to lack of numbers. It is very disappointing to wake up docked at a beautiful Caribbean island to find a letter shoved under your door declaring that low attendance has necessitated the tour operator cancelling your booking. Independent operators don't cancel tours because their profit margins are slight and they have a reputation to maintain by offering you a fantastic day.

The majority of cruise ports have independent tour operators who will have a good selection of accessible tours to suit mobility-challenged and elderly guests, and in the unlikely event that you need to cancel or the ship has to miss the port, the majority will offer up a no quibble refund. Most reputable independent companies, like Shore Trips (*shoretrips.com*) and Cruising Excursions (*cruisingexcursions.com*), offer collection from the quayside and a guarantee that you will either get back to your ship on time or they will pay to get you to your ship's next port in the unlikely event that you miss sail away because of them.

Viator (*viator.com*) has tours designed especially for cruise passengers, with dates and times that coincide with your itinerary. They tend to have the largest inventory of excursions available in the most popular cruise ports, with hugely competitive prices and pick-ups right from the ship. Their 'Worry-free Shore Excursion' policy ensures your timely return to the ship, and if a rogue occurrence causes you to miss your boarding time, Viator will arrange and pay for your transportation to the next port of call. In addition, if your ship gets delayed or misses the port altogether, the company will automatically refund you. With a low-price guarantee, a 24-hour live phone support system and a no-penalty refund policy if cancelled at least seven days in advance, there's pretty much no downside.

Accessible Island Tours (*accessvi.com*) specialise in disabled-friendly excursions on the island of St Thomas. Their tours are fully equipped for guests with limited mobility, with each of their vehicles accommodating up to five wheelchairs and come equipped with a lifting device.

With more than 4000 underwater educators in over 45 countries, the Handicapped Scuba Association (*hsascuba.com*) is dedicated to enabling people with disabilities to receive the same quality training, certifications and dive adventures as the able-bodied population.

Disabled Accessible Travel (*disabledaccessibletravel.com*) design accessible tours for visiting cruise ship passengers on Mediterranean, Greek, Baltic and British Isles itineraries, and all their tours are private and guaranteed. Booking a private tour has many advantages, as you can liaise and request changes to an itinerary, extend the duration of the tour or add extra stops.

## Private Tour Guides

If you're someone who hates crowds and having to make multiple pitstops in one journey, each of which involves having to wait for 60 other people to have a toilet break before the bus can leave, you might benefit from hiring your own private sightseeing tour guide. Viator (*viator.com*) and ToursByLocals (*toursbylocals.com*) only list travel guides with professional licenses or tour guiding certificates. The most significant benefits to booking a private guide is that you get to set your own schedule and receive real insight into the country from someone who knows the area like the back of their hand. Also, hiring a qualified, knowledgeable tour guide will help you make the most of your limited time in port, as not only will they know where best to show you, but they'll know plenty of time-saving, and perhaps even money-saving, tips.

## Going It Alone

Venturing off on your own in foreign lands is an exciting but often intimidating prospect, especially in countries where you don't speak the language. However, many ports in Europe and the Caribbean are ideal for independent exploration because the main attractions are often close to the ship, taxis are widely available, and a lot of the locals speak English; as such, choosing to 'go it alone' can be a rewarding decision.

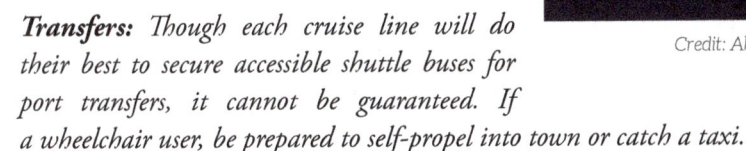

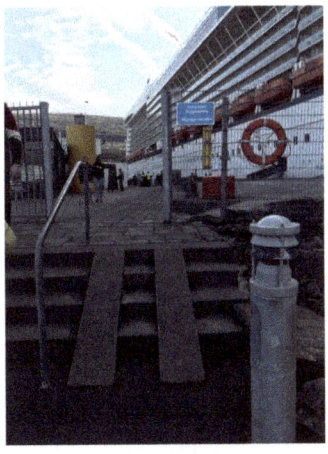

*Credit: Akureyri, Iceland*

***Transfers:*** *Though each cruise line will do their best to secure accessible shuttle buses for port transfers, it cannot be guaranteed. If a wheelchair user, be prepared to self-propel into town or catch a taxi.*

Exploring a port independently could mean coping with steep inclines, stairs, cobblestone streets and high thresholds in shops and restaurants, so it is important to investigate all your options before arriving. That being said, it's important to make sure the research you are doing is accurate. For example, a lot of people rely on the internet for all their information and take what they read online as gospel, but it's not uncommon to find that an article is out of date. There is no point in arriving in Venice expecting to use the wheelchair bridge lifts when in fact they were taken out of service years ago. The main takeaway here is that if you plan on exploring a port independently, make sure your sources of information (guidebooks, brochures, the internet, etc.) are fully up to date.

# The Autonomous Cruiser

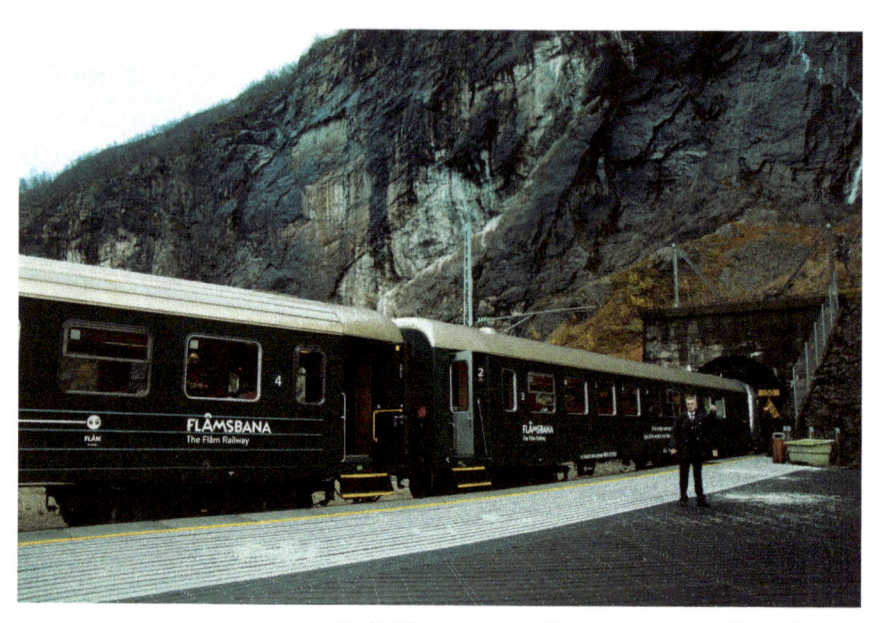

Credit: Flåmsbana train at Kjosfossen, Norway - W Alan, Unsplass

***Tour Tip:*** *Monuments and historic sites can be closed for repairs, renovation, or a public holiday on the day you are visiting that destination.*

***Wheelchair User Tip:*** *A host of museums across Europe offer free or discounted entry to wheelchair users and their caregivers.*

You can book the Flam Railway in Norway independently, but some cruise lines offer it exclusively by booking the whole train for their passengers on the day it will be in port. One guest was excited at the money she saved by booking the train herself, but what she didn't realise was it didn't return the same day! Don't just assume a train will make a return journey.

You might find you're better off booking through the ship or an independent tour company if a port is miles away from the main tourist area. Paris, Florence, and Rome are prime examples, being between one and three hours away from the 'local' port terminal, so a first-time cruiser might well prefer to leave the logistics to someone else. It's worth noting that a lot of cruise lines will also offer services like 'Rome on Your Own', a return transfer (guaranteed by your cruise line) to a central meeting place in a given city that gives you the luxury of being able to explore on your own for a set number of hours.

***Cruise Tip:*** *Before booking any tour or activity, check TripAdvisor and Cruise Critic for unbiased reviews and opinions from past patrons.*

If your only plans for the day are to venture to a popular local beach, you may be better off going independently. If you go with your ship you'll probably pay over the odds for transport, you may be charged too much for sun loungers which are either free or incur just a small local fee, and the whole outing typically only lasts three hours from start to finish. Apart from having to stand on the quayside while the tour bus loads, and the nuisance of waiting for any latecomers, most tours only give you two full hours of beach time - not much time to fully enjoy the sun, sand and ocean. As an example of the benefits of going it alone, a water taxi from just outside the cruise terminal in Grenada takes you across to Grand Anse beach in just 15 minutes. You're dropped right on the sand with sun loungers and facilities aplenty. Furthermore, St Lucia's Rodney Bay offers all the beachfront and water sports you could ask for and is only a 20-minute ride away from either of the ports you might dock at. If you're spending the day with a couple of friends, splitting the cab fare will cost about $5 each. Taxis are readily available in most ports around the world, as well as the Caribbean, and with an average port stop of eight hours, a short cab ride will give you the option of spending most of your day basking in the sun.

In La Palma there is a gorgeous black volcanic sand beach directly opposite the ship's berth, Samil Beach in Vigo is just a short 15-minute taxi ride from the port. Belgium's Blankenberge Beach is a skip and a jump by bus from the port, and Warnemunde Beach in Germany is right on the cruise terminal's doorstep.

It's often far more cost-effective to explore on your own, and outside nearly every port of call you'll find eager taxi drivers hoping to get your business. You will have full control over how you spend your time in port, and the locals will know the area better than anyone. They can help you structure your day based on your wish list and perhaps even give you tips to avoid the crowds. They'll also know what time the ship's tours visit an attraction and will ensure you go either before or after the hordes have gone. Plus, on a ship's excursion you can't hold up the bus because you want to watch the buskers on Barcelona's La Rambla (aka Las Ramblas) or you're hungry for some gelato in a picturesque piazza, but going it alone allows time for pottering.

# The Autonomous Cruiser

Supplying commentary in several languages, Hop-On-Hop-Off bus tours are an excellent way of getting a quick overview of a city, and as the name implies, you can get on and off as many times as your day allows. City Sightseeing (*city-sightseeing.com*) are one of the leading open-top bus tour operators worldwide, with locations in over 100 cities on five continents, and most of their buses are wheelchair-accessible (by wheelchairs measuring up to 28" (70 cm) wide, 47" (120 cm) long and 53" (135 cm) high). Each of their buses can, however, only accommodate one chair, so if the space is already taken, you would need to wait for the next bus. If your chair is larger than specified above, contact the company for more advice. Practically all City Sightseeing Hop-On-Hop-Off destinations have vehicles which allow service dogs for people with impaired sight, but it is always best to check with the city you are visiting.

The other major player offering Hop-On-Hop-Off bus tours across 20 cities is Big Bus Tours (*bigbustours.com*). Their open-top buses offer 360-degree views across the city, and although not every destination has vehicles with wheelchair accessibility, most do with a dedicated space onboard the vehicle.

Isango (*hop-on-hop-off-bus.com*) is a specialist retailer of tours, experiences and attraction tickets in over 300+ destinations, with their own Hop-On-Hop-Off bus tours in some of the most popular destinations around the world and all their vehicles are wheelchair-accessible, however, service dogs are not allowed on their buses.

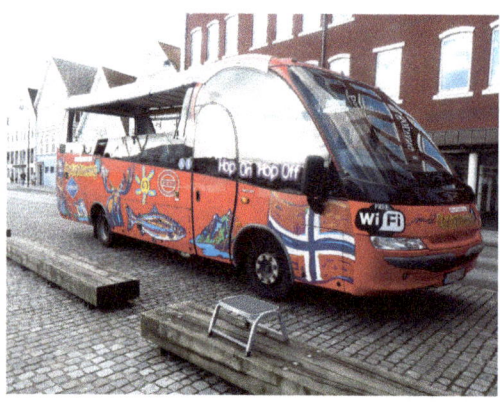

In certain ports, the Hop-On-Hop-Off companies stop at the cruise terminal as part of their route, especially for cruise passengers. For example, in Copenhagen and Lisbon, the tour buses are directly across from the port gates.

Another area where cruise lines have made cutbacks in recent years is with shuttle buses, which in the past were offered free of charge but now typically cost around £10 per person (charged to your onboard account), though this does often include multiple trips. On some ships, you can purchase shuttle tickets onboard, while on other lines you will have to queue outside the terminal. In some ports, it may be compulsory to board your cruise line's shuttle bus to the port gate because of health and safety reasons, but in these cases, the service will be complimentary. All the information you might need about your ship's shuttles will be in your cruise planner the night before you arrive in port.

It might also be quicker and cheaper to take a taxi than to pay for multiple tickets on the ship's shuttle. In Madeira, for example, four people paying €12 each for the shuttle into the town's central hub means a cost of €48, plus the inevitable queue to buy your ticket and the wait to board a bus with available space. On the other hand, a taxi will charge just €15 for all of you each way, a saving of €18, plus you'll have the advantage of being dropped off exactly where you want.

***Transport Tip:*** *There are always generous amounts of taxis to be had at Madeira cruise terminal, with a queue for a straight transfer and a separate one for day tours.*

The ships' port guides usually list the nearest beaches and shopping areas, but they are generally not available until the night before you dock, so you'll have a hard time pre-planning your day in port if you don't seek your own information before your cruise.

***Translation Tip:*** *Learning the phrase "Where is the port?" or "Please take me to the cruise ship port" in the local language could help you grab a taxi back to the ship. It's also worth carrying your ship's daily planner as it will have the name and details of the port you are docked at.*

Going it alone lets you experience the pure joy of falling in love with a destination having arrived with no expectations, whether it be through a picnic on a secluded beach, an amble through a museum's exhibits or a short stop to watch street performers while you eat a freshly baked local pastry.

Spending time in port certainly doesn't have to mean shelling out vast amounts of money on shore excursions or private tours. Every port in the world will have plenty of free activities to enjoy, whether you're out on your own, with a close friend or with your whole family. Some ideas are:

- Visit the beach - go swimming in the ocean, build sandcastles, collect shells

- Visit a public garden or park - go for a picnic (grab food from the morning buffet), read a book on the grass
- Build a snowman and have a snowball fight
- Go on a bird walk
- Look for local hiking or walking trails
- Explore an old church
- Enjoy a puzzle day with crosswords and Sudoku
- Create a journal or travel blog
- Attend a local festival or carnival
- Visit a national museum or gallery
- Spend the day at a local library
- Tour the city's landmarks
- Browse local markets
- Attend a religious service
- Catch local live music
- Go on a photographic scavenger hunt
- Enjoy a nearby river or creek
- Get close to local wildlife by exploring the local woods
- Sit by a river and write poetry
- Draw, sketch or paint a local scene
- Visit the local town hall and learn about the history of the city
- Watch street performers
- Go in search of street art
- Watch a craft demonstration
- Explore a National Park
- Watch local fishermen haul in the morning's catch
- Play backgammon or chess with a local
- Join the world's largest treasure hunt and Go Geocaching - there are millions of people participating worldwide, just create an account and track the treasure by its GPS coordinates (*geocaching.com*)

## Local Customs

If you intend to visit sacred monuments or buildings whilst in port, you'd be wise in ascertaining what their local customs and cultural practices are. In certain countries, it is culturally offensive to expose the skin on your arms or legs, and many religious sites have strict dress codes, especially for female tourists. Women should avoid miniskirts, bra tops, short-sleeved shirts, shorts and cleavage-bearing necklines. It's also wise to cover your knees, shoulders and hair if you want to visit a sacred place, so carry a cardigan, scarf or pashmina with you. Most temples and mosques will also require you to take your shoes off at the door, but it's best not to leave them outside, as they might not be there when you return.

It's not just religious sites that have imposed stringent dress codes. ItIs illegal to wear high heels or stilettos around Greecess historic sites as they can damage the monuments, while in Majorca and other parts of Spain you could face a fine of up to £500 if you wear swimwear anywhere other than the beach. On the other side of the world in Victoria, Australia, once the clock has struck noon on Sunday, it's against the law to appear in public places wearing pink shorts. Also, wearing any form of camouflage print clothing (of any colour) is illegal in many cruise destinations throughout the Caribbean, as well as in Nigeria, Oman, Saudi Arabia, South Africa, Uganda, Zambia, and the Philippines (uniforms only).

Chewing gum in Singapore will incur fines of $1000 and it's best to avoid clothing sporting religious or military insignia, national flags or emblems, as they are also deemed illegal unless a specific exemption is granted. Finally, a sizable fine will be imposed on anyone feeding the pigeons in Venice's St Mark's Square, as the city deems the birds a health hazard.

## Local Events

Foreign shores are tempting enough to explore as it is, but your visit could be further enriched if you find your ship will be in port the same day as a local festival, tournament, exhibition or sporting fixture. Below are few notable examples to whet your appetite, but of course there are literally hundreds of annual events taking place worldwide, so be sure to check out what's happening in the ports you'll be visiting and immerse yourself in a cultural experience like no other.

> **Don't Ask:**
> *Does this lift go up or down?*

**The Carnival of Venice** takes place every year just before the six-week Catholic religious observance of Lent. It's a wonderful event of street parades, masked balls, and shows on the city's famous waterways, and locals and visitors are encouraged to dress up, wear masks and show off their fabulous costumes.

**The Copenhagen Jazz Festival** is a must on Denmark's music calendar. You'll find more than 1000 separate performances in clubs, cafés, concert halls, and open-air destinations over a two-week period. Visitors can enjoy live music in the historical streets of Copenhagen, which has been known as one of the jazz capitals of Europe since the 1950s.

**Keukenhof: Amsterdam's Tulip & Flower Festival** sees more than 500 flower growers and bulb suppliers show off their prowess over a 200-hectare site known as the 'Garden of Europe'.

**The Stars of the White Nights Festival** is St Petersburg's annual summer calendar event. Run throughout the season of the midnight sun, the arts fair is one of the most popular musical and cultural events in Russia. Most cruise itineraries enjoy an overnight stop in the city so visitors can enjoy music, opera, ballet, film and outdoor celebrations, including a fantastic fireworks display.

**The Fiesta de San Isidro** honours Madrid's patron saint. It's the annual highlight on the springtime calendar, and for several days the city becomes a festive riot of Latin culture, with more than 50 music, theatre and dance concerts taking place in locations throughout the city.

## Getting to the Cruise Terminal

Plan your journey to and from the cruise terminal in full. If you plan on driving yourself to the terminal, book yourself a spot in a nearby car park well in advance as some ports have limited spaces. If you're not driving, consider a train or coach to a station near your port of choice, or even a door-to-door taxi transfer.

## UK Cruise Ports

Detailed information on each cruise port in the UK and their facilities is provided in the 'UK Cruise Ports' section of the Directory.

## Pier Transfers

Some cruise lines and tour operators include a transfer to the port within your holiday package. If you did secure the service, which must typically be reserved two weeks before sailing, a representative will meet you outside the customs area and once you have claimed your luggage, you will be escorted to a designated coach. If a transfer is not included in your holiday cost, the cruise line is often willing to organise travel for you.

## Luggage Services

Wouldn't it be nice to have your own personal valet, letting you bypass the long queues at the airport, avoid paying the penalty for excess luggage and sidestepping baggage claim when you travel? Getting your bags to the cruise terminal is the last hurdle before starting your holiday, but it doesn't have to be difficult. There are now a number of established luggage delivery services that offer you peace of mind, safe in the knowledge that your belongings will be waiting for you in your cabin when you arrive on the ship, and that they will be delivered back to your home when your holiday is over. Even if your travel plans do not involve flying, you can enjoy a stress-free journey and avoid the hassle of having to contend with weighty cases. You might even have plans for the days after your cruise and do not want to drag your luggage around with you - now you don't have to. Also, in the unlikely event that your bags are delayed, most companies will refund the delivery fees and offer a tidy sum back as compensation. The luxury of travelling hands-free isn't cheap, but for some, especially those travelling with a service dog or with limited mobility who have a hard enough time as it is travelling through airports, the added convenience is worth the extra cost.

*Time Factor: If you have booked a fly-cruise, all your luggage must pass through customs, whether you are travelling with your suitcases or not. Unaccompanied luggage can arouse suspicion from custom officers, and an in-depth search could cause delays. Baggage handling services are powerless to intervene, so safeguard against this unexpected problem by building in a little extra time by sending your belongings earlier rather than later.*

Depending on where you are travelling to and with whom, you can either book a luggage delivery service through your cruise line when you make your booking, or you can contact the baggage companies directly. Cunard has recently withdrawn their own White Star Luggage Service, instead partnering up with Luggage Forward. Several other companies have also retired their own luggage services and followed Cunard's directive, including Crystal Cruises, who have chosen Luggage Concierge as their new baggage handling provider.

If you're not sure as to whether your cruise line offers their own service, it's best to just call up and ask.

**Baggage Handling Company (***thebaggagehandlingcompany.com***)**
A family-run business specialising in transporting your luggage to and from your cruise ship. Serving the ports of Southampton and Portsmouth, the company also deals with unaccompanied baggage for world and sector cruising. All luggage is insured up to £250 per bag, but additional cover is available should you need it.

**Direct Baggage (***directbaggage.com***)**
Direct Baggage takes the hard work out of travelling by offering a bespoke luggage service to and from most countries, including cruises from Southampton. The company takes the sting out of paying an airline to transport your cases and saves you time at check-in and in baggage halls. This door-to-door service might not be the cheapest, but they guarantee the quality of their assignment and offer next day delivery within the UK and most European cities.

**Disabled Cruise Club (***disabledcruiseclub.com***)**
Disabled Cruise Club are committed to providing the perfect accessible cruise holiday, arranging exclusive sailings, disabled equipment, adapted excursions, port assistance and their own home to cabin luggage delivery service. For Dover, London and Southampton departures, your suitcases will be collected from your address and delivered to your cabin on the day of your cruise, with the service reversed on your return.

**Excess Luggage (***excessluggage.co.uk***)**
Excess Luggage is a leading name in baggage handling. They provide a UK, domestic and international concierge service that will ensure you enjoy a stress-free journey to and from your cruise ship without the burden of taking your luggage. Your suitcases will be collected from an address of your choice, whether your home, hotel or office, and delivered to your cruise cabin.

**First Luggage (***firstluggage.com***)**
First Luggage will arrange for your suitcases to be secured from any destination worldwide and then delivered to your chosen address without any stress,

inconvenience, tedious airport queues or inflated airline baggage costs. The bespoke concierge service allows you to relax, safe in the knowledge that your bags are tracked from the pick-up address right through to your cruise cabin ready for your arrival.

**GAC Baggage UK** (*gac.com/cruise*)
Exclusive port agents for Fred Olsen, GAC Baggage UK has the global resources, expertise, and integrated services to ensure your suitcases enjoy a smooth journey to and from your home. For Dover, Liverpool, Newcastle and Rosyth departures, your bags will be collected from your address three days before your cruise and delivered to your cabin on the day of embarkation. For bookings ring 0191 431 8976 and quote 'Fred Olsen'.

**Luggage Concierge** (*luggageconcierge.com*)
Benefit from the freedom and ease of travelling without suitcases with Luggage Concierge, the exclusive partner of Crystal Cruises. The six-star door-to-door luggage service will ship your bags to and from your destination, providing a stress-free travel option and giving you the luxury of moving through airports without the misery and aggravation of carrying anything other than your carry-on. Luggage Concierge offers the best insurance in the industry, providing up to $5000 coverage per bag as standard.

**Luggage Forward** (*luggageforward.com*)
With more than a decade of experience behind them, Luggage Forward has forged partnerships with a worldwide network of shipping specialists, ensuring thousands of pieces of luggage have reached their destination in a timely manner. The company will deliver your luggage directly to your cruise ship in more than 200 territories and countries, backed by a full refund plus a $500 on-time delivery guarantee.

**Luggage Free** (*luggagefree.com*)
For the more discerning traveller, this white-glove concierge service company offers the convenience of carrying, checking and claiming luggage on your behalf from 150+ countries worldwide. Enhance your cruise experience by securing a door-to-cabin on-time guaranteed delivery service with bags of any size or weight. Your luggage is tracked from pick up to delivery, and you'll be sent an email confirming the person who took receipt. Luggage Free

offers complimentary insurance cover of up to $1000 for each shipment, with additional coverage should you need it.

### Luggage Mule (*luggagemule.co.uk*)

Experience a low cost, maximum convenience service with this worldwide door-to-cabin luggage delivery company. Luggage Mule will collect your unaccompanied cases, allowing you up to 30 kg per piece without excess baggage charges, and deliver them to any cruise ship departing from Southampton or Barcelona using a fully trackable online service.

### Princess Luggage Valet (*https://app.luggageforward.com/book/princess*)

Offered in partnership with Luggage Forward, Princess Cruises' preferred baggage handling company guarantees safe and timely deliveries of your personal belongings. Whatever port you are embarking in, the company will deliver your luggage directly to your cruise ship backed by a full refund plus a $500 on-time delivery guarantee.

### TEfra-bag (*tefra-bag.com*)

TEfra-bag now offers its door-to-ship luggage delivery service in the UK. For Bristol, Dover, Portsmouth, Southampton and Tilbury departures, your suitcases will be collected from your address and delivered to your cabin on the day of your cruise, with the service reversed on your return. TEfra-bag offers a clear-cut pricing structure together with the added bonus of cover up to £1000 per bag on each journey.

## Door-to-Door Cruise Transfers

Start your holiday in style with your own private transport service to the airport or cruise terminal. Just sit back, relax, and enjoy the first-class service of your driver and rest assured you'll arrive stress-free, on time, and ready to start your vacation.

***Take Note:*** *It is an offence under the Private Hire Vehicles (Carriage of Guide Dogs etc.) Act 2002 for the operator of a private vehicle to refuse to take a booking because of a disabled person being accompanied by a guide or service dog, or to impose an additional charge for carrying the dog.*

## Before You Go

**Ports Direct** (*portsdirect.co.uk*) - *0843 0843 003*
Ports Direct has been a market leader in the cruise transport industry since 2007 and fully understands the logistics of planning, booking, and managing safe transportation for cruise passengers. They provide comfort, safety and affordability and will drive you to and from any seaport or airport in the UK, as well as offering tours. Wheelchair-accessible vehicles are available and must be confirmed at the time of booking.

**Titan's VIP Home Departure Service** (*titantravel.co.uk*) - *0808 274 2725*
Your holiday starts the moment you step outside the front door with Titan. There is no need to fret about taxi fares, train timetables or having to lug your bags onto public transport – Titan will take care of the whole journey for you. There are no mileage limits or supplements to pay as the service covers every UK address (with the exception of the Scottish Islands and Sark). The company's vehicles do carry collapsible wheelchairs, and they provide a step for their clients with limited mobility.

**Free Door-to-Door Transfers** (*fredolsen.co.uk*) - *0800 690 6654*
On certain sailings, a Fred Olsen representative will come to your door, pick you up and drive you to your ship, and at the end of the cruise, the chauffeur will collect you from the port and drive you home. If you live within 90 miles of the port, these transfers are completely free of charge. If you live further away, you can simply pay a top-up to allow your holiday to begin and end at your front door. A Fred Olsen representative will liaise with a local supplier to ensure the vehicle meets your mobility needs if you require wheelchair-accessible transport.

**Travel Management Solutions** (*cmacgroup.co.uk*) - *03333 207 100*
With a nationwide network of vetted or approved suppliers, Travel Management Solutions offers a punctual, reliable transfer service. An agent will pick you up from your home or other convenient address and deliver you to your chosen destination (port, airport, station). Their drivers will be happy to help with your baggage and offer any assistance that may be required. With access to a wide range of vehicles, including standard, executive and wheelchair-friendly options, their team will ensure all your needs are met.

**Cruise Transfer** (*cruisetransfer.com*) - *0800 069 6090 or 01895 622 226*
Cruisetransfer.com is offered by Central Chauffeur, a group of companies

specialising in professional ground transportation services and cruise or airport transfers. The group prides itself on its principles, which aim to provide top quality cars, knowledgeable drivers and excellent service. Cruisetransfer.com offers a fully comprehensive transfer service throughout the UK, including all major airports. The company does not have wheelchair-accessible vehicles.

***Twelve Transfers*** (*twelvetransfers.co.uk*) - *0203 479 5700 or 07514 354 474*
Travel in style and comfort! Choose from a wide range of services for groups of up to eight passengers (larger groups can be accommodated in multiple vehicles). Because Twelve Transfers has over six years' experience in providing private transfers between all major UK seaports and London airports, you can rest assured that your journey will be handled by professionals and planned to the last detail. The company does not have wheelchair-accessible vehicles.

***Saga VIP Travel Service*** (*travel.saga.co.uk*) - *0808 250 2517*
Saga includes their VIP door-to-door travel service on all their cruises, so whether you're travelling to an international or domestic airport, or your UK departure point, you can relax knowing that your travel details will be taken care of by one of their handpicked partners. An experienced chauffeur will collect you from your home, or other convenient address, so you can enjoy a relaxing journey to the airport or cruise port, and on your return to the UK, your chauffeur will be there to greet you ready for your trip home. If you are travelling with a wheelchair or scooter, or any other mobility aid or equipment, Saga will ensure a suitable vehicle is arranged.

***Wheelchair Travel*** (*wheelchair-travel.co.uk*) - *01483 237 668*
With 35 years' experience, Wheelchair Travel provides excellent transport exclusively for wheelchair and scooter users either resident in or visiting the UK from overseas. Offering 'meet and greet' airport transfers, cruise transfers to Southampton, Dover and Tilbury, and local and long-distance taxi services, Wheelchair Travel provides an unrivalled service to travellers who are mobility impaired. The company also has a network of overseas agents specialising in travel for special needs clients.

## Coach Transfers

Coach travel is a popular option for travelling across the UK especially for large groups. It is also a more 'greener' form of travel, with reduced fossil fuel usage and lower emissions per traveller. Travelling by coach is also cost-effective, more spacious than a car with extra legroom, reclining seats, air-conditioning and onboard toilets.

***Cruise Connect*** (*intercruises.com*) - *0131 226 8524*
Cruise Connect provides a coach transfer service for Cunard, P&O Cruises and Princess Cruise passengers to and from their cruise ship. There are 50 collection/drop-off points in the UK, and since the service started in 2001, they have never missed a sailing. Wheelchair access is available, but you need to advise the Cruise Connect team during the booking process of your special needs. If you are travelling with oxygen, supplies must be in hand-held bottles.

***Eavesway Cruiselink*** (*eaveswaytravel.com*) - *01942 727985*
With over 40 years' experience catering to cruise passengers, Eavesway Cruiselink is the premier coach travel service for sailings from Southampton, Dover and Newcastle. The company offers transport for the leading cruise providers from major towns and cities across the UK. Wheelchair access via a demountable ramp is available at all collection and drop-off locations, just advise the company at least 21 days before departure of your special needs. Liquid oxygen is allowed in the seating area, but pressurised containers must be placed in the hold.

## Airport Lounges

Flying can be stressful, so why not take advantage of an airport lounge to while away the time after check-in but before you have to board the aircraft? Lounge access provides a sanctuary away from the crowds in the terminal and often includes comfortable seating areas, free drinks and snacks throughout the day, television, free Wi-Fi and a selection of newspapers and magazines. Gone are the days when you had to travel in business or first class to gain access to these exclusive areas; several airlines now offer a day pass so you can sit back and enjoy the facilities, but they vary in what they offer - some

> **Don't Ask:**
> What do you do for a real job? (said to crew member)

have fabulous facilities, such as massage and facials at Heathrow Airport's Virgin Atlantic Clubhouse, while some are basic rest stops. Priority Pass (*prioritypass.com*) and Lounge Pass (*loungepass.com*) offer pre-bookable airport lounge access on both the outward and homeward legs of your journey.

Download the LoungeBuddy app (*loungebuddy.co.uk*) for information on the lounge facilities at your chosen airport, including the number of hours you can stay as well as reviews and photos. If you don't have a mobile phone, you can access lounge reviews on *skytraxratings.com* or *loungeguide.net* before investing your money.

## Must Have Buys

We all have our favourite and essential items that we like to take away with us such as a power bank that can charge our mobile phone multiple times and a worldwide travel adaptor, but while you may think you have everything you might want or need, here are just a few things that you might have overlooked that could come in very handy. Although I have suggested a company that sells each item, it may be possible to find it cheaper if you shop around.

*Pressure Relief Memory Foam Vinyl Wheelchair Seat Support Comfort Chair Cushion* (Sold by Allcare Medical Ltd and fulfilled by *ebay.co.uk*)
Designed specially to make your ride more comfortable, these wheelchair cushions have a wipe-clean vinyl cover with foam inner and a memory foam topper. The cushion fits most types and sizes of wheelchair and comes with integrated ties that secure it to the wheelchair frame.

*UK Foam Comfort Donut Ring Chair Seat Cushion* (Sold by Sheng Yan and fulfilled by *ebay.co.uk*)
The donut ring provides comfort and gentle support while reducing the pressure on tender areas when seated. Perfect for pain and pressure relief from haemorrhoids, hip bursitis, and general coccyx pain. The air mesh cover can be removed easily for cleaning.

*Wheelchair Shock Absorbing Caster Forks* (*froglegsinc.com*)
Frog Legs is a worldwide expert in wheelchair suspension. With over fourteen years of experience, they manufacture the original and best wheelchair shock

absorbing caster forks available, absorbing 76% of jolts and vibration that affect the ride of a user's wheelchair.

### Wheelchair Tire Covers (rehadesign.com)
Certain museums, churches and historic buildings insist on wheelchair tyre covers to keep dirt and germs from transferring to clean floors. Specially designed so there is no slippage, these covers are machine washable and go on your manual wheelchair in seconds. There are three types available: Wheelchair Slippers which cover the rear wheels, Mud Eaters which are water-resistant and also cover the rear wheels, and Wheelchair Socks which cover the small front caster wheels.

### *Personalised Luggage Tags with leather strap* (*zazzle.co.uk*)
*Custom luggage tags from Zazzle are sturdy and weatherproof, and will stand up to the travel demands of any cruise warrior or adventure seeker. Your designs, text, and photos are displayed in vibrant clarity and brilliant colours.*

### *Personalised Passport Holders* (*zazzle.co.uk*)
*Keep your most important travel document protected and looking new with a variety of custom passport holders. They also safeguard your identity by shielding your information, keeping you secure in public.*

### Bags of Love 'Design Your Own Suitcase' (bagsoflove.co.uk)
This personalised suitcase is a travel essential and easy to spot amongst other generic luggage on the carousel. Both the suitcase and carry-on size feature TSA approved lock technology, four wheels for easy manoeuvring and are printed with your own photos, design or name.

### MYCARBON Travel RFID Money Belt (mycarbon.cc) (amazon.co.uk)
Travel safely and securely with a radio-frequency identification blocking security travel pouch with multifunctional pockets for your passports, tickets, credit cards, cash, phone and more. Designed for wearing under your clothes, the innovative material protects you from unwanted scans and hi-tech pickpockets, and ensures your money and credit card information remain secure and safe.

### Pacsafe Metrosafe LS120 Hip Bag Black (addnature.co.uk)
These bags have the advantage of being hands-free so you can propel your

wheelchair or use other mobility aids without worrying that your money is vulnerable to thieves. The bags have RFID protected pockets that keep thieves from scanning the magnetic strips on your credit cards and passport. Invisible to the eye, the bag has a flexible, lightweight, stainless steel wire that is integrated into the adjustable straps, preventing bag slashers from cutting through and running off with your belongings.

### *Secrid Slimwallet (secrid.com) (slimwalletjunkie.com)*
A sleek minimalist wallet which blocks radio frequency identification (RFID) theft, prevents card clash and stores business cards, banknotes and up to 11 credit cards.

### *Kindle Paperwhite (amazon.co.uk)*
Perfect for those with vision impairment, the Kindle Paperwhite enables you to adjust the text size and font shade for maximum readability while Whispersync lets you switch between reading and listening mode without losing your place The thinnest, lightest version of this popular device now lasts weeks on a single charge and is even waterproof so you can listen to your audiobooks at the pool, by the beach on in the bath. Pair Bluetooth headphones or speakers and you're ready to go.

### *The Lifemax Pill Box Reminder (lifemaxuk.co.uk)*
This pill box features an integral timer that is simple to pre-set for an easy-to-see-and-hear reminder. It has a flashing light and audible alarm that sounds for one minute when your medication is due. It also features two storage compartments and a real-time clock with hours and minutes.

### *Talking Time Big Digit Alarm Clock (completecareshop.co.uk)*
A lightweight, compact, battery-operated talking travel clock recommended especially for people with sensory loss. The clock has a large and clear digital display, but can also speak the time and temperature. There is also a sound-controlled backlight and projection display.

### *Trendform® Stainless Steel Magnetic Hooks (amazon.co.uk)*
Cruise ship cabin walls and doors are made of metal, so these fabulous brushed stainless-steel magnetic hooks are perfect for hanging items up to 250 g in weight, such as windbreakers, scarves, hats or handbags, when you need more space.

### Before You Go

***Shoe Organizer, 24 Large Mesh Pockets Heavy Duty Over the Door Hanging** (amazon.co.uk)*
Even on the newest ships, your stateroom could be lacking in storage space. A hanging organiser can be used to swallow up toiletries, charging cables, medication, bottles and sterilisation tablets easily, freeing up potentially much needed space.

***Key Chain Personal Alarm** (completecareshop.co.uk)*
A disability can make you feel vulnerable at times so a simple but effective protection alarm, which can act as a useful deterrent against mugging, assault or harassment, can bolster your confidence when out and about. This police-approved alarm can be attached to a keychain, belt, bag or similar by its metal key ring. When you press the button or pull the metal pin from the device it activates a very loud continuous alarm.

***WIWO Sandal Flip Flop Towel Clips** (amazon.co.uk)*
These clips remove the annoyance of sun lounger towels falling down or blowing in the wind. Use them beside the swimming pool, at the beach, or even at home in your garden!

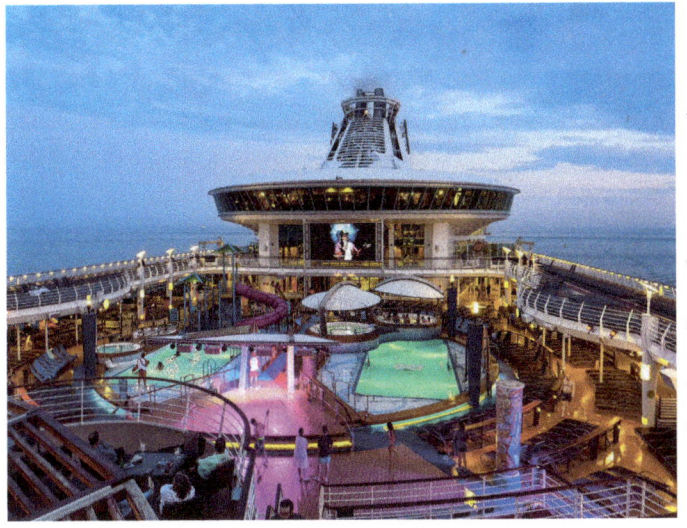

*Credit: Royal Caribbean - Miguel Angel Sanz, Unsplash*

## Cruise Apps

The majority of cruise lines now have their own dedicated apps, designed for you to use before and during your cruise to add to your experience. Most of the apps will include your cruise itinerary, deck plans, daily planner, shore excursions, menus and tour and spa reservations, while others give you access to your shipboard account and even a chat service.

Walkie Talkies were the age-old method of being able to communicate with your friends and family during a cruise. This dated technology has been abandoned in favour of communicating through your cruise line's app; though each varies slightly, invariably they enable holidaymakers to use their smartphone to stay in contact with other people on the same ship. The good news is that these do not require an internet package and for the most part are free while onboard, though there might be a small charge to use the text messaging service.

Search your phone's app store for your cruise line's app and get set up as soon as you can so you can get as much use out of it as possible. While you're on the app store, check out some of these more general cruising apps that could also help make your trip easier.

**Cruise Finder by iCruise**
This award-winning cruise app provides detailed information on 40 different cruise lines, 350+ ships (including stateroom photos and deck plans), 25 destinations, and 32,000+ itineraries complete with route maps. Review cruise calendars, port information, and weather. Set the cruise countdown clock to your departure date and share your favourite photos via email, Facebook, and Twitter.

**Cruise Ship Mate**
This is the only cruise app you can use before, during and after you sail and it works on every cruise line, not just one. It offers detailed information on deck maps, port excursions, cruise price alerts, ship trackers, and a countdown to your cruise. It provides tips, photos and reviews for the destinations you'll be visiting, and you can also use 'ship chat' to ask other shipmates for advice.

## Cruise Ship & Port News

This app provides updates on the newest ships, port information, and individual cruise companies, including Celebrity, Carnival, Royal Caribbean, NCL, Princess, and Holland America. Discover interesting articles and hints that will help you save money and make your cruise even more enjoyable.

## CruiseMapper

This app allows you to search by cruise line or ship name, locate itinerary schedules, check shipping forecasts and will relay any shipping news. Regional trackers will enable you to see which ships are at sea and which are in port. You can also access cruise ship reviews, special features, technical details and even deck plans.

## VesselFinder Free

Features include real-time positions of over 100,000 ships every day, searchable by ship name, IMO (International Maritime Organisation) number or MMSI (Maritime Mobile Service Identity) number. Access ship details including their name, flag, type, destination, arrival time, draught, course, speed, gross tonnage, year of build, and size.

## Ship Finder Lite

This app covers most of the world, tracking 30,000+ ships simultaneously. Simply tap on a vessel to see its name, type and destination. Colour coded icons make identification easy too. The full version includes additional features, including route history, search, filters, bookmarks, photos, and the ability to add your favourite ships.

# Dress Codes

Information on each cruise line's dress code will be available in their brochure, on their website, and within your final cruise confirmation documents, giving you an indication of what to expect when you arrive on board and helping you plan what to pack for your trip. Typically, cruises of six nights or more will have at least three casual, two elegant and one formal evening, but you can always choose to opt-out and eat in the buffet restaurant for a more casual dining experience on any evening. In general, cruise ship dress codes only apply in the evenings, with most restaurants, bars and theatres adopting the policy from around 6pm. The ship's daily planner advises on what the dress code is that day, and when and where it will be enforced.

## Taboo

Swimwear is not permitted in any ships' lounges, theatres or restaurants at any time. Also, most cruises do not allow bare feet, robes, jeans, baseball caps, flip-flops, shorts, tank tops, and torn or ripped clothing in public areas during the evening.

As of 1 January 2018, P&O do not allow any fancy dress or novelty clothing on their cruises unless it is for an official P&O themed night. *"In addition to the fancy dress policy, clothing personalised with images/slogans, and/or clothing that features offensive language, images or slogans, will not be allowed on board at any time."* The cruise line's brochure stipulates that they reserve the right to deny embarkation to guests who they deem are inappropriately dressed.

## Daywear/Casual

When it comes to your day outfit, the general rule of thumb is to use the same principles that you would use on any land-based holiday: lightweight shirts, shorts or trousers, and swimwear are all ideal for hot weather, with a jumper or jacket on top if it's a little cooler out. Remember that, while we all love our jeans, some lines such as Crystal and Swan Hellenic do not allow them in any of their restaurants, irrespective of how expensive they are.

Even on the most exotic itineraries you might find yourself a bit chilly, particularly in the evenings and on American lines that have air-conditioning, so it is a good idea to pack a warm cover up or lightweight jacket, or even a coat in case of the occasional shower. Decks can often get slippery, so flat rubber-soled shoes are somewhat of a necessity. Sports activities feature on most ships so you might consider bringing trainers, shorts, track pants and gym attire.

## Freestyle Experience

Some cruise lines, including Norwegian, have a 'freestyle' system, with no formal dress code in place. Casual clothing is acceptable throughout the cruise, including summer dresses, skirts, shorts, jeans and tops for women, and khakis, jeans, shorts and collarless shirts for men.

Other lines that also have a totally relaxed atmosphere when it comes to clothing are Carnival, Disney, MSC and Royal Caribbean, all of which are family-friendly with a dress down option available throughout their ships. They do all offer a formal evening, but there is no need to don a tuxedo or wear a ball gown, and they can be by-passed altogether if the mood does not strike.

**Smart Casual**
Smart Casual (or elegant/evening casual) is, as you might guess, somewhere between normal daywear and formal attire. Stylish resort wear is ideal, including informal separates or dresses for ladies, and long trousers and open-necked shirts for men.

**Cruise Elegant/Evening Chic**
Some cruise lines, including Celebrity, have done away with traditional formal wear and offer a more relaxed alternative in the evening. Elegant is the keyword, with men donning blazers, chinos and enclosed shoes, and women in simple trouser suits or cocktail dresses.

**Black Tie/Formal Nights**
Tradition dictates a touch of glamour and a real sense of occasion that will see guests donning their finery for special gala nights at sea. Men generally stick to dinner jackets, tuxedos, formal Highland wear, formal national dress and military uniforms (ceremonial blades are not allowed), while women usually wear ballgowns, cocktail dresses and trouser suits.

**Themed Nights**
Many lines host special events that range from a Black/White Ball, Pirate Night, Caribbean/Tropical Night, and even a Hoedown Country Night. Passengers who enjoy participating are encouraged to dress according to the theme, but don't worry if you have come without, you can usually find something on a market stall when you venture ashore. The number of themed events will be in the cruise literature that is sent out several weeks before the start of your holiday.

## The Ultimate Cruise Packing List

Your holiday is looming and all that is left to do is tackle the packing, some travellers' worst nightmare. The fear of forgetting something and having to buy it at double its normal price on the ship or in a foreign country is a lot to bear, and that is if you can find it at all. As such, a comprehensive packing list is essential.

You won't need everything listed below, just tailor it to your own needs, including factors like the length of your cruise, your ship's dress code, the climate of your destinations, any planned excursions or activities and your luggage limitations.

It's best not to pack expensive jewellery for your trip, as tourists are common targets for thieves; criminals look for people who stand out, swathed in flashy watches and expensive trinkets. When packing your belongings at the end of your cruise, keep any valuable items you bought while on your cruise in your carry-on luggage.

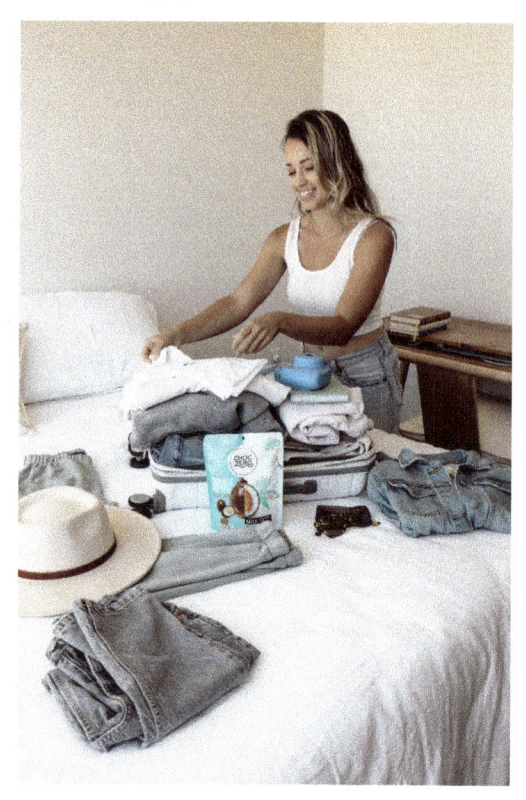

*Credit: Tyler Nix, Unsplash*

**Cruise Tip:** *Several ships have self-serve laundry and ironing facilities in addition to the cabin laundry service. This service is particularly useful if you've booked a fly cruise - it makes more sense to do a load during the cruise rather than paying for excess luggage with an airline.*

Make sure you print off any luggage labels you might need, which should include your name and stateroom number. If you have a hard-sided case, you can place a sticker on it with your details as a precaution, or buy a set of flexible silicone labels that can be used several times over and aren't as easily ripped off. Make sure you have padlocks for all your bags, as not securing them might void your insurance policy, plus it's always better to be safe than sorry.

# Before You Go

***Luggage Essential:*** *Divide your parties' items throughout several suitcases so that if one case goes astray you will all still have something to wear.*

## Crucial Items

- Airline tickets (physical or digital)
- Hotel reservations
- Hotel and port directions
- Cruise documents: boarding passes, cruise loyalty card, land transfer documents, tour confirmations
- Government-issued ID: passport or other proof of citizenship
- Visas
- Vaccination certificates
- Birth or marriage certificates
- Driver's licenses, auto insurance cards, Blue Badge - quad biking excursions or car rentals will require your driving license (check the expiry date as people have been known to find out their license has expired when they need it most)
- Travel insurance papers, medical cards, medical history
- UK Global Health Insurance Card (GHIC)
- Copy of medication and optical prescriptions and a list of all medicines you are taking
- Credit and debit cards (call your bank and credit card companies before travelling so they can document where and when you are away - doing so will make them much less likely to lock down your account, thinking the card has been stolen)
- Contact numbers for reporting lost or stolen credit and debit cards
- Prepaid international SIM card for mobile phone
- Sterling cash
- Foreign currency for all ports
- Emergency home phone numbers
- Emergency holiday numbers (travel agent, cruise line, excursion companies)
- Wallet or purse
- Valuables (don't bring expensive jewellery, especially on excursions)
- Watch

# The Autonomous Cruiser

***Essential Documents Tip:*** *Keep a digital and physical copy of your important documents when travelling, and leave a copy at home with a trustworthy person, including your passport, airline tickets, cruise tickets, itinerary and any confirmed shore excursions. It is unlikely you'll ever need them, but it's better to be safe than sorry.*

***Driver's License Tip:*** *Some countries require an international driver's license if you want to rent a car or go quad biking. These are available from the Post Office and most last 12 months.*

***Travel Money Tip:*** *Do not leave changing money until the last minute. Poor rates at airports and on cruise ships can lose you a small fortune. If you do run short of time, buy your travel money online and have it delivered to your door. There are 11,500 Post Office branches across the UK offering competitive exchange rates, 0% commission, buy-back and next day delivery. Up to 80 currencies are available, and if you order before 3pm on a working day, you will get your holiday funds the next day.*

***Cash Tip:*** *Take as much money for this trip as you deem necessary and then some, as it is better to have too much than too little. Exorbitant ATM fees both onboard the ship and in foreign ports can leave a nasty taste in your mouth.*

## Reading Material and Miscellaneous

- Glasses, contact lenses, lens cloth and cleaner
- Extra reading glasses
- Hearing aids and batteries
- Guidebooks and other information on your ports of call
- Foreign language phrase books and dictionaries
- Maps
- Books and magazines (though most ships have well-stocked libraries)
- Journals or notebooks
- Pens (also helps avoid queuing to borrow a pen when it comes to filling in embarkation, disembarkation or excursion forms)
- Highlighters to accentuate activities on the daily planner and for marking excursion options
- Home and email addresses of friends and relatives

# Before You Go

**Electronics**

- Plug adapters and converters
- Mobile phone, charger, selfie stick (your phone can be used as an alarm clock, media player, or radio - make sure to program a contact into your phone in case of emergency)
- Headphones
- Tablet or eReader and charger
- Laptop and charger
- Portable power bank (for charging items whilst ashore)
- Digital camera and charger, spare batteries, extra memory cards, tripod
- Underwater camera and charger (for snorkelling or diving)
- Extension cord and non-surge power strip with multiple plug-ins (most cabin only have one power outlet)
- MP3 player
- Hairdryer (most cruise ships provide one but you may find they are not powerful enough to meet your needs - if you're fussy, bring your own)
- Travel alarm clock and spare batteries
- Binoculars (invaluable for dolphin and whale spotting)
- Nightlight
- Walkie talkies (a great tool if cruising with children or travelling companions so you can keep in touch easily and for free)
- Luggage Tiles (a tiny Bluetooth tracker to help you find your luggage if it gets lost)

***Electrical Essential:*** *American electrical equipment runs at 110 volts and should never be plugged into a 220-volt outlet.*

***Clock Tip:*** *Most cabins do not have alarm clocks. Although wake up calls can be booked through your cabin phone system, having an alarm clock next to your bed is a better option than padding across the room to answer the phone at the crack of dawn.*

# The Autonomous Cruiser

***Outlet Tip:*** *Cabins typically have only one or two electrical sockets. If you find you need more, check out your in-cabin television, as newer models often have a USB port, which you can utilise as an extra outlet to charge your devices.*

***Power-Up Tip:*** *Cabins that have energy-saving light switches can be annoying as all the outlets and lights in the cabin are powered by your cruise card, and when you leave the cabin, the card comes with you. For cruisers who wish to charge up a device while out of the room, simply use another wallet-sized card, like a British driving license, library card or store loyalty card, and it will work just as well.*

## Medical Emergency Kit

- Prescription drugs and other essential medications (pack in hand luggage)
- Earplugs (some cabins aren't ideally sited, such as being near a nightclub, the engine room, lifts, a laundry room, or busy walkways)
- First-aid kit (bandages, plasters, Q-tips, Vaseline, antiseptic cream, diarrhoea remedy, cortisone cream or tablets for allergies, pain reliever of choice (in original packaging), bite or itch cream, throat soothers, blister plasters, headache remedy, antacids, cold and cough remedy, eye drops, saline nasal spray, sinus drops, alcohol wipes)
- Motion sickness prevention (seasickness pills, acupressure wristbands, ginger tablets or capsules - some ships provide seasickness pills free of charge)
- Antibacterial hand gel
- Sanitising wipes
- Face masks
- Emergency dental kit
- Insect repellent
- Thermometer

**Don't Ask:**
*Do all Australians speak English?*

***Cruise Tip:*** *A visit to the sickbay can be expensive, so carry a well thought out first-aid kit. Also, items are often not easy to find in port, and products could be unfamiliar, written in the local language and cost a fortune. Once you have prepared your first-aid kit, check it regularly to ensure items have not passed their sell-by date.*

***Seasickness Tip:*** *Aurora Expeditions suggests the use of medication to help prevent or treat seasickness. Recommended medicines include promethazine (Phenergan, Avomine), hyoscine (Kwells, Travelcalm, Scopolamine patches), and dimenhydrinate (Dramamine). Less sedative medications include cinnarizine (Stugeron) and meclizine (Antivert). It is important that before a trip, travellers speak to their doctor or pharmacist regarding suitability with other drugs and medical conditions.* **Important note:** *prochlorperazine (Stemetil) or metoclopramide (Maxolon) are not effective for managing motion sickness.*

***Cruise Tip:*** *Remember to take seasickness medication at least two hours before you sail, as preventing symptoms is easier and more effective than curing them.*

## Wheelchairs

- Charger and adapter
- Tyre patches, lever and pump
- Cushion and extra cushion cover
- Repair kit (spare parts like inner tubes and fuses, simple tools)

***Wheelchair Tip:*** *Buy a cheap poncho to keep you and your wheelchair batteries dry in the rain.*

***Wheelchair Essential:*** *If you have a variable voltage charger, you only need a plug adapter when travelling abroad.*

***Wheelchair Tip:*** *Take a door wedge with you as it can be difficult to get a wheelchair in and out of your cabin if the door is not propped open.*

## Toiletries

Your cabin will typically provide soap, shampoo and shower wash, but some people prefer to bring their own.

- Hair: hairstyling appliances, shampoo, conditioner, hairspray, gel, bobby pins, ponytail bands, brush, comb, shower cap (also great for protecting your camera if caught in the rain)
- Hygiene: soap, deodorant, shaving supplies, perfume, aftershave

- Teeth: toothbrush, toothpaste, mouthwash, dental floss, denture bath, denture adhesive and tablets
- Feminine hygiene: tampons, sanitary towels, feminine wet wipes, incontinence wear (incontinence pads can be extremely difficult to buy on the ship or ashore)
- Contraceptives
- Face: makeup bag, makeup and remover, mirror, tweezers, cleanser, moisturiser, lip balm or salve
- Skin: body lotion, sun protection, after sun, aloe vera (a gentle breeze while cruising can belie how intense the sun really is - your sunblock should have a high UV protection rating and you should use it liberally)
- Eyes: eyedrops, sunglasses with full UV protection, contact lens solution
- Hands and feet: nail polish and remover, nail file, clippers, nail scissors, nail glue, hand and foot lotion (anything sharp must be packed in checked luggage)

***Cruise Tip:*** *You can free up valuable suitcase space by leaving your towels at home as they are provided on all cruise ships, not just in your cabin bathroom, but also beach towels that you can use at the pool, in ports of call and on tour excursions. Some ships have check-out stations on the pool deck, in which case you will need your cruise card to take them out.*

### Miscellaneous

- Duct tape (emergency luggage repairs, remove particles from clothes, identify your bags at the terminal, fix a hem, secure curtains in the cabin if there is a gap that lets in light)
- Extra plastic cable ties for securing luggage for your return trip
- Extra luggage name tags (in case yours get lost on the outbound trip)
- Luggage locks
- Ziploc bags for dirty or wet clothes (you can also place your credit cards or cash in one to keep them safe in your swimwear)
- Multi-gadget tool (be sure to pack in checked luggage)
- Small umbrella
- Travel pillow for long flights or coach journeys

- Sports gear
- Shoehorn
- Sewing kit and scissors (pack in checked luggage)
- Travel-size detergent, stain remover
- Dryer sheets (pack a couple to eliminate odours in your luggage)
- Clothes pegs
- Tote bag (for souvenirs or the beach)
- Water bottle for taking drinks ashore
- Hot water bottle (invaluable for keeping the chill off on deck)
- Hats, caps, visors
- Insulated coffee mug
- Shoe polish
- Lanyard for cruise card
- Magnets (a great way of displaying the daily schedule on the walls or doors of your cabin as they are metal-based)
- Compression stockings (prevents swollen ankles if flying)
- Extra hangers (some people pack their clothes on hangers so they can simply unpack items and hang them straight up, but your cabin steward will always provide more if asked)
- Walking stick
- Wrinkle releaser (essential, as travel irons aren't allowed in cabins anymore)
- Post-it notes (for leaving messages for your steward or family members)

***Cruise Tip:*** *Take a deodoriser, such as Neutradol, as older ships can suffer from unpleasant smells from plumbing systems, poor ventilation, diesel fumes, fresh paint and leftover smoke. Note, inside cabins don't have the luxury of opening windows to let fresh air in.*

***Smoker's Tip:*** *Smokers beware, most ships do not sell lighters or matches anymore.*

## Women's Clothing

- Bras (including strapless if needed for evening wear)
- Underwear
- Stockings, tights, socks
- Sleepwear, dressing gown, slippers

- Camisole, slip
- Swimwear, cover-ups
- T-shirts
- Shorts, trousers, jeans
- Skirts, dresses
- Blouses, short-sleeved, long-sleeved, sleeveless tops
- Sweaters, sweatshirts, fleeces
- Workout clothes and sports bra
- Crossbody bag or bum bag (for sightseeing)
- Bags (day and evening)
- Belts
- Scarves
- Jewellery, watches
- Walking, hiking, athletic, casual shoes
- Sandals, flip-flops
- Water shoes or aqua boots (good for water sports and ideal foot protection in the water)
- Evening or dress shoes
- Formal wear
- Waterproof windbreaker jacket
- Warm coat with hood
- Waterproof poncho
- Hat, scarf, gloves for cold weather cruises

*Packing Tip:* To save space, roll your clothes rather than fold them.

*Packing Tip:* Pack dresses on hangers to save time when unpacking.

*Judaism Essential:* Candles have deep symbolic meaning in the Jewish religion and are usually lit prior to every Shabbat or before sunset on Friday evenings. However, naked flames are prohibited in staterooms, so you will need to get battery-operated candles instead.

## Men's Clothing

- Underwear
- Undershirts or vests

- Day socks, dress socks
- Sleepwear, dressing gown, slippers
- Swimwear, cover-ups
- T-shirts, casual shirts
- Shorts, slacks, jeans
- Sports jacket
- Sweaters, sweatshirts, fleeces
- Workout clothes, joggers
- Travel pouch (for port sightseeing)
- Backpack (for port sightseeing)
- Jewellery, watches, cufflinks, studs
- Belts
- Walking, hiking, athletic, casual shoes
- Sandals, flip-flops
- Water shoes or aqua boots (good for water sports and ideal foot protection in the water)
- Evening or dress shoes
- Tuxedo (or dark suit)
- Dress shirts
- Tie, suspenders, cummerbund
- Waterproof windbreaker jacket
- Warm coat with hood
- Waterproof poncho
- Hat, scarf, gloves for cold weather cruises

***Cruise Tip:*** *Shoes are bulky, but you can put them to good use when packing. Fill your footwear with all the small items that clutter up your case, like socks, underwear, ties and small toiletries.*

***Cruise Tip:*** *Keep an extra pair of socks on you when hiking or visiting a glacier, just in case your first pair gets wet.*

**Baby, Toddlers & Kids Toiletries Kit**
Refer to the 'toiletries' and 'medical emergency kit' sections but also include;

- Calpol (suitable for the age of the infant)
- Teething tablets or gel

- Nappy rash cream, baby powder, baby wash, baby shampoo
- Bug spray and bite cream
- Antiseptic cream
- Antihistamine cream
- Thermometer
- Washproof plasters
- High factor sunscreen, lip balm, after sun
- Fingernail clippers

***Infant Sun Protection:*** *The US Food and Drug Administration does not recommend sunscreens for infants under six months old because of the risk of side effects such as a rash.*

***Waterproof Sunscreen Advice:*** *There is no such thing as waterproof sunscreen. They may be advertised as 'waterproof resistant' but they will eventually wash off and need reapplying. The label is required to inform you how long the sunscreen will remain effective for and directions of when to reapply it.*

***Child Health Cover:*** *Each member of the family requires their own UK Global Health Insurance Card (GHIC), whatever their age.*

**Kid's Stuff**

- Underwear
- Nightwear
- Socks
- Swimwear, goggles, floaties, cover-ups
- Shorts
- T-shirts
- Short/long-sleeved shirts
- Dresses, skirts
- Trousers
- Sweatshirts, fleeces, cardigans, sweaters
- Coat
- Footwear

**Sun hat** (*wool hat, scarf, gloves for cold weather*)

- Sunglasses
- Travel journal and pencils
- Books, sticker book, colouring book and crayons
- Electronic games device, charger, batteries, headphones
- Books
- Kid's cup

***Cruise Tip***: *Pack a small backpack full of snacks, activities, and swimwear, so your child is kept busy while waiting at terminals, on tour buses or around the pool. You can buy them ready-made from* keepemquiet.com.

**Baby & Toddler Items**

Most cruise lines do not supply consumables for babies and require you to bring anything your child might need, though most lines do provide cribs at no extra charge (do not assume they will provide one, make sure to request one in advance) and high chairs are available in most dining areas. I have not included infant clothing but other things you might need are:

- Baby carrier or baby sling
- Lightweight umbrella stroller
- Adult sized disposable poncho (great for keeping baby and stroller dry in the rain)
- Nappy bag and changing pad
- Disposable nappies, pull-ups, swim nappies
- Baby wipes
- Nappy sacks for disposing nappies
- Breast pump and accessories
- Bottles, nipples, caps
- Baby formula, food, snacks
- Bottle brush and detergent
- Baby spoon
- Disposable bibs, burp cloths
- Dummies
- Teething ring
- Sippy cup

- Comfort blanket and cuddly toy
- Nightlight
- Inflatable infant pool (most ships do not allow non-potty-trained infants in the pool, so this is a clever way for babies to splash around, also ideal for bathing your child as most cabins have showers)

**Cruise Tip**: *Check whether you can hire baby equipment onboard.*

**Storage Essential**: *Take an over-the-door clear plastic organiser - they're a great way of organising bottles, dummies, sunscreen and the like. Everything is easily accessible and it saves on valuable vanity or counter space.*

**Did You Know?** *Most cruise lines will only allow a child to travel with them if they are at least six months old on the day of embarkation. This increases to 12 months old if you are sailing transatlantic or transpacific. The age restriction is put in place for medical reasons: given the special care needed for infants, cruise lines do not want children of the most vulnerable ages to be stuck at sea. MSC is the only exception to this rule, accepting babies of any age but they do require a medical 'fit to travel' certificate for babies below the age of 12 months.*

## Hand Luggage

With the crew trying to deliver thousands of bags to passenger cabins, the items in your carry-on might be the only things you have on your first day onboard, and in the case of lost luggage, they may be the only things you have all trip. As such, if you have prescription medication that you need to take daily, do not let them out of your sight, as the medical centre is not a fully-fledged chemist that can easily refill your supply. Other things to pack into your hand luggage are:

- Passports, ID, cruise documents, travel insurance papers
- Credit cards and cash
- Camera (you may want to take photos of your sail away)
- Mobile phone (you can send texts and chat to friends and family as normal while you can still access land-based mobile networks)
- Laptop and other valuables
- Swimwear, sunscreen, a cover-up, flip-flops and a book (to enjoy some pool time straight away)

# Before You Go

- Change of clothes (the first evening's dress code is typically casual, so if your luggage is lost or delayed, you can still freshen up)
- Sunglasses, reading glasses
- Baby supplies (nappies, nappy sacks, pull-ups, wet wipes, kiddie snacks, bottles with formula, dummy, teddy bear or favourite toy, change of clothes)

*NEVER leave your carry-on bag unattended.*

***Cruise Essentials****: Make sure your mobile phone is in 'Airplane Mode' or is turned off before you sail, otherwise you could end up with hundreds of pounds in data roaming charges if your phone performs automatic updates or downloads new emails.*

***Turn Data Roaming off:*** *It's true that there are no roaming charges within the European Union for calls, texts or internet usage, but only when in port. At all other times, turn roaming off to avoid potentially huge charges.*

## Restricted and Dangerous Items

There is a comprehensive list on each cruise line's website of items that guests are not allowed to bring onboard. The main cause for concern is items such as alcohol, illegal drugs, flammable liquids, explosives, dangerous chemicals and any item that can interfere with the safe operation of the vessel or could present harm to people or property. The examples below and other similar objects will be confiscated on sight:

- Firearms and ammunition (including realistic copies, whether toys or otherwise)
- Sharp objects, including knives and scissors (safety razors are allowed, as are scissors with blades of less than four inches)
- Any illegal drugs or substances
- Candles or incense
- Coffee makers or hot plates
- Clothes or hair irons
- Baseball or cricket bats, hockey sticks, bows and arrows
- Skateboards, surfboards
- Martial arts equipment

- Self-defence items, including handcuffs, pepper spray, nightsticks
- Lighter fluid or fireworks
- Ham radios, drones
- Dangerous chemicals, including bleach and paint

Dive knives or similar must be reported to the ship's personnel at the time of boarding. They may be permitted, but held in safe custody by the ship's security staff when not in use ashore.

Most companies do not allow guests to bring alcoholic beverages aboard their ships, with the exception of embarkation day when guests on certain cruise lines may be allowed to bring two bottles of wine (subject to a corkage fee) per stateroom. Security may inspect containers, including water bottles, soda bottles, mouthwash, canteens, etc. at any time and dispose of alcohol concealed in such containers. Alcohol that is purchased from onboard shops or ports of call (which must be presented to security upon re-boarding) will be secured by the ship's personnel and returned to guests just before the end of the cruise. Guests who are under the legally permitted drinking age will not have their alcohol returned to them.

Be careful when packing as wearing camouflage is illegal in some parts of the world, including the Caribbean, South America, the Philippines and Oman. You will be required to go back to the ship and change, or worse, the offending item may be confiscated, or you could even be arrested.

## Leaving Home Checklist

Doublecheck that you have adequate home insurance in place and that your policy won't lapse while you're away. Also, read the small print and make sure there are no exclusions that might apply during the time you are away; some policies only provide cover for a certain number of days away from the property or will void the cover if a non-family member is house-sitting.

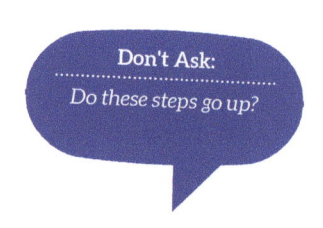

> **Don't Ask:**
> Do these steps go up?

- Take durable hard-sided suitcases and make sure your luggage labels include your name and phone number. Opt for a bright coloured case as it is less likely to be a target for thieves at airports and cruise

# Before You Go

terminals. Also, decorate the handle with neon ribbons to make it easier to locate in the baggage hall.

- Take photographs of the inside and outside of your luggage. Doing so will make it easier to identify your belongings to a cruise or airline official if they get lost. It's also a way to prove there was no damage to your cases before embarking.
- Place a card with your name, address and contact number inside your luggage, as well as on the tags on the outside, as they can get ripped off.
- Weigh your luggage if flying, and make sure they conform to the airline's weight allowance. If your bags are overweight, always book extra bags in advance rather than at the airport as waiting will cost you more.
- Inform your neighbours you are going away so they can keep an eye on your home. Leave them a set of keys so they can access your property if needed.
- Distribute your cruise contact details to friends and relatives in case they need to get hold of you urgently.
- Leave copies of your passport and credit cards with a family member of trusted friend.
- Doublecheck your passport and travel tickets are in your hand luggage.
- Take a photograph of your contact details on your camera and your phone, so that if you happen to lose either and they are found by someone honest, they will be able to contact you.
- Keep any valuables out of sight, but avoid obvious hiding places that burglars are wise to.
- Have a neighbour or the Post Office hold your mail. Royal Mail's Keepsafe service will hold any parcels or post for up to 66 days and will deliver them to you once you are home again.
- Water your plants or take them to a neighbour or friend.
- Set up standing orders so bills are paid on time and avoid incurring any late charges.
- Arrange pet care.
- Arrange transport to the airport or cruise terminal.
- Charge all electronics that you intend to take with you in hand luggage, such as a laptop, mobile phone, kindle, camera, or iPad.

It is now an extra security requirement that all electrical items are sufficiently charged so they can be powered-up if requested. Failure to comply can result in the item being confiscated.

- Download any films or programs onto your tablet or laptop to take away with you so that you can access them without an internet connection. It's a great way to while away the time on a shuttle or tender transfer.
- Set your TV to record your favourite programs (do not unplug these appliances if you wish to utilise them).
- Set your answerphone.
- Set light timers for indoor lights.
- Stop the newspaper or milk delivery
- Clean out your fridge of anything that will go off before you return.
- Take the rubbish out.
- Disconnect your water supply to avoid leaks or frozen pipes while you're away.
- Turn off the gas.
- Turn your heating, boiler or thermostats down or off.
- Except for the fridge, unplug your appliances and electrical equipment to reduce the risk of fire.
- Doublecheck that all your doors and windows are locked, including the garage and shed.
- Set the burglar alarm.

Although tempting, try not to advertise the fact that you're going away. If you tell friends on social media sites such as Facebook or Twitter, make sure you don't post the information publicly as you will also be informing strangers.

***Cruise Tip***: *Go through your handbag or wallet and take out anything you won't need whilst on holiday, like store cards, money vouchers, library tickets, etc.*

***Electronic Packing Helper***: *If you would rather have an electronic 'packing list', download an app that tells you what to put in your suitcase. PackPoint offers packing suggestions based on your answers to a few questions and allows you to customise your own checklists. After inputting your gender, where and when you are travelling, and what activities you might be considering, it will retrieve the weather forecast for your travel dates and create a list of suggested packing items.*

This clever little packing helper even suggests pieces you can wear more than once and whether or not laundry services will be available.

***Security Tip****: Always carry a spare padlock or cable ties in case you do buy a cruise holdall, as you shouldn't rely on the padlock that comes with the case. The holdalls are stocked on several cruise lines and the keys are generic and will open any identical holdall.*

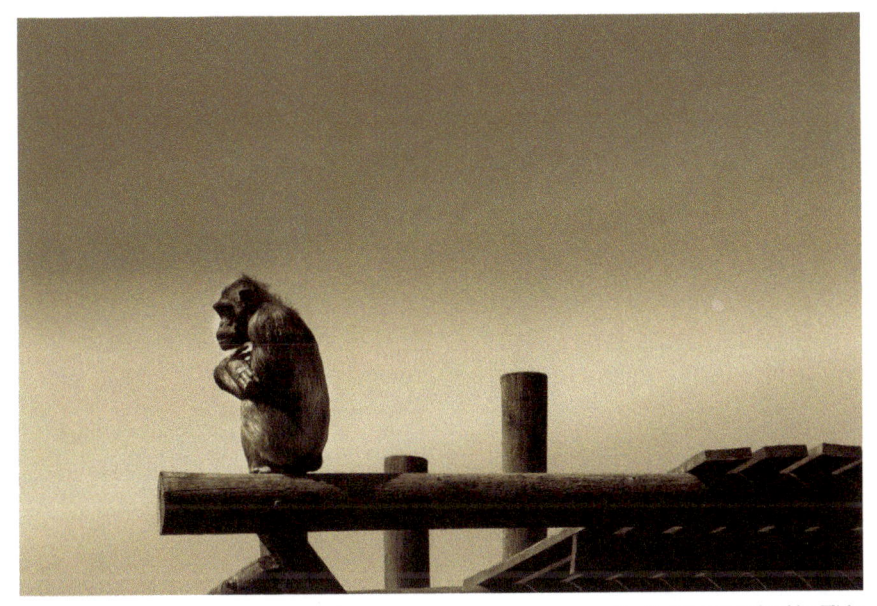

Credit: Edward Dalmulder Flickr

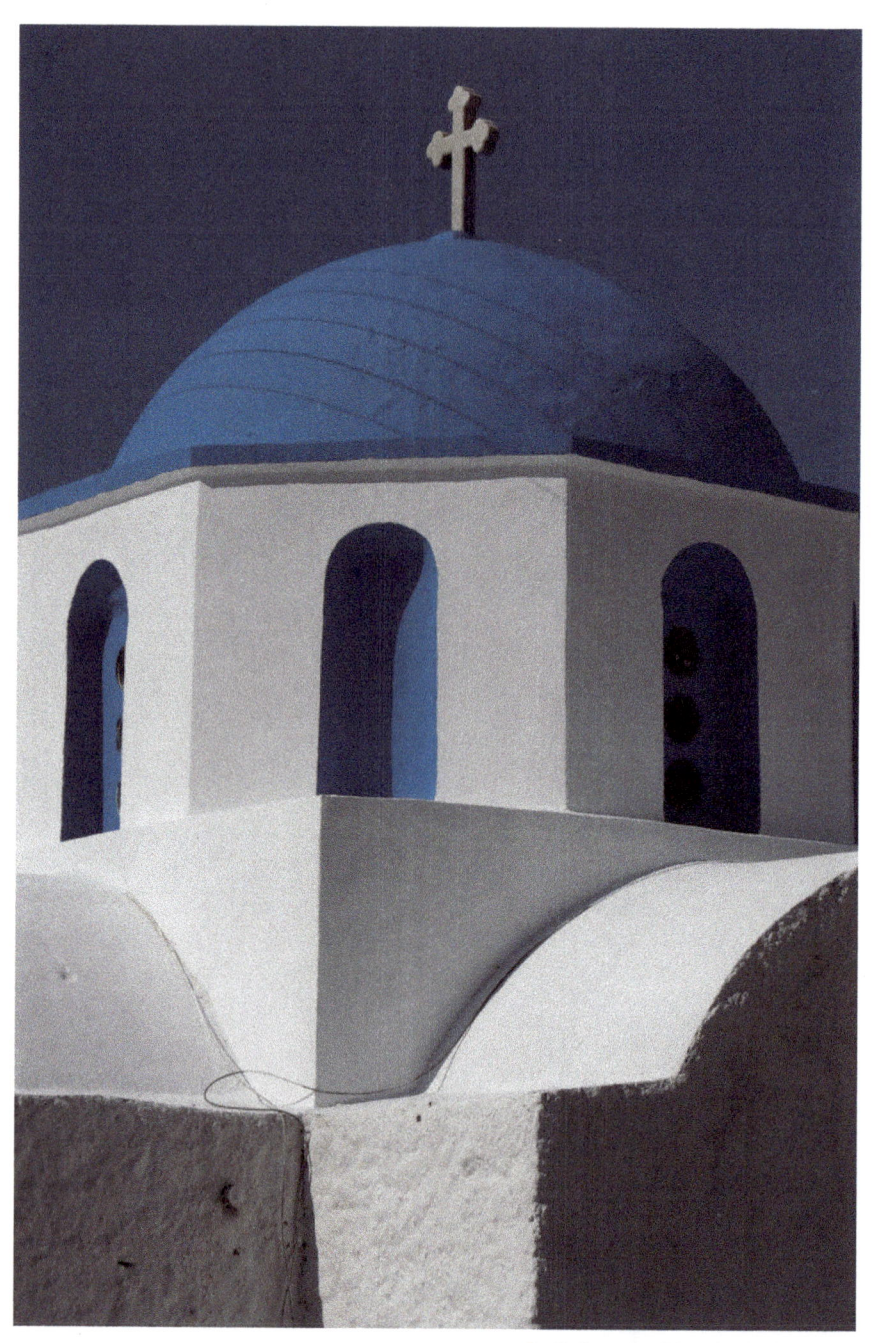

Credit: Santorini, Edward Dalmulder, Flickr

# Life Onboard

## Embarkation

First things first, make sure you leave yourself plenty of time to get to the airport or cruise terminal especially if you have a long journey. Why get stressed before your holiday starts? If you're driving to the port, don't put all your trust on a route planner to estimate your time of arrival, as it might not take into consideration congestion, road works or maintenance. It's best to listen to traffic updates before leaving home, especially if sailing from Dover; the Kent police, in conjunction with Highways England, use a procedure called Operation Stack that forces thousands of lorries and freight traffic to queue (or stack) on the M20 motorway until they can be loaded onto trains or ferries if the services across the English Channel are crippled due to bad weather, industrial action, migrant activity, or fire, electrical failures or derailments in the tunnel. In effect, it closes large parts of the M20 and uses it as an enormous parking lot. All other traffic is diverted to alternative routes which gridlock quickly.

***Delayed Arrival:*** *If bad weather, a motorway accident, mechanical breakdown, or flight delay impedes your arrival at your embarkation port, ring your cruise line, travel agent or port terminal to inform them of your delay. Whichever company you speak to will do their best to make sure you join your cruise.*

Arriving at the port, you will be directed to drop your luggage off in a designated area, from which it will be sent to your cabin. Your luggage should be affixed with labels with your full name, the name of your ship, your cabin number and the departure port on them. If you drove to the terminal, there will be plenty of port staff on duty to direct you to the parking bays; most of which will be a short walk away, but if not, a shuttle will be laid on to transport you back to the terminal.

# The Autonomous Cruiser

***Disabled Drop Off:*** *If arriving at the port terminal by taxi, get the driver to state that they have a disabled passenger and port security will allow the vehicle to go directly to the main entrance of the terminal, rather than the designated drop-off area.*

While you might have forgotten your cases for the moment, security won't have. All personal belongings checked onto the ship undergo the same rigorous security checks that are implemented by the airlines. Your bags will be subject to x-ray screening, metal detectors, sniffer dogs and sometimes physical searches to ensure that nothing dangerous or prohibited slips through the net. You might think you've snuck a couple of bottles of alcohol aboard, but you will probably find they've been confiscated before your cases are delivered to your cabin.

Your cruise documentation will state your allocated embarkation time. It's best not to arrive too early as you might have to endure a long wait if the departing passengers from the previous cruise are still being processed or because security is prohibiting early access. The mega-liners are brilliant at turning around their ships quickly, and some such as Celebrity will welcome you to use all the ship's facilities as soon as you're onboard, though you'll usually have to wait until around 1 pm until you can access your cabin. Smaller lines, such as Saga and Fred. Olsen, are not quite as adept in this department, meaning you might have to wait a little longer to enjoy all the facilities of your ship, and cutbacks have even seen some of them do away with lunch on embarkation day. On the other end of the scale, government regulations regarding the departure manifest require all guests to be on board the ship no later than an hour before the ship's departure time, or they will not be permitted to sail.

***Hand Luggage Tip:*** *Some smaller ports won't let you access the terminal early, and you will be forced to wait outside. Ensure you have a sweater with you in case the climate is colder than you are used to.*

***Time Essential:*** *As with airline procedures, if you arrive even just a few minutes after check-in has closed, security will not allow you to embark.*

Some cruise lines provide wheelchair assistance for embarking passengers, and upon entry to the terminal, those who have booked the service will find staff ready and waiting to take them through to the ship. If you haven't booked, you will need to find a cruise line representative who will place your name on a first-come-first-served list and in the interim you will be directed to a seating area. Once an attendant is available, you will be taken through the pre-boarding process and dropped off in a public area of the ship if you arrive before the cabins are ready. The wheelchair will not be left with you after boarding as it will be needed to bring other passengers onboard that are waiting back in the terminal.

Some cruise lines or ports have security rules in place that won't permit a ground handler onto the vessel, so they'll only take you as far as the entrance to the ship. If that is the case, you will be required to transfer from the shoreside wheelchair to an oceanside chair, and a member of the crew will take you the rest of the way.

***Mobility Rental Essential:*** *If you've booked a wheelchair or scooter to use onboard, as per the terms of your rental contract it should be delivered to your cabin at around 2 pm, but it could be later as ship supplies take priority at the loading zone. There will be no wheelchair assistance provided by the ship from the public area to the cabin. If the disabled party is unable to walk, someone in their group will need to go to the cabin and bring their wheelchair or scooter to them. At a designated time at the end of the cruise, those that have booked disembarkation wheelchair assistance will be directed to a waiting area at a central pick-up point; an attendant will not pick you up from your cabin.*

***Mobility Aids:*** *If a disabled passenger usually uses a cane, crutches or a walker, they should still bring them onboard, regardless of having rented a wheelchair or scooter. Electronic mobility equipment is not allowed on tenders, so having a walking aid may provide the stability needed if you want to get off at a particular port.*

***Online Check-in:*** *Cruise lines require you to complete online check-in before your departure date, as doing so expedites the verification process. Those that have not complied will be subject to delays at embarkation.*

The advent of norovirus has meant that cruise lines issue a medical disclaimer on arrival which you will need to fill in before proceeding to the check-in desk. Once at the counter, you'll go through the formalities of showing your passport, your cruise paperwork and registering your credit card for onboard charges as your cruise ship is a cashless resort. If you would prefer to settle your account with cash at the end of your trip, you'll be required to pay a deposit to cover any charges onboard.

The recent outbreak of coronavirus (COVID-19) saw the cruise industry suspend operations and adopt protective protocols in an attempt to safeguard the public. Now, in an effort to regain the trust of their clientele and reintroduce ocean holidays, a reduction in the number of guests onboard, self-check-in and online health questionnaires have been introduced across the industry, along with allocated arrival time slots to manage passenger flow. Physical distancing has been implemented on arrival at the cruise terminal, and masks are mandatory in situations where distancing is not possible, especially in narrow corridors and lifts.

Temperature checks and new medical testing procedures has been introduced at all cruise terminals and at each port of call, every time a guest or crew member gets on or off the ship, and anyone exhibiting a marked temperature over 37.8°C will likely be subjected to a secondary screening by medical staff.

The Royal Caribbean Group is replacing the need for group gatherings at the muster drill with an innovative app program 'Muster 2.0™'. The new protocol, which will initially be available on all Royal Caribbean, Celebrity Cruises and Azamara ships, will be delivered to each guest through their mobile phone with a visit to their assigned assembly station completing the process. The patented technology has also been granted to TUI Cruises, Norwegian Cruise Line, Oceania Cruises and Regent Seven Seas.

It's early days as cruise lines wait for government and health organisation clarification before finalising their health, safety and sanitation protocols, but some have forged ahead, eradicating air recirculation with a commitment to ventilation systems only using 100% fresh air mix. If a vessel cannot completely eliminate recirculation, ventilation systems onboard are being equipped with new efficient HEPA filters designed to remove at least 99.95% of airborne pathogens.

Each cruise line has brought in elevated sanitation and cleaning protocols, and extra sanitiser stations are available throughout their ships. As is the procedure with an outbreak of norovirus, self-service will not be permitted; instead, the ship's crew will be posted at all buffet stations to serve food to passengers.

All entertainment venues have reduced their audience numbers and stage extra performances, while spas might dispense with close-contact areas such as steam rooms, saunas, hot tubs and shower facilities. Those vessels having libraries could suspend self-service book-lending and either staff the venue or offer reading materials through digital apps.

Tour excursions will run with limited numbers and vehicles will be sanitised before passengers board them. Most cruise lines have gone one step further and will only allow guests to disembark in port if on a ship's shore excursion.

Ships have equipped their medical centres with COVID-19 diagnostic kits, and medical services are free of charge for any passenger displaying flu-like symptoms or breathing difficulties. A response plan is activated if a suspected case is identified, including dedicated isolation cabins and a transfer to a land medical facility.

Certain safety measures may be relaxed once the pandemic is considered contained, but it is still likely that a lot of these preventative measures will remain in place indefinitely.

Before checking in for your cruise, you will have to go through the same security measures as you would in an airport. You will have to remove any electrical items before placing your hand luggage on a conveyor belt which will take it through an x-ray machine while you walk through a metal detector. Don't be surprised if you have to remove your coat, belt or shoes as an added precaution.

> **Don't Ask:** What happens to the ice carvings after they melt?

For those travelling with a cognitive, intellectual or developmental disability, it's best to board the ship later rather than earlier, as the queues are generally much shorter. If you don't need any special assistance then you might want to go straight to security. The screening process can be daunting for companions or caregivers travelling with someone prone to exhibiting physiognomies of anxiety and meltdowns in unfamiliar situations, but it's important to keep as calm as possible so that your angst doesn't transfer to the person you are travelling with. Hopefully, by preparing them for change, their fears and negative behaviour can be reduced. Once you've dealt with security you will be directed where to check-in, a huge bay decked out in wall to wall registration terminals. Ground staff will be on hand to direct you to the correct desks. Loyalty Club members and suite guests will usually be provided with priority boarding - there will be clear signage to direct you to those allocated check-in desks. Also, most cruise lines offer priority boarding for guests with special needs.

***Passport Tip:*** *Some lines will retain your passport for the duration of your cruise in order to expedite the ship's arrival procedure in each port. Each time the ship docks,* *immigration officials come aboard the vessel and check the ship's manifest and the passports of each passenger and crew member before allowing anyone ashore.*

To complete the check-in process, and for the benefit of security, your photograph will be taken and attached to your onboard account, mainly so it can be displayed on a computer terminal every time your cruise card is swiped when boarding or exiting the ship to confirm your identity. Some lines also print the photo on your cruise card as an added security measure. Your check-in agent will then issue your Sea Pass card, which acts as a cabin key and as a means of charging to your onboard account. If you want a completely separate account to those you are travelling with, you'll need to register a second debit or credit card to the cabin. Children will be issued with their own key card which will in turn allow them to make purchases; it is possible and perhaps wise to set a spending limit so you can monitor their outgoings. Depending on the volume of traffic in the terminal, you might be able to walk straight on or you may be given a number and have to wait for it to be called before you can board.

In the larger cruise terminals, the ship's crew will have set up stands advertising extras that your cruise has to offer. Here you might be able to buy a drinks package, book a spa treatment, reserve a table at one of the specialty restaurants or register for the youth programme, if you haven't done so already.

**Accessibility tip:** *Most of the busier cruise port terminals throughout the UK are wheelchair-friendly, with full access walkways and entrances, accessible lifts, and disabled toilets.*

Cruise lines love to take your photograph at any given opportunity, so don't be surprised if a photographer asks you to stand in front of a picture of the ship during the boarding process. Your shots will usually be available to view later that evening in the Photo Gallery, but you are under no obligation to buy them. If you do want to keep one as a special memory of your cruise, you can charge it to your shipboard account.

A final cruise card swipe at the entrance to the ship will complete the embarkation process, and your holiday can officially begin. Cruise staff are usually lined up just inside the hull who, depending on the cruise line, might offer you a welcome glass of champagne, while nearby stewards will relieve you of your hand luggage and direct you to your cabin if it's ready. If you have to wait for your stateroom, you are free to explore the ship, grab lunch or have a swim.

In your first hours exploring the ship you'll likely encounter all the same promotional tables that were on display in the terminal, and now is the final time to decide if any are suitable. Bonus minutes on internet packages, special spa rates and 2-for-1 in a specialty restaurant will usually only be available on embarkation day. There are also usually a number of free classes at the gym offered on the first day, so sign up quickly as they only accept a limited number of people.

***Dollar Bills:*** *Don't be miserly when it comes to tipping the crew, especially if you have a lot of luggage, or need wheelchair assistance onto the ship - it is only the lowest wage earners that provide these services. Dollar bills are accepted by the crew even on a British ship, as most ports will take the currency.*

Once the announcement is given that your cabin is ready, it's worth going down to it to help you become familiar with the route and to drop off your hand-luggage, coats or items you don't need with you all day. Being cashless, you won't need your wallet, purse or credit cards, and you won't need your passport or keys, so as soon as you get to your cabin put them in the safe along with any jewellery. If you have downloaded your cruise line's app, it might be worth keeping your phone with you so you can check your cruise planner, book restaurants, spa visits, or browse excursions. If you don't have the app, turn off your phone and stick your mobile in the safe too.

There are a few tricks in order to make the most out of potentially limited cabin space. First off, most cabin furniture can be moved around, and with a bit of tweaking, you could gain valuable extra space or a layout which better accommodates your disability; your steward will be happy to help you rearrange the furniture if you can't do it on your own. Also, make use of the storage areas beneath the settee, behind a vanity mirror, above your bed or on the window sills beneath a porthole. Utilise the area under the bed to hide away your suitcases, and if space is at a premium, use the empty cases as extra drawers or a laundry area. All cabin walls are made of metal, so you can utilise magnetic hooks to hang scarves and belts up, to gain extra space.

Your minibar or fridge may well be fully stocked, but you'll be paying a premium for anything you eat or drink, as these items aren't included as part of most cruise packages. The items are counted each day and charged to your onboard account.

Your room steward will be extremely busy on embarkation day, but their name and contact details should be displayed on the vanity unit, together with your dining confirmation. When you do finally meet them, introduce yourself and make any special requests you may have, like extra hangers, more towels or a second cruise planner each day. Another popular request is to empty the minibar so you can fill it with your own sodas or medication. If you have pre-ordered any tours, the tickets will be waiting in an envelope in your room. Don't worry if your luggage hasn't arrived once you have access to your cabin, as it can take up to five hours depending on the size of the ship. Finally, your cabin will have a copy of the ship's daily planner and instructions regarding the time and place of the safety drill.

***Disposal Tip:*** *Ask your cabin steward for a sharps bin if you need to dispose of needles and syringes safely.*

Long corridors and generic doors can make finding your cabin for the first time quite the challenge, and finding it throughout your cruise can be difficult for those with memory impairments. Consider decorating your cabin door to make it distinguishable from others, such as using photo magnets of familiar people. For less than £2 you can purchase an audible door mini alarm (Sealants & Tools Direct) that will alert you if the cabin door is opened.

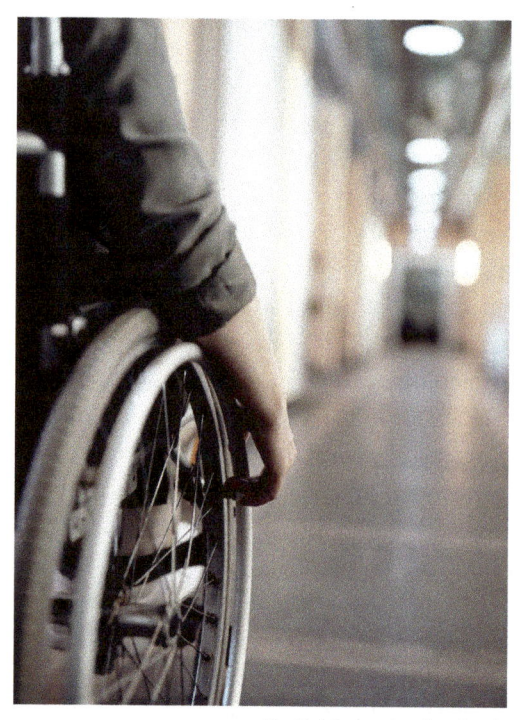

Credit: Marcus Aurelius, Pexels

Maritime law dictates that every passenger attends a mandatory safety or muster drill on embarkation day, regardless of whether you have sailed before or are on a back-to-back cruise. Also, following the *Costa Concordia* tragedy, the drill

## Life Onboard

must now take place either before leaving port or immediately thereafter. The location of your muster station is written on your cruise card and on the back of your cabin door. Your steward should have laid out lifejackets on the bed in your cabin, but if not, they can often be found in your wardrobe or under the beds. The general emergency alarm (seven or more short blasts followed by one long blast of the ship's horn or whistle) will signal the start of the safety drill and is when you should head down to your Assembly Station. Life jackets may or may not need to be worn, depending on your ship, but there will be a demonstration of how to put them on properly during the drill. A check-in procedure will be in operation at your muster station, and your cruise card will be scanned to mark your attendance. If passengers appear absent, the crew will call out the applicable cabin numbers to ensure they haven't slipped under the radar. If you miss the drill you may be invited to attend another one, however the cruise line will be within their rights to disembark you from the ship; if the vessel has already sailed, you may be offloaded at the next port and will have to pay for and organise your own passage to get back home. The drill will prepare you for the safe evacuation of the ship in the event of an emergency - the 20 minutes of 'practise' could save your life.

Muster drills can be very crowded and clamorous. If loud noise is a problem for you or your loved one, a pair of noise cancelling headphones can go a long way to helping. Also, some cruise ships allow families to attend a 'quiet muster' which is held separately from the main one. Also, make sure the crew knows if you have a physical infirmity that may hamper a speedy exit from your cabin, so that in an emergency, a crew member can be dispatched to assist you.

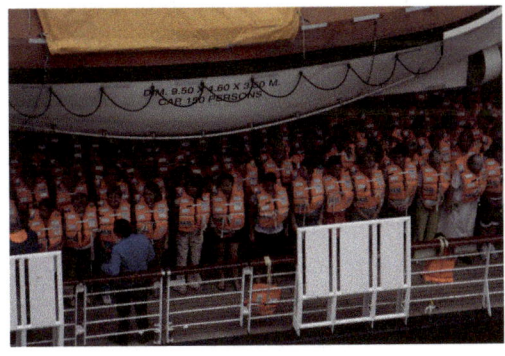

*Credit: Safety/Muster Drill - Mike. W, Flickr*

***Cruise Essential:*** *Set your watch and mobile phone to the ship's time, as it may be different from the local time in your ports of call.*

If you intend to keep your phone on and with you during your cruise, one of the most important things to do before sailing away from port is to adjust your phone's settings to avoid crippling fees, as it will automatically connect to the ship's network when at sea unless you turn your data roaming off. Also, mobile phones are always updating apps in the background, which will cost a fair amount of money if you are connected to the wrong network, so it's best to also disable 'automatic app downloads.' If you want your phone for uses that don't require a network connection, like for reading or playing games, simply enable 'Airplane Mode' to ensure you are not charged unexpectedly.

**Smartphone Tip**: *You can still use Wi-Fi if your phone is in 'Airplane Mode'.*

If you're travelling with someone with a cognitive disability, such as autism spectrum disorder or Alzheimer's, it might be a good idea to create your own safety plan with them once you're onboard, as many people with autism suffer from communication difficulties and are prone to wandering, and so may struggle if they find themselves on their own in an emergency. Review your plan often, perhaps at each new location, asking your companion to repeat back to you what they must do if they get lost, where they should wait and who to ask for help. Inform the key members of the crew that you are travelling with someone with a disability and inform your steward of any special instructions for the cabin. If your ward is prone to wandering, examine the cabin locks and make sure they are in fully working order on the main door, room connector and balcony if you have one. Always use the security lock on your cabin door at night, and if there isn't one available consider using a chair to block the exit door. A door alarm is sometimes necessary so you as a carer can relax and rest at night.

It wasn't that long ago that you would reward your steward, table server or anyone else that had earned your admiration by discreetly giving them an envelope filled with cash at the end of your cruise. Now, most cruise lines have taken to adding these gratuities automatically to your account, though you can request that these charges are removed from your bill by visiting reception, which seasoned cruisers tend to do on embarkation day. On some cruises, however, tips are part of your fare and so can't be removed from your account.

**Guest Relations:** *Stop by Guest Relations in the early morning or late evening to avoid long queues, especially on embarkation day, unless of course your problem is urgent. They are open 24/7.*

*Cruise Tip*: *Make sure you book your hairdressing appointments for formal nights on embarkation day as the slots sell out fast. You can always cancel (often without penalty) a couple of days before if you decide not to go.*

Now that you're onboard and settled in, it's time to have fun and enjoy your floating hotel, taking the time to search out all the things that the brochure boasted about. The first big event is the sailaway, which is typically built around a party that coincides with the departure of the ship; if the weather allows, it will be held on deck, so come with your cameras ready to capture the first of a million holiday memories.

**Guest Relations**
Similar to a hotel reception desk, Guest Relations' main role is to make guests feel welcome and ensure total passenger satisfaction through a consistent personalised service. As well as printing and issuing guest cruise cards, they are responsible for all broadcast announcements, cabin changes, foreign currency exchange, onboard accounts and the ship's daily program. They should always be your first point of enquiry if you have any questions, concerns or complaints.

Lost and found is also located at Guest Relations, so you can check with them if you lose something. Most unclaimed items are donated to charity after a three-week grace period, so keep checking with the cruise line even after you've disembarked.

## Cruise Ship Etiquette

There's no doubt that you deserve a fantastic holiday, but it's important to make sure it's not at the expense of others. Cruise ships can be like small cities and, like any metropolis, it's home to a culturally diverse set of people that have to live and work in harmony. It's important to respect other people's differences. Cruise ship etiquette is important, so spare a thought for your fellow cruiser who might want to enjoy their holiday in a completely different way to you, but who ultimately, like you, just wants to have a good time.

## All Aboard Time

Make sure you return to the ship in a timely manner on port days, as dock space, landside crew and pilot slots are booked up to 18 months in advance, and every extra minute in port is an added expense. Don't be complacent - the captain won't wait.

## Balcony Railings

The conduct policy on most cruise lines bans 'standing, sitting, laying or climbing on, over or across any railing of the ship, whether interior or exterior.' One woman on Royal Caribbean's *Allure of the Seas* climbed over a balcony railing to capture herself in the perfect Kodak moment, and after being caught, she was removed from the vessel when it next docked. The ruling does not only pertain to your body, but - it also applies to anything you want to hang out to dry. While your bikini might dry quicker over your balcony railing than on the feeble clothesline in the shower, it could still present a fire threat if left unattended, and you will be grateful you kept it indoors if a high wind blows up that would have seen your favourite swimsuit heading towards Miami! It's also against the rules of your cruise (and often even the law) to throw anything off the balcony, not least as the item could easily be sucked back into the ship and damage a propellor, block a vent, or cause a fire.

## Behaviour

Cruise lines can refuse to carry anyone if they are deemed unruly, unfit to travel or a danger to other passengers. The lead booker of any party is responsible for their whole group. If any action results in damage to the ship, causes a delay or affects the enjoyment of other guests, the cruise line reserves the right to terminate your entire group's holiday, right then and there. If the ship has already sailed, you will be removed at the next port and left to make your way home at your own expense. If the infraction is severe, the offender will be sent to a small room that is assigned as the 'brig' and which is where unruly passengers are detained. On a small ship, offending guests will be confined to their own cabins, and a security guard will be posted outside their door for the duration. The guests will be held and offloaded at the first possible port to the care of port authorities.

## Children

Don't allow your children to run around the pool, jump in it, splash people or hog the hot tubs. These activities are not allowed and can be dangerous as decks can be very slippery when wet. Most hot tub temperatures are set to 104 degrees which can scald young skin. It is recommended that children should not be allowed in a jacuzzi unless their heads are completely out of the water when they stand on the bottom of the hot tub, and even then, only for short periods.

It is difficult to curb a child's enthusiasm especially after making new friends, but discourage them from using lifts as their private playgrounds, dripping water on the carpets, shouting along the corridors at night and generally being a nuisance. Register them into one of the fabulous kid's clubs and ensure their behaviour doesn't spoil other people's enjoyment.

***Lift Tip:*** *Although cruise line policies vary, children should be at least ten years old when exploring the ship on their own, especially on the outdoor decks by the pools. There have been several cases of children drowning despite having their parents near to them. Hot tubs are every bit as dangerous as pools, with drowning under the age of six the most common.*

## Complaints

If you have a genuine complaint, go and speak to Guest Relations, but don't expect your fellow passengers to be interested or to care - one lady found out that doing so can sometimes backfire. She never stopped bending the ears of other guests, and kept lodging letters of complaint to the front desk. On the fifth day, she received a letter confirming an appointment with the captain who sympathetically listened while she reiterated her upset. He apologised that the cruise wasn't measuring up to her expectations and told her that, as she was obviously not enjoying her holiday, he had arranged for her to be disembarked the next morning. The captain only relented under the condition that neither he nor his crew or any passengers heard any further complaints. Worked like a charm.

## Crew Areas

Entering a crew area is against the rules, and doing so could result in you being disembarked at the next port. For what it's worth, it's mainly just a myriad of corridors known as 'I-95' that runs nearly the length of the vessel, allowing the crew to access any part of the ship without passing through passenger areas. These corridors also lead to housing, welfare, accounts, uniform stores and the officers' cabins, as well as the crew laundry room, library and bar.

Every member of the crew works exceedingly hard, for long hours and little pay; the crew areas are the only place where they don't have to wear a painted smile and can let their hair down away from the demands of awkward and over-demanding passengers. Don't go down to the staff areas or gate-crash a crew party, even if you are invited.

**Dress Code**
Every evening the ship's planner is delivered to your cabin, giving details of the next day's activities and dress code, which generally kicks in at 6 pm. It's simply impossible to be overdressed on a cruise ship, and formal nights are something some cruisers really look forward to. The dress code will be enforced in most public areas, especially the formal dining rooms and theatres; if you'd prefer to dress down, eat at the buffet, enjoy a mostly empty deck or find some peace and quiet in your cabin.

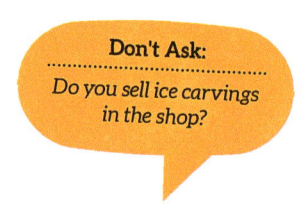

> **Don't Ask:**
> Do you sell ice carvings in the shop?

**Drunken Behaviour**
Holidays are a time for letting your hair down, but everything must be enjoyed in moderation. Most accidents that require onboard medical attention involve excessive drinking, and a lot of people are surprised to find out that their medical insurance will not pay out because they were intoxicated. The ships have a 'zero-tolerance' policy on unruly behaviour due to alcohol. There have been plenty of occasions when drunken behaviour has gone too far, and there is no second chance, no time to apologise and no amount of pleading that will help - your entire group will be taken off the ship, even if you were not involved personally.

**Embarkation and Disembarkation**
Don't be the person in the long snaking queue in the terminal that, upon finally getting to the check-in desk, doesn't have their documents at hand. The same applies when getting on or off the ship in port: have your cruise card ready for security to scan. Long lines are frustrating at the best of times and rifling through your bag for your card does not go down well with the rest of the guests.

# Life Onboard

Don't block the hallways and stairwells while waiting to disembark - just because the ship has docked doesn't mean you can jump off straight away. As annoying as it might be, you will have to wait until the vessel has been cleared by local authorities, after which an announcement will be made advising guests they may go ashore. While everyone wants to be the first off the ship, loitering in areas the crew have announced need to be kept clear will only delay the process and cause congestion. This applies more so when a tender is in operation, as the disembarkation process is even slower. If you wait until your number is called before going down to the tender station, it makes the process go quicker and doesn't compromise the safety of a fellow passenger.

**Excursions**
Don't hold the ship up because of thoughtlessness, especially on an excursion. Allow yourself plenty of time to get to your tour bus as keeping people waiting is annoying and curtails the time that they could enjoy in port.

**Fire**
Fire is one of the biggest risks at sea. One prime example was when 79 cabins were condemned after a fire broke out on *Star Princess* in 2006. It started on a cabin balcony, and in the 90 minutes it took to extinguish it, the fire had spread over five decks. The fire claimed the life of one passenger, 13 were treated for smoke inhalation, and 218 cabins were damaged by fire, smoke or water. It was thought to be caused by a discarded cigarette. Royal Caribbean banned balcony smoking as of 1 January 2014, and the majority of other cruise lines followed suit. Other notable cases were the fires that broke out in the engine rooms of *Carnival Splendor* in 2010 and *Carnival Triumph* three years later. Both fires disabled their respective ships, ending with them needing to be towed back to the States.

There is a long list of forbidden items that could cause fires, ranging from travel kettles and irons, to candles and surge protectors. Don't break the rules - not only is it highly unsafe, but you could be subject to substantial fines (up to $500), or sometimes disembarkation, for violating them, even for simply lighting up in a no-smoking zone.

## Gym

If you intend to use the gym facilities on the ship, you need to wear appropriate clothing and footwear for your own safety and wellbeing. Also, wipe the equipment down after use so others can equally enjoy their time working out.

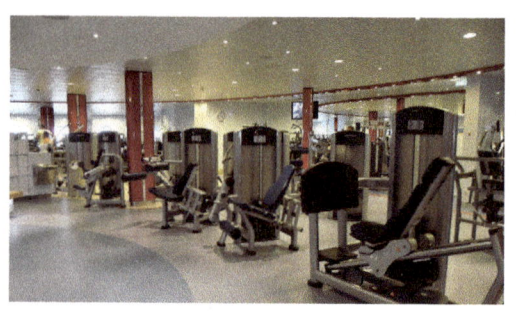

*Credit: Royal Caribbean Allure of the Seas - John Ostrom, Flickr*

## Hallways and Corridors

Not everyone goes to bed at the same time. There will be someone resting at all times of the day, so try to avoid shouting from one end of the corridor to the other, and don't let your cabin door slam. Sound carries a long way in narrow corridors, and you will undoubtedly disturb several people if you make a lot of noise.

## Hygiene and Norovirus

One of the most common stomach bugs, norovirus causes cramps and nausea at first, followed by vomiting and diarrhoea. The virus is most commonly caught by touching contaminated surfaces or by consuming compromised food or water. There is no treatment for norovirus, also known as the 'winter vomiting bug', but it typically runs its course within 72 hours.

Norovirus can run rampant in enclosed spaces like a cruise ship, living on surfaces for weeks, fabrics for up to 12 days and in water for months, making it difficult to eradicate. The easiest and most effective way to prevent the virus from spreading is to wash your hands after using the bathroom, before and after eating, and once you return to your cabin, as the infection spreads easily on surfaces like handrails, door handles, and lift buttons. Use the hand sanitisers posted throughout the ship, not as a substitute to washing your hands but as another preventative measure. If there is evidence of the virus, use your own bathroom rather than the public ones, avoid the hot tubs, saunas and lifts, and minimise your direct contact with other guests.

If you are taken ill with norovirus, food poisoning or other gastrointestinal illness, you should notify the ship's medical centre immediately, confine yourself to your cabin and limit your interactions with other guests to help prevent it from spreading. In the unlikely event there is an outbreak on board, the medical team will immediately begin procedures to mitigate its spread,

# Life Onboard

and the crew will implement comprehensive cleaning and sanitising programs to control its reach.

**Jogging Track**
The daily program indicates when the jogging track is open. While you might think it should be available at all times, you need to spare a thought for a sleeping passenger whose cabin is directly below the jogging area.

**Lifts**
While waiting for a lift, a few people can turn into a crowd very quickly. It is especially busy after the safety drill, a show or a port arrival. Let people out before you try and squeeze in, and always give priority to wheelchair users and the elderly, as they have no choice but to use the lift.

**Nudism**
Sunbathing nude in public areas is against the rules of most cruise lines and will often upset other passengers. Enjoying the sun and ocean breeze on your 'private' balcony without clothes might seem appealing, but there are security cameras everywhere and you could give one of the junior officers quite a scare. Also, a lot of guests like to lean over the railings with their binoculars or video cameras, and it is quite easy to see into the adjoining balconies, so it might be more prudent to cover up.

**Pool Loungers**
Just like some hotels, cruise ships can be a victim to those that get up at 6 am to lay out their towels or personal belongings on prime sunbed real estate, and then go elsewhere for extended periods. While it is perfectly acceptable for someone to leave a sun lounger to use the bathroom or grab a drink from the bar, it isn't fair to take up the poolside space and then disappear for the rest of the day. Only save a chair for your partner or family member. This is a common gripe among passengers and most pool attendants now remove belongings if a chair is unattended for more than 30 minutes.

**Punctuality**
Don't be late for dinner, especially if you are on the first sitting - there is a limited amount of time for the serving staff to take orders, get the food out and turn the dining room around ready for the next set of diners. It is also

very inconsiderate to the other people on your table who might have to wait to place their order until everyone is seated.

**Saving Seats**
While it is acceptable to save a seat for one or two people, reserving entire rows in show lounges or several tables on deck for a party is strongly frowned upon. If your friends want seats together, they need to arrive early and grab their own spaces.

**Smoking**
All cruise ships have clearly designated areas for smoking.

**Sound Levels**
MP3 players, iPods, and any other portable gadgets should be used with headphones and not played aloud in public spaces. Sound carries across the decks, and not everyone wants to hear Pavarotti at full blast. You should also try to keep your volume at a reasonable level in your cabin, and whilst it's understandable that someone with hearing loss might need the volume up quite high, perhaps it's best to use subtitles or limit your use of the TV to the day time.

**Tipping**
You should always have money earmarked for additional gratuities for baggage handlers, tour guides and room service deliveries, as well as for your cabin steward. If a member of the crew has gone the extra mile to make your cruise a trip to remember, you could also consider writing a note to the onboard hotel director or head office as it could help them earn a sought-after promotion or bonus.

**Toilets**
Don't flush tampons or nappies in the onboard toilets as you may block the entire system and leave your neighbours without working toilets. The plumbing on ships works on a vacuum system rather than relying on gravity and is easily blocked, and it doesn't help if you place something in the toilet bowl you shouldn't have. In 2019, after sending down an engineer to deal with a blockage, the captain on Celebrity Silhouette revealed that the culprit was a pair of jeans! Don't underestimate the suction power of these vacuum powered toilets - never flush while sitting on them.

# Life Onboard

## Bon Appétit - Cruise Ship Dining

Shipboard dining in one of a ship's elegant restaurants is the highlight of the day for many travellers, and cruise lines pride themselves on the dining experiences they offer. That being said, dining on cruise ships has changed dramatically over the years compared to the limited options available 'back in the day'; today, most cruises have dozens of eateries, with alternative dining options and open seating, and with this improved flexibility passengers are now spoilt for choice.

As you would expect, the degree of accessibility of onboard dining venues is mainly dependent on the age of the ship, with smaller crafts (including river cruises) often not suitable for those in wheelchairs. On the other hand, the majority of larger, post-2015 vessels have excellent dining accessibility for mobility challenged passengers, with entrances wide enough for wheelchairs, and even though some have gradual inclines, restaurant routes are manageable and include lifts where needed.

If for some reason your assigned table in the main dining room doesn't work for you, speak to the maître d' who will arrange a table as near to the entrance as possible and the dining venue's staff will be happy to move furniture to create an easy route to your table. If you need to stay seated in your mobility aid, dining room chairs will be removed to give you access to the table. You can also speak to the maître d' if you'd rather have a table to yourselves, perhaps if you're travelling with someone with dementia who doesn't enjoy the company of strangers, and they will do what they can to accommodate your request. Establishing a good daily routine with the same meal times and dining locations will help passengers with learning and developmental needs, as well as those suffering from dementia and the like.

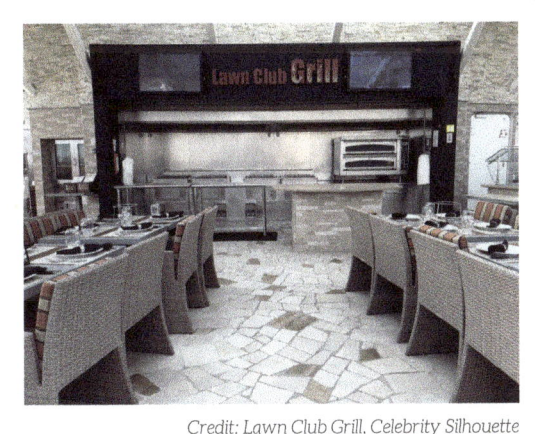

*Credit: Lawn Club Grill, Celebrity Silhouette*

Service dogs are allowed to accompany their owners in all public areas of a ship (excluding pools, whirlpools and the spa), including the dining rooms,

# The Autonomous Cruiser

but they must be on a leash, harness or other restraining device. The maître dt can arrange a convenient table in the dining room with space for your animal if you make a special request in advance, but under no circumstances should your dog be fed under the table. Also, some ships offer menus in large print or braille, and if for some reason they are unavailable, your waiter will happily discuss that evening's food options.

***Dedicated Seating:*** *Some ships have dedicated seating for wheelchair passengers in their buffet restaurant, and staff are trained to anticipate the needs of a passenger, especially those with a mobility or audio-visual handicap. If a sight-impaired guest is travelling alone, most crew members will be happy to assist with food selection and carry their choices back to the table for them. Always ask a staff member for assistance if you need it, they will be happy to help.*

## Breakfast Options

The main dining room on most ships will offer seated service for breakfast, but if you only fancy something quick and simple, pop to the buffet restaurant instead. Like hotels, a continental breakfast is usually available for early risers, as well as a typical 'fry-up' if you'd prefer. Some ships also have specialty items like an omelette station, fresh pancakes and waffles, and even the firm favourite of bagels, cream cheese and smoked salmon. For the most part, trays have been dispensed with, but if you need help, one of the staff will be happy to assist you. Using the buffet also gives you the option of eating out on deck. Your other main option for breakfast is to order it from room service to eat in your cabin or on your balcony.

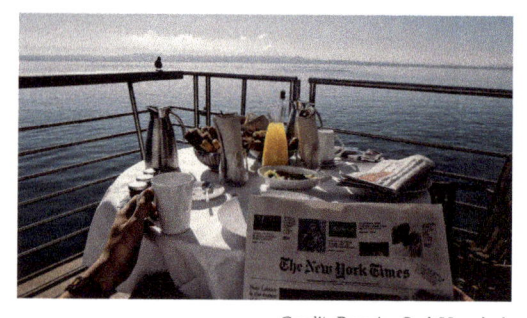

*Credit: Reynier Carl, Unsplash*

## Lunch Options

Dining on cruise ships is all about diversity and lunch is usually no different, offering up umpteen casual and specialty dining venues. The main dining room offers a stylish alternative to open-deck dining, with freshly-prepared dishes and impeccable service, but if you'd prefer to stay in your swimwear, poolside grills serve favourites like pizza, burgers and hot dogs. Most ships also have a self-serve buffet with a staggering amount of options, from hand-tossed pizzas to a fully laden salad bar. To finish off lunch, visit the cheeseboard, complete with all the trimmings, and finally the dessert section, with its delicious pastries, decadent cakes and mounds of ice cream - that is, if you have any room left.

*Pizza Feast:* Instead of just grabbing a slice, order a whole pizza for your family or friends. It might take a few extra minutes, but it will be piping hot and all yours.

### Snacks

Fruit, ice cream and freshly baked cookies are typically available in most of the ship's coffee shops or in the buffet. If, however, you want to make your snack more of an event, don't miss afternoon tea, typically at around 3 pm, where you can find delicious finger sandwiches, scones with whipped cream and jam, and much more.

Most lines have dispensed with late-night food options to cut back on costs, but some like Carnival, Disney and NCL still put on lavish late feasts at least once during your cruise. On the larger cruise ships, self-service hot drink dispensers are available 24/7, and a lot of lines offer kettles in the cabin.

### Dinner Options

Traditional cruise ship dining is still available on virtually every ship. There are usually two different options when it comes to the time of your sit-down dinner, the more popular early sitting (typically 6.00pm) and the late sitting (typically 8.30pm). You will have been asked for your preferred time and table size at the time of booking, with table sizes usually ranging from two to ten people; tables for two, however, are extremely scarce as they use the space in the dining room least efficiently. You'll be assigned to a specific table with the same tablemates and the same waiting staff for the entirety of your cruise, unless for some reason you request to be moved - this can be difficult, but your best bet is to speak to the restaurant manager as early on in your trip as possible. Confirmation of your dining sitting will be waiting for you in your cabin upon boarding the ship.

*Picky Eaters:* If nothing on the menu tempts you or doesn't comply with a dietary requirement, ask your waiter if they can get you an alternative. It might take longer but the crew can usually offer up different options.

# The Autonomous Cruiser

Flexible, freedom or anytime dining gives you the option of eating when and where you want - you simply turn up at the restaurant when you are ready to eat. Some ships will give you a buzzer that vibrates when your table is ready, others will just have you make a reservation. Your waiting staff will also be different each night, so those with special dietary needs will have to relay this information nightly.

***Seconds:*** *If you can't choose between some of the menu choices, just order one of each! Waiters are more than happy to accommodate your request.*

***Temptations:*** *Menus are usually posted outside the restaurant's entrance if you want a preview of the day's meals.*

***Autism Tip:*** *Some people on the autism spectrum have a problem occupying themselves in 'dead' time, such as when queuing outside the dining room or waiting for food, and subsequently get irritable or stressed. To combat this, plan your meal times to be similar to those at home, and if anything in particular provides them with comfort, like a favourite television show or toy, take it with you into the restaurant to act as a distraction.*

For those passengers that want an alternative to traditional cruise dining, the buffet is always popular and included in the cost of your cruise. Buffet dining often offers similar dishes to that of the main dining room, as well as an array of crowd-pleasing favourites and regional dishes. Freshly baked breads, a loaded salad bar and a profusion of desserts will always be waiting to tempt you. Themed evenings are also offered on occasion, with foods reflecting that of the port visited that day; for example, you might find a poolside Caribbean buffet on your cruise planner.

A buffet isn't always your only alternative as most ships now offer several specialty restaurants, ranging from Asian-fusion to the finest French cuisine. Though typically not included in the price of your cruise, you might have something special to celebrate or just want a romantic dinner in a more intimate setting on a table for two, so the extra cost may prove worth it. Specialty venues usually only serve dinner, but some do also offer a lower-priced lunch option on sea days. Some larger cruise lines tempt food lovers

> **Don't Ask:**
> How small does your face have to be for a mini facial?

with a specialty dining package that offers meals at multiple restaurants on different evenings for a more competitive price. In all cases, you will still need to make a reservation, either online before sailing, on embarkation day at one of the reservation stations, on your phone if you have your cruise app downloaded, on your stateroom's television or by phoning the venue once onboard. As well as superb food, specialty restaurants also allow your party the luxury of being allocated your own table. If the dining venue is nearly full, instead of being turned away, you might be offered the option of sharing.

***Specialty Deal:*** *If your itinerary features an overnight stay in a port or a late sailaway, you can usually get a discounted reservation in one of the specialty venues as the maître d won t want empty tables.*

Some luxury lines have partnered with Michelin-star chefs, and their food will take you on an ever-evolving culinary adventure that will thrill from the first moment to the last. Flawless silver service showcases the finest seasonal ingredients with both classic and ground-breaking culinary techniques, but you will certainly need a reservation to sample these extraordinary menus.

Nearly every ship offers room service or in-suite dining for those that don't fancy leaving their cabin for dinner, and while the facility is free on most ships, some have taken to charging for handpicked dishes on the menu. Smaller ships generally have a more limited choice, while the larger vessels might even serve the same menu as the dining room. The food choices are usually offered 24/7 except for the night before disembarkation, and there is no limit to the number of items you can order. It might be the perfect time to try something new without feeling embarrassed if the dish is not to your palate.

***Dietary requirement:*** *Every ship offers vegetarian and vegan options on their menus, and most dietary requirements can be accommodated for, including gluten-free, low sodium and low sugar options. If you requested a special meal with your agent at the time of booking, inform your table server once onboard.*

You would think that all these options would satisfy even the most exacting foodie, but for those looking for something especially extraordinary, look into booking a seat at the Chef's Table. The evening offers the rare opportunity of enjoying an intimate dinner in a private setting, savouring an evening of memorable sights, tastes and conversation hosted by the executive chef.

The specially created multi-course menu is not offered anywhere else on the ship and might include a showcase of native ingredients from a recent port. Detailed explanations of the distinct flavours and cooking techniques accompany each course, with specially selected wine complementing your meal. Prices vary by cruise line and limited seating at this elite event means you'll have to reserve your spot on the first day of your cruise, otherwise you'll most certainly miss out.

## That's Entertainment

The price of your cruise doesn't just include travelling to exotic havens and nonstop dining, but also incredible entertainment opportunities. It isn't just about the fabulous Broadway-style extravaganzas, ice shows, acrobatic feats or quick-fire comics that entertain every night, there is also an abundance of daytime activities to sink your teeth into. Sea days are when you can really take advantage of what the ship and its entertainment team have to offer. Though the main areas of the vessel can be crowded on sea days, with sun loungers at a premium, there will always be a quiet nook to unwind in or a group activity you can try before your next port. Most modern ships have public areas and pool decks that are spacious and accessible, making it easy for wheelchair users to participate in most of the activities that take their fancy.

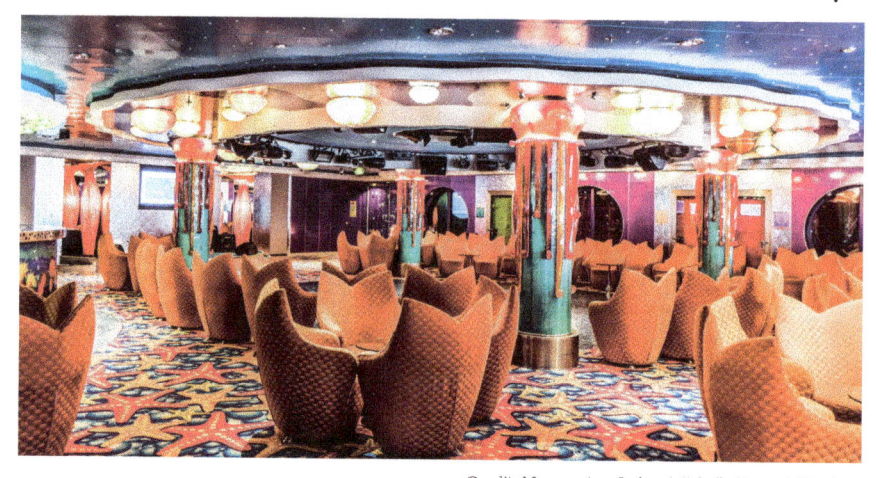

*Credit: Norwegian Jade – Michelle Raponi, Pixabay*

# Life Onboard

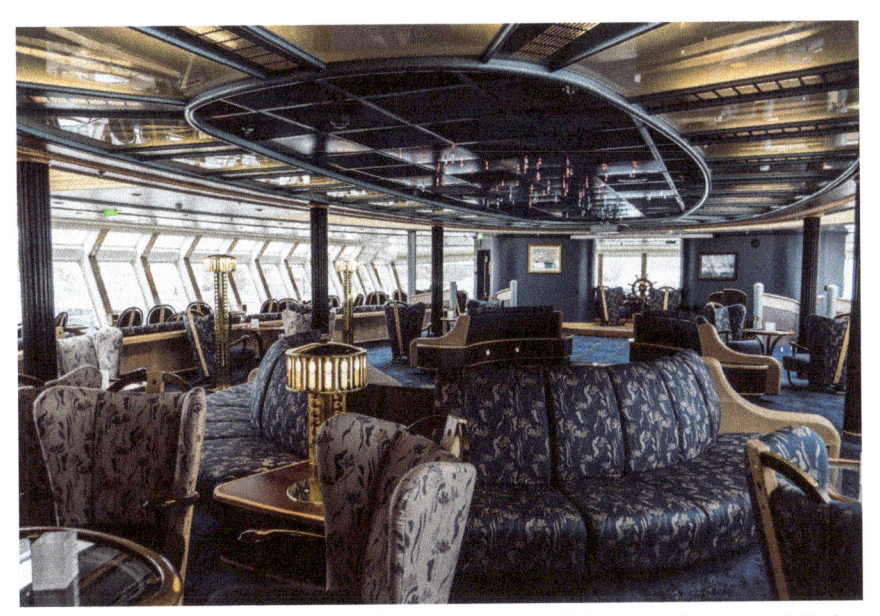

*Credit: Hurtigruten – Michelle Raponi, Pixabay*

Your steward will deliver the ship's daily planner to your cabin each night when they are doing their evening rounds. It provides a breakdown of all things pertinent to the following day, including the sunrise and sunset times, suggested dress codes and the opening times of dining venues, shops, the spa, the library and the countless bars. More importantly, it also contains a rundown of all the next day's activities and entertainment, so you can plan ahead and use your time optimally. The majority of onboard activities are free, but there are a few, like wine tastings and arcade games, that will carry a charge - your daily planner will highlight these. Several of the larger liners now also have downloadable apps for your phone that act as an alternative to the printed program. On port days it will even give you information on your arrival and back onboard times, the port agent's details in case of a problem and the weather forecast.

# The Autonomous Cruiser

## The Library

Some ships still offer an onboard library, but a reduction in the number of new book deliveries and a clear shrinking of the space devoted to a ship's reading room has been obvious over recent years. The libraries often have reference material and travel guides for your ports of call, but unfortunately, a lot of them will be out of date as they have been left on the ship by past cruisers. Of those libraries that do exist, some stay open 24/7 with a librarian on hand, however others may only be open for a few hours a day, with books needing to be checked out manually. The libraries on P&O, Cunard and Crystal ships provide audiobooks and DVDs for their guests, which is especially useful for those with limited or impaired vision.

Not only is the square footage afforded to the libraries decreasing steadily, the bookshelves are also fighting for space with computer terminals that line one wall and jigsaw puzzle tables. What is traditionally missing is a ship's globe and world maps that always used to grace these spaces. You might, quite rightly, expect a library to be a quiet zone onboard, but that isn't always the case; for example, Celebrity's Solstice class ships and Seabourn Odyssey have sited their reading rooms in central hubs which tend to be busy and loud areas at certain times of day! Cunard, on the other hand, has upheld the seafaring tradition of a fully stocked library across its fleet of three - QM2 has the most extensive library at sea, holding an inventory of some 10,000 tomes.

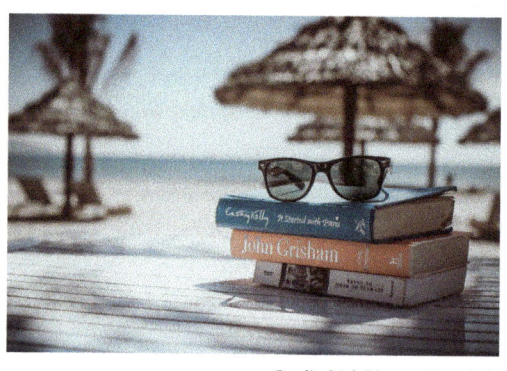

Credit: Link Hoang, Unsplash

Most onboard theatres have a designated area, often towards the front or rear of the venue, for people who are full-time wheelchair users, with nearby seats provided for travelling companions or caregivers. The smaller lounges should all be accessible too, but spaces cannot be reserved in advance for any entertainment venue so you will need to get there in good time to guarantee a spot for your whole party. The main theatres, show lounges and cinemas offer aisle seats for those with service dogs. If a night in the casino is your preferred choice of entertainment, there are lowered blackjack tables and slot machines on several ships.

## Life Onboard

The majority of ships have some type of assistive listening device for individuals with residual hearing, with most offering induction loop systems in most of their onboard entertainment venues. Some have adopted the most up-to-date technologies, with Carnival offering Listen Technologies infrared-based headsets for those with a hearing impairment - they work by amplifying the sounds of live performances in their main showroom.

Sensory overload is a real threat for autistic passengers. Get seats at the back of a theatre or showroom so you can make a quick exit if needed. A set of earplugs can also be useful for dampening the sound whilst still allowing the full visual experience. More 'tailor-made' experiences are often available, for example, Royal Caribbean provides specially designed films that reduce anxiety and create a supportive atmosphere for people with autism spectrum conditions, learning disabilities and other sensory and communication disorders. The lights and sound levels are lowered, and guests are encouraged to walk about and talk during the films.

***ASL Tip:*** *On cruises departing from and returning to the US and Canada, Disney, Azamara and Royal Caribbean (among others) provide their guests with an American Sign Language (ASL) interpreting service on request for a variety of onboard shows and entertainment.*

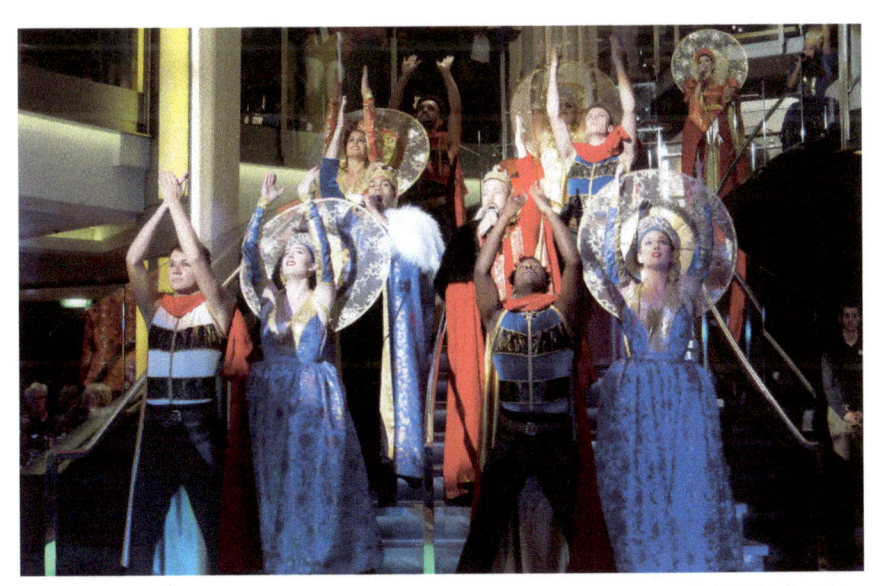

Credit: Celebrity Eclipse

# The Autonomous Cruiser

In nice weather you might be treated to a musical performance around the pool, an ice carving demonstration, or you could take part in one of the traditional outdoor cruise games like shuffleboard, deck quoits or bocce, which is closely related to British bowls. If the weather is inclement, the entertainment team may organise indoor carpet bowls, napkin folding classes or a culinary demo. Quizzes are held frequently and are always popular, offering the chance to show off your general knowledge and maybe even win one of the ship's sought-after branded keyrings!

The mega-liners are continually trying to outdo each other in offering the newest, biggest and best activities on the market, enticing thrill-seekers with ziplining, rock climbing, skating, skydiving, and even FlowRiders, a surf simulator that supports traditional surfing and boogie boarding.

From port talks and specialised guest speakers, to watercolour tutorials and photography workshops, there is quite literally something to suit everyone. However, if you want to slow down the pace you could simply watch the sun set over the ocean or stargaze on deck. Once dinner is over you can relax with a live game show, sit in a piano bar with the cocktail of the day, spin the roulette wheel, take part in karaoke, or collapse on a lounger with blankets and popcorn for a Movie Under the Stars. As the evening settles in your ship starts to come alive with an air of expectation as music wafts through from the various lounges onboard and if you love dancing, you can listen to the resident band while your partner twirls you around the floor, or let one of the dance hosts show you the latest moves. Ships have upgraded their dated sound and lighting systems in favour of state-of-the-art technology, enabling revolutionary magic shows, dazzling productions and full out extravaganzas. If you're still not ready for bed you can have fun at the silent disco or get caught up with the frenzy on nights that are themed around different music eras and genres.

Aside from the 'standard' entertainment offered on a day-to-day basis on your cruise, you may find a host of one-off special events, including:

**Captain's Welcome Reception**
Traditionally held on the first full sea day of the cruise in the main show lounge, each guest is invited to an evening cocktail party hosted by the captain, who will introduce themselves and their officers and welcome you aboard, all while you enjoy a free glass of champagne and a nibble or two. The event also happens to fall on the first formal night, with the dress code observed by close to 100% of guests.

# Life Onboard

*Captain's Welcome Reception*

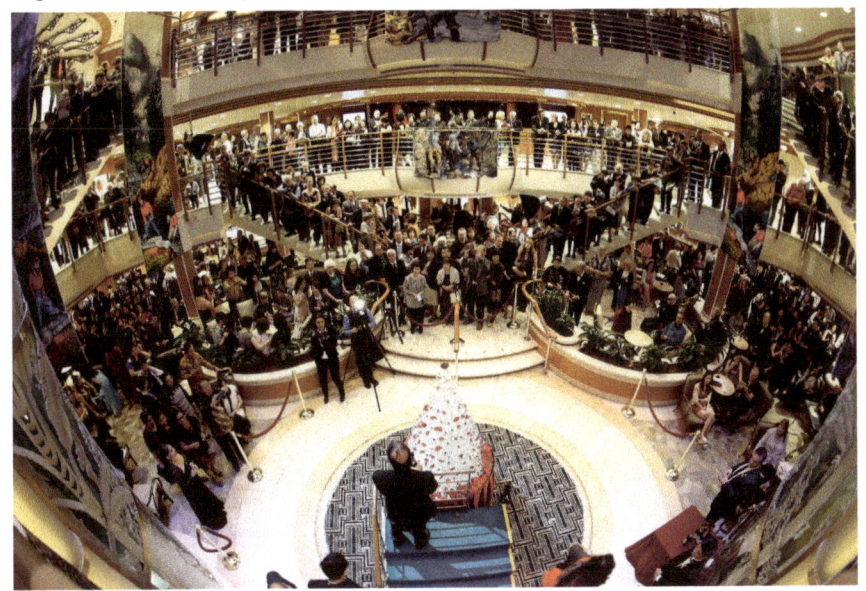

*Credit: Watcharapong Tunpornchai, Unsplash*

### Farewell Gala Night
This is the one dinner that you don't want to miss in the main restaurant, usually held on the penultimate night of the cruise with the Head Chef and their team pulling out all the stops. The captain is usually in attendance for photo opportunities so you can take home the perfect cruise memento.

### Solo Travellers' Mingle
All cruise lines welcome solo travellers and most include a single's coffee morning, lunch or cocktail party, giving guests the opportunity to meet other independent cruisers looking for fun and friendship. It's the perfect opportunity to arrange port outings, find dinner companions and perhaps even someone to share amazing cruise experiences with.

### Loyalty Cocktail Party
If you travel multiple times with the same cruise line your loyalty is often rewarded with exclusive perks, such as a private member's cocktail party. For top-tier members, a special lunch may also be arranged.

## The Captain's Table

Every cruise ship has a Captain's Table in the main dining room, usually in the centre of the room and set for 10-12 people, though seats are by invitation only. Most ocean guests consider an invitation to the Captain's Table a privilege and hope for the golden ticket opportunity. Invitees can include the captain's friends, company officials, loyalty members and retired military personnel.

## The Chef's Table

This private epicurean feast usually takes place at an evening meal with a small number of guests seated at an exclusive table. The experience starts with a champagne and canapé reception before moving onto multiple courses of gourmet dishes that aren't available on the ship's regular menus. Each course is accompanied by a thoughtful wine pairing selected by the sommelier, and ends with a visit from the executive chef at the end of the meal. This is always a very popular event, so the limited number of spaces fill quickly.

## Themed Nights

Several cruise lines lay on lavish theme nights, like Mardi Gras, White Night, Colourful Tropical, Caribbean and Bollywood, at which the food and entertainment are theme-appropriate. Some crew members may even dress in their traditional attire, and though cruise guests are strongly encouraged to participate, it is not compulsory.

> **Don't Ask:**
> What time is the midnight buffet?

## Silent Disco

You'd be forgiven for not hearing the phrase 'silent disco' before, but the last few years have seen the event gaining a lot of attention from cruise ships. Guests wear wireless headphones with the option of several channels with different music, almost like your own private DJ in your head. No longer do you have to lose your voice shouting to be heard, as you can simply take the headphones off and chat freely at a normal volume. It also makes for a hilarious sight as legs and limbs are flailing to different beats and tempos that only the dancer can hear. This silent party option has allowed partygoers to dance long into the night without disturbing other cruise ship guests.

## Passenger Talent Show

There is always a rich and diverse collection of performances by passengers who sign up for this event during the cruise. If the show is oversubscribed, then auditions take place first, and for those who qualify, the final will be presented in the ship's theatre or show lounge and often on the cruise TV channel. All you have to do is decide which of your many talents you are going to showcase.

Introduced in the spring of 2016, Princess Cruises' onboard version of ITV's talent show *The Voice* has been a hit with passengers since its inception. Participants are voted into the final by fellow cruisers in a gruelling public audition, with finalists performing in the ship's theatre for the coveted 'Voice of the Ocean' trophy. This is the ultimate competition for karaoke lovers, so if you fancy your chances, make sure you don't miss out! Some cruise lines have become more inventive and host their own versions of *The X-Factor* or *American Idol* with contestants being accompanied by the ship's house band.

## Passenger Choir

These usually take place on cruises of two weeks or longer so that there are plenty of sea days available for rehearsals. The music is easy to sing, and you're encouraged to harmonise if you are able. Participants are required to dress up (some ships stipulate formal wear) for two performances that take place towards the end of the cruise. This is an ideal opportunity to make new friends, and the concerts are always a big hit with passengers.

## Strictly Come Dancing

If you are a fervent fan of the hit BBC show, then you'll love P&O's *Strictly Come Dancing* themed sailings. As well as celebrity guests to mingle with, such as Craig Revel Horwood, who often makes up part of the judging panel, you can enjoy taking part in a good old-fashioned dance competition. Hosted by the cruise director, this popular event is staged in the ship's main theatre. Other cruise lines host dance contests such as Carnival's Nationals at Sea, which sees one of the largest dance competitions on the water. Keep an eye on your daily planner to see what your cruise line is staging.

## Inaugural Sailings

There are plenty of choices for those that like inaugural or maiden sailings and, as you would expect, the big brands like Celebrity, Carnival, P&O and Virgin all have new vessels they want to show off, but the lesser-known Ponant, Ritz-

Carlton and Havila also deserve a look in. It's hard to comprehend some of the newest things coming to cruising, like how lavish the new suites are, some with their own plunge pool, or innovative features like cantilevered platforms, a Skydome with a retractable stage for aerial performances, a Nordic-themed spa, virtual balconies, and BOLT, the first roller coaster at sea.

# Meetings

### Friends of Bill W
Bill W refers to Bob Wilson, the co-founder of Alcoholics Anonymous, whose primary focus was on bringing together a society of members dedicated to helping each other achieve and maintain sobriety. These meetings are a lifeline for many recovering alcoholics, and most cruise lines provide a meeting area as a service to members who like to meet during their cruise.

### Friends of Dorothy
Dorothy is, at least officially, a reference to Dorothy Gale, the character played by Judy Garland in *The Wizard of Oz*, though some say it instead refers to Dorothy Parker, the well-known American poet, writer, critic and satirist who often included gay men in her social circles. Initially set up as a positive social space for gay men, this has now expanded to include the entire LGBTQ+ community.

### Community Boards
Special events planned by cruise passengers will not be listed in your daily cruise planner, though they may still be open to everyone. Check the community notice board located by Guest Relations for times and meeting locations of passenger-led group gatherings, such as a veterans' meet, a chess club, a singles event or a bridge tournament.

# Bridge Visits

Bridge visits have generally been stopped for safety reasons, though some cruise lines include it as part of a 'Behind-the-Scenes' tour, which will be advertised in your ship's daily planner and needs to be booked. If you want to be among those that visit some back of house areas that are considered the heartbeat of cruise operations, including the engine room, main galley, laundry room and the theatre's backstage area, typically finishing with a glass of champagne with the captain in his command centre, a large fee will be charged to your onboard account for the privilege.

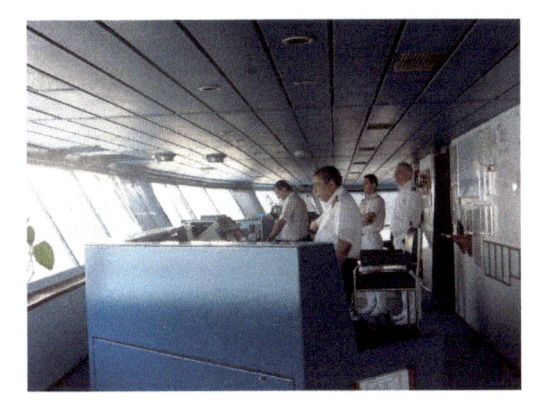

## Children's Clubs

Most cruise ships provide age-appropriate children's clubs included within the price of your cruise, so you can grab some much-longed-for alone time while your kids enjoy making new friends and participating in their very own activities schedule, which will be waiting for you in your cabin on embarkation day. First-time cruisers are often reluctant to leave their children in a club, worried they might not enjoy themselves, but with trained crew offering endless activities, pool parties, and special tea times, it is usually the child that is reluctant to leave. Some ships allocate entire decks as a space for children, housing all the clubs, activity areas, splash zones and themed pools - Royal Caribbean's Oasis Class ships dedicate 28,000 square feet to youngsters. Night nurseries and babysitting services are all on offer but do incur a fee; the majority of lines will only accept babies from six months old, but MSC is the only line not to have a minimum age limit.

If you didn't pre-register your child into the children's club before sailing, some cruise lines have a desk in the terminal on embarkation day, or you can do it once aboard the ship. Most clubs are limited in how many children they can accommodate on each sailing, so you'll need to register as soon as you embark so they are not excluded from the program. Similarly, any special events like character Meet & Greet opportunities get booked out fast despite their additional cost, so be sure to secure your family's place early. Finally, note that children may only participate in the club designed for their age group. To register your child, simply take them along to the appropriate club to meet the team and to familiarise them with the facilities, fill in any relevant forms and speak to one of the clubs' youth staff. You will also have to inform the staff if you wish to authorise other adults to sign your child in and out of the club, or if you're okay with your child signing themselves in or out (depending on your child's age and your cruise line).

Carnival Cruise Line encourages parents of special needs children to work with them so they can integrate the child into a program they will enjoy. Register early as 'KultureCity Sensory Bags' are issued on a complimentary, first-come-first-served basis and contain items to help calm, relax and manage sensory overload including comfortable noise-cancelling headphones, fidget tools, a visual feeling thermometer, and a KultureCity VIP lanyard to help staff quickly identify a guest.

Most modern cruise ships are equipped with a comprehensive range of facilities and staff to accommodate less mobile or disabled guests. If your child has a special need, advise the youth team and they will make every effort to accommodate them, though they are generally not allowed to offer one-on-one supervision, change nappies, bottle feed, or administer medication. If your child can't or doesn't want to go to the children's club, ask staff to give you any activities and crafts that can be done in a quieter area or your cabin under your supervision.

## Swimming Pools

All cruise ships, save a few expedition vessels, have at least one pool, and in recent years, with cruise lines taking delivery of new ships on a regular basis, the pool designs have become bigger and more extravagant. Pools generally take centre stage on deck, surrounded by rows of sun loungers and overlooked by the floor above. Most cruise ships still use seawater which passes through a filtration and desalination process before reaching the pool. Some of the larger cruise lines such as Azamara, Celebrity, Cunard and Holland America also provide an indoor pool. Carnival *Splendor*, MSC *Meraviglia* and P&O *Ventura* have retractable roofs so they can be opened as soon as the warm weather appears, or closed if it's raining.

# Life Onboard

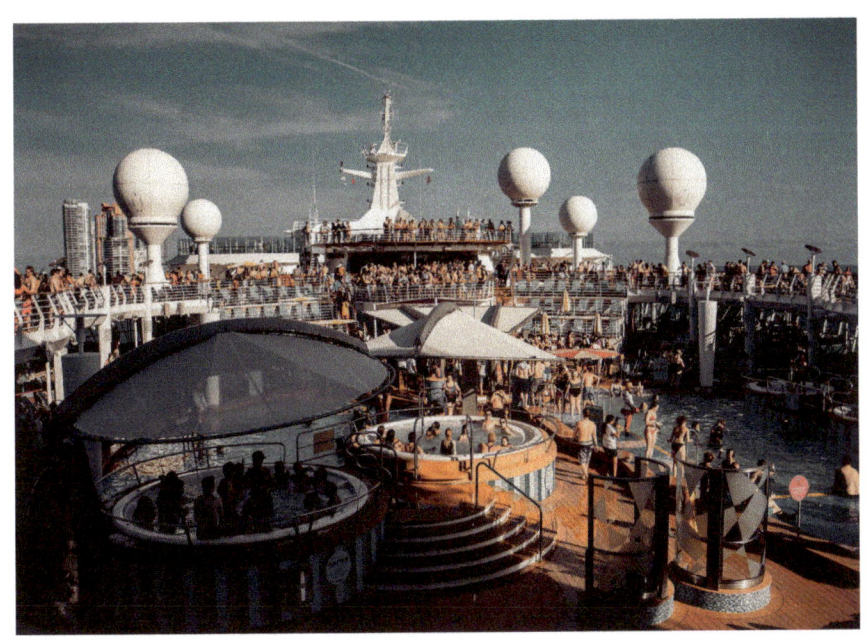

*Credit: Royal Caribbean - Colin Lloyd, Unsplash*

Trained lifeguards are only employed by a handful of cruise lines while others have life-guard certified attendants but they don't advertise the fact as they want to promote active parental supervision. Complimentary floatation vests are typically available on ships that offer family pools, including Carnival Cruise Lines and Celebrity Cruises.

## Spa Centres

Spas are big business at sea, with nearly every cruise line offering their unique wellness menu across the oceans, capitalising on sea days where a relaxing session in a ship's spa is sometimes too strong a temptation to resist. Decked out in natural materials like dark wood, marble, limestone, black slate and oodles of glass, the opulent décor is clever in promoting a sense of wellbeing before youSve even started. The waiting areas, fitted with deep-seated leather chairs, tend to lead through to changing rooms with showers, toilets and lockers.

Restorative treatments are aimed at nourishing, toning and revitalising your body, with treatment rooms often affording the best sea views through floor-to-ceiling windows. The largest spas incorporate thermal suites, thalassotherapy pools, relaxation areas, couple's rooms, fitness centres, personal trainers, barbershops, hair salons, nail therapy areas and makeup rooms. Not content to just indulge the face and body, treatments have now expanded to acupuncture, teeth whitening, Thermage or Q-Frequency (a radio frequency skin-tightening treatment), and chiropractic care. Select ships even offer medi-spa services which provide Botox and dermal fillers, such as Restylane, Perlane and Dysport.

**Skin Tip:** *For those suffering from eczema, grab some natural yoghurt from the breakfast buffet and spread it over the offending area. It might be messy until it dries, but the results after three days will be worth it.*

It is not just women who line up for appointments - most ships offer a complete menu of services for men too, including grooming treatments, facials, massages, manicures and pedicures. Not wanting to miss a trick, Royal Caribbean, Celebrity and MSC are also catering to the teenage brigade, offering acne treatments on top of their more standard options. Also, hair salons no longer limit their offerings to a simple wash and blow-dry, a tint, perm, or highlights. Instead, menus now incorporate scalp rituals, hair gloss treatments, lash and brow tinting, waxing services and liquid golden tans.

**Diabetes Alert:** *People with diabetes need to take extra precautions when getting foot treatments. "Any break in the skin, potentially from the aggressive trimming of a callous or cuticle, can increase the risk of foot infections called cellulitis," says Sharon Horesh, MD, an internal medicine doctor with Emory University's Department of Medicine.*

**Wheelchair Tip:** *Most of the newer cruise lines have accessible spa facilities for wheelchair users. For example, you can stay seated in your chair when having your hair washed and styled as the wash units swivel over to you and are height adjustable.*

Once relegated to a tiny room, gyms have now expanded into spacious fitness centres bedecked in state-of-the-art machines and weights, and which host Pilates, aerobics, kickboxing, spinning, yoga, stretching and body sculpting classes. The inclusion of access to the gym within your cruise fare is standard on most cruise lines, along with a selection of free fitness classes. Their generosity also extends to the use of the sauna and steam rooms, with the exception of Costa, Norwegian and Seabourn, who all charge for using their thermal suites.

***Sauna Tip:*** *Saunas and steam rooms with moist heat can improve sinus congestion, asthma, and allergies, but avoid them if you have a heart condition, as the sudden change in temperature can put a strain on your heart.*

Nearly every cruise ship spa is operated by either Steiner of Miami or Canyon Ranch. With little competition, these companies have adopted their own pricing structures which has seen costs soar in recent years. A range of signature treatments are peppered throughout the tariff, a reflection of the spa's most popular restoratives. Canyon Ranch has also branched out with branded menu items in the dining room on select Regent Seven Seas and Cunard ships.

***Don't Forget:*** *Port days offer reduced spa treatment prices, sometimes by as much as 50%. The deals will be advertised in your ship's newspaper delivered to your cabin the night before, and prices remain in force all day regardless of the time the ship sails.*

The Elemis Experience, offering luxurious facial and body-spa therapies, is now available in more than 100 of the world's finest state-of-the-art cruise line spas, with programs designed to deliver the best treatment experience your money can buy. Elemis therapists make it personal, performing transformative treatments, tailored to the ever-changing nature of your skin. The feel-good factor can even be taken home, as a range of their products are also available to purchase.

## Spa Cabins
A new addition to contemporary cruise ships, this category of cabin is usually sited close to the spa and features enhanced perks which could include unlimited access to the spa's thermal suites, plush bathrobes, a rainfall shower, superior toiletries, pillow menu, and complimentary fitness classes. Although more costly, these living spaces offer health-conscious guests a more holistic holiday experience.

## Thermal Environments
The larger spas have impressive fragrance-infused thermal suites which can include aromatherapy steam rooms, saunas, heated ceramic-tile loungers, therapeutic salt rooms, whirlpools, sensory showers and hydrotherapy, plunge or thalassotherapy (saltwater) pools, all designed to offer relaxation.

You will need to buy a daily, weekly or cruise-long spa passport if you plan to make regular use of the thermal environments, as they are very rarely offered as part of your cruise fare. If you want to use these areas every day, you should make your purchase on embarkation day as spaces are limited.

**Treatments**
Looking through the treatment lists, you could be forgiven for being confused as to what it all means, but in general, procedures can be broken down into four main areas: massages, facials, wraps and body scrubs.

**Massages**
Massages are by far the most popular treatments on any cruise ship, and spas will offer up several types named after their respective countries of origin, such as Swedish, Thai, or Balinese, as well as staunch favourites like hot stone, bamboo, deep tissue and reflexology. With heavenly smelling aromatic oils designed to stimulate circulation, dissolve tension and soothe aching muscles, a massage offers the ultimate in relaxation. Massages aren't just confined to the neck and back, with most spa menus also offering dedicated scalp, hand and foot treatments as well. While it isn't possible to dissect everything on offer, the onboard spa concierge will be happy to explain all of your options, or you can pick up the treatment list which will provide a full description of each service.

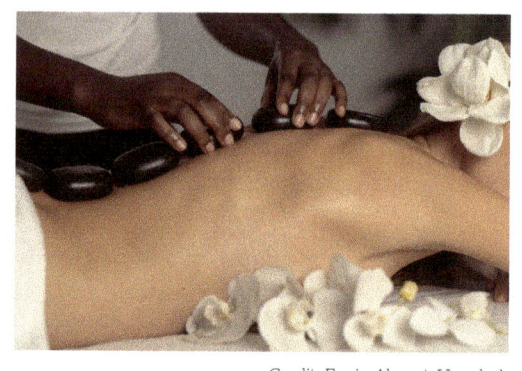

*Credit: Engin Akyurt, Unsplash*

The newer ships usually provide adjustable treatment tables in the spa which make it possible for most wheelchair users to enjoy one of the pampering regimens on offer. Some ships will even send a massage therapist to your stateroom or suite, while cruise lines that incorporate a private island visit into their itinerary may also deliver beach massages.

If you suffer from back pain, conditions like fibromyalgia and osteoarthritis, or need ongoing physiotherapy to help ease aches and pains, a daily massage might help. Massages help relax muscle tissue and aids circulation, which in turn enhances the delivery of oxygen and nutrients to muscle and tissue cells. It can improve stiffness, flexibility, reduce pain caused by muscle tightness and help manage sleep disorders. Massages also release endorphins, the feel-good chemical, and can alleviate stress and anxiety.

A hot oil head massage helps to improve blood circulation and can help a variety of conditions, including reducing blood pressure, stress, headaches, and migraines. An Indian head massage can help you feel better physically, mentally, emotionally and spiritually by massaging the pressure points around the neck, head and shoulders gently. It is an excellent treatment if suffering from alopecia as it is also said to stimulate hair growth.

*My Pick - Elemis Aroma Stone Therapy:* *Small heated stones are placed on the body's key energy points to release tension in the muscles, while Frangipani Monoi Body Oil is massaged into the skin for the ultimate in relaxation.*

### Facials
Where once a facial simply meant a thorough soap and water workout, treatments are now made unique with the addition of gemstones, plant extracts, precious minerals and even 24- carat gold leaf. Whether you are trying to reduce the effects of ageing, fine lines, acne scarring, sun damage, age spots, or uneven skin pigmentation, just one treatment can help to rejuvenate the skin and leave it feeling radiant.

*My Pick - La Therapie Hydralift Facial:* *Treats causes of skin ageing, sun damage, pigmentation, acne, sensitivity, enlarged pores and rosacea by using medical-grade ingredients to polish away dead cells and enhance your skin's natural ability to repair and resist everyday damage, right down to your fifth layer of skin.*

### Wraps
Typically employed to detoxify the body and lose inches, treatments involve your body being encased in mud, clay, seaweed, hot wax or even chocolate, then wrapped in foil or cling wrap and finally in blankets. Some enhance the session with a sensory dry float. Ionithermie cellulite reduction goes one step further, adding galvanic stimuli (electrical stimulation) once plastered and wrapped. It's said you'll see weight loss after just one session, but a course of three sessions during your cruise will deliver optimum results.

*My Pick - Euphoric Detox Wrap:* This purifying wrap uses pure essence of rose, which is bursting with vitamin C and other natural antioxidants, together with natural rhassoul clay, leaving skin supple, clean and glowing. A touch of moisturizing tangerine fig cream at the end seals in all the benefits.

## Scrubs

Primarily used to exfoliate the skin and get rid of impurities and dry skin, organic salt scrubs are very popular, as are lime and ginger salt rubs, and olive and coffee firming polishes. P&O and Princess Cruises have even incorporated a DIY Scrub and Shine Bar, where a spa mixologist will create a bespoke salt or sugar scrub tailored to your skin type.

*My Pick - Elemis Exotic Lime & Ginger Salt Glow:* This exotic exfoliation ritual will invigorate, cleanse and polish your skin. After a light body brushing, warm oil is dripped over your body before the sublime salt glow is applied. An application of Elemis Exotic Island Flower Body Lotion finishes the treatment, leaving your skin replenished and vibrant.

## Rasul Ceremony

A centuries-old Arabian favourite, this cleansing ritual pools the health-enhancing properties of heat, steam and mud for a totally relaxing skin conditioning treatment in a private, sensory setting with glimmering lights and fragrant vapours. The coloured chakra muds and scrubs are lavished on your skin and dried by the herb-infused steam that fills the room. The ritual ends with warm water raining down from sprinklers to wash the muds away, leaving beautifully soft and supple skin underneath.

## Vinotherapy

MSC, in partnership with Bocelli Wines, have included this beauty therapy process at their spas. A therapist creates a concoction of grape skins, seeds and stems, and rubs it into your skin as part of a massage. This brand-new therapeutic treatment uses the antioxidant properties of red wine by applying it to your skin to help rejuvenate the body. The pulp is said to have fabulous exfoliating qualities and help reduce the problems associated with ageing. Look out for this on other cruise lines in the near future.

### Acupuncture

A key component of traditional Chinese medicine, acupuncture is used as a supplement to assist more conventional medicine, said to be effective in the treatment of over 300 ailments, both chronic and subtle. This alternative treatment approach has many facets, for example, Elemis offers facial rejuvenation, pain management, weight loss, stress-free, detox and kick-the-habit options. A complimentary tongue and pulse analysis are usually included in your first acupuncture treatment to help determine the best course of treatment.

Some cruise lines offer up the option of pre-booking your spa treatments online weeks before your travel date, but for the most part, appointments are usually booked at the spa desk once onboard the ship. Seasoned cruisers opt to visit the spa before even unpacking so they can grab the prime slots, such as the hairdressing services on formal nights, as they always book up extremely fast. For those occupying suites or spa cabins, your concierge or butler can secure these appointments for you.

### Deals

If you are looking to have more than one spa treatment, you might find a bundle offered for less on embarkation day, either in the port terminal or once onboard; one of the most popular and worthwhile deals is the common 10-20-30 promotion: the percentage discount on your first, second and third treatments while onboard. Embarkation day will also see a complimentary spa tour on the schedule, with the offer of a free raffle to entice guests. Daily treatment seminars will often require a model to demonstrate their services on and so are always a good way of bagging a quick freebie. Although the workshops are designed to try and sell you something, they do sometimes give away money-off vouchers at the end of the talk. Larger ships may also have therapists on deck offering a complimentary ten-minute taster, but a word of warning - it can be hard to walk away without making a booking. Finally, special spa promotions are advertised in your ship's daily planner, but you'll also find countless flyers delivered to your cabin.

The spa staff are pushed into hard-sell techniques because they work on commission, irritating many cruise-goers. If you don't want a pushy sales talk at the end of a fabulous relaxation treatment, pre-empt the pitch by telling your therapist that you'd rather not discuss products before, during or after your appointment. Also, be aware that most lines add an automatic 15-20%

service charge to your bill, and though the invoice will leave space to add a gratuity, you are not required to do so.

***Did You Know:*** *Because of outlandish prices and hard-sell tactics, onboard spas are the single largest source of complaints from cruise guests.*

***Spa Tip:*** *Price drops are usually seen on port days, where the mass exodus of passengers going ashore can see the spa devoid of paying clientele. Port day prices extend to closing time so you can still go ashore and nab a 'bargain' once you return.*

# Shopping

The new breed of mega-liners don't miss a trick when it comes to making money, with ships now having several high-end shops, exclusive shopping arcades and premium boutiques onboard, all designed to part you from your money. The major players supplying the cruise retail sector are Starboard Cruise Services, Harding Retail, Gebr, Effy, Heinemann and Dufry Ltd., and they are allocated a significant area of any ship. Marble corridors showcase branded designers who get a shop all to themselves including Bvlgari, Rolex, Breitling, Omega and Michael Kors. From perfume and jewellery to innovative gadgets, there will be something to tempt you and provide the ultimate holiday souvenir.

The main boutique will have an array of brands such as Swarovski, Ray-Ban, Marc Jacobs, Kate Spade and Gucci, as well as cruise apparel. You are also likely to find books and kiddie-friendly plush toys, as well as a convenience section with essentials like shampoo, toothpaste and sunscreens. Another area will house sweet treats and savoury snacks, but you would be wiser to buy these ashore as it will probably be a lot cheaper.

***Shopping Temptation:*** *Throughout your cruise there will be daily 'specials' which will be advertised in your cruise planner.*

All shops onboard promise duty-free prices, and the ever-popular beauty emporium is filled with well-known skincare and cosmetic products, from Estee Lauder and Clinique to Lancôme and Dior. and the latest perfumes and aftershaves on the market, including favourites like Chanel and Hugo Boss. Some of these stores even offer free make-up consultations.

The shipboard hosts will deliver port shopping talks so you can make the most of your time ashore. Avoid buying at front-line port shops as their premium rent costs will be passed onto you; instead, head to the city centre for more reasonably priced gifts.

***Green with Envy:*** *Don't be tempted to buy what looks to be a great deal on an inch of gold. In most cases, it isn't real gold but is actually layered or plated, and has been known to turn green.*

## Duty-free

There are no duty-free shops at any of Southampton's cruise terminals or at any embarkation cruise terminal in the UK, so you'll have to wait until you're onboard before you can start shopping.

The duty-free shops will open shortly after setting sail, as they are not allowed to open while in port, but only if your ship is visiting at least one non-EU destination. Duty-free has a good selection of cigarettes and alcohol, but bear in mind, on most ships, any alcohol purchased from the shop cannot be consumed onboard and will be held until the last night of your cruise.

***Cruise Tip:*** *Most ships do not sell lighters onboard.*

At the end of 1999, UK travellers lost the right to purchase duty-free goods within the European Union after the single market was introduced. Leaving the EU could mean its return, though travellers will probably only get a paltry tax-free allowance. Whatever changes come to pass, the current rules will continue to apply during the 21-month transition period.

Spain has now adopted a 'use and enjoyment' rule on bar and restaurant services enjoyed onboard ships which are berthed or sailing in Spanish waters (within 12 nautical miles of the coast), and on entire itineraries which start in Spain and only call at EU ports. You may have to pay up to 10% extra for any onboard drinks purchases, depending on what cruise line you are with; for example, AIDA and TUI do not pass this fee onto their passengers, as they include VAT in the prices shown onboard.

*Cruise Essential*: *If your cruise visits at least one non-EU destination, such as Gibraltar, Morocco and the Canary Islands, the Spanish tax will no longer be applied for the length of the cruise, just when berthed or sailing in Spanish waters.*

*Spanish Query:* *Even though the Canary Islands are part of Spain, they are outside both the Spanish VAT regime and the EU customs union.*

If your cruise originates from a Spanish port, a 21% IVA tax is applied to all purchases made in the ship's shops, photo gallery and spa. For cruises starting from Italy, the IVA is 22%, and if sailing from Malta, an 18% VAT charge is applied.

*Tax Tip*: *If you have purchased a drink's package in advance, you shouldn't have to pay the Spanish IVA tax.*

*Duty-free Essential:* *Some duty-free shop staff have been known to give out false information, telling guests there are no restrictions on the amount of duty-free goods they can take home, in order to hit their sales targets, knowing that cruise ships do not generally inform guests of their duty-free allowance until the night before disembarkation.*

*Cruise Tip:* *Most ships don't sell loose tobacco and only offer certain brands of cigarettes. A limited number of single packets should be available at the bars onboard.*

## What are the duty-free allowances for British cruisers travelling within the European Union?

You do not have to pay tax and/or duty on goods brought in from the EU as long as you transport them yourself, they are for your own consumption, and tax and/or duty has been paid in the country where you bought them. Technically, there are no limits on the amount of alcohol and tobacco you can bring into the UK from EU countries, but you are more likely to be asked questions if you have more than the amounts listed below:

- 800 cigarettes
- 200 cigars
- 400 cigarillos
- 1 kilogram tobacco
- 110 litres beer

# Life Onboard

- 90 litres wine
- 10 litres spirits
- 20 litres fortified wine (e.g. sherry, port)

***Customs Essential:*** *For the sake of clarity and customs purposes, The Canary Islands, the north of Cyprus, Gibraltar and the Channel Islands are not included as part of the EU.*

**What are the duty-free allowances for British cruisers travelling outside the European Union?**

HM Revenue & Customs stipulate the following allowances if you are transporting goods to or from a country outside of the EU:

- 1 litre of spirits or strong liqueurs over 22% volume **or** two litres of fortified wine (such as port or sherry) **or** sparkling wine **or** any other alcoholic drink that's less than 22% volume
- 200 cigarettes or 100 cigarillos **or** 50 cigars **or** 250 grams of tobacco
- In addition, you may also bring back both of the following:
- 16 litres of beer
- 4 litres of still wine

You can bring in other goods, including perfumes and souvenirs, worth up to £390 without having to pay tax and/or duty. If you are transporting more than €10,000 in cash or cheques outside of the EU, then you must declare you're doing so.

Allowances are subject to change. For more information, contact HM Revenue and Customs on 0845 010 9000, or go to *gov.uk/duty-free-goods*.

***Duty-free Essential:*** *When entering Singapore, if your last port of call was Malaysia, there is no duty-free allowance on alcohol or tobacco.*

Regardless of how lucky you might have been on past holidays, don't believe the myth that customs never bother with cruise ship terminals. There is always a chance of being stopped by customs, wherever you enter the country. Southampton is one of the ports where spot checks happen quite frequently in Southampton, especially following itineraries that visit the Canary Islands, Gibraltar and the Caribbean.

## Photo Gallery

All ships have a team of photographers who happily snap away at every opportunity, from when you first board the ship, to deck parties, formal nights and on the pier at every port of call. Their gallery displays all those photos in the hope that you will want one as a memory of your cruise. Aside from their regular photos, you can book private sessions, either in different areas of the ship or in the dedicated studio. These sessions are often free, and you only pay for the photos you want. Most of the galleries also sell a limited selection of cameras, memory cards and tripods, though, as well as having more choice, it is usually cheaper to buy ashore.

## Onboard Savings

One of the perks of cruising is that you'll never be caught short without your purse or wallet while onboard as all ships operate a cashless system, so any purchases you make will be charged to your onboard account through your SeaPass card. The exception to this is in the casino, where the cashier or dealers will accept cash to purchase chips. The downside to this cashless system is that it's easy to hand over your card unconsciously, without realising how much you are actually spending. The cruise line's main objective is to part you from as much of your money as possible by offering you hundreds of extras while at sea. Of course, you are on holiday, and you don't want to be overly frugal, but you might want to take heed of a few money-saving tips so as not to go overboard with your spending.

**ATM Fees**
ATM fees can add up quickly if you're using your debit or credit cards abroad, but there's an easy way to avoid them if you need cash to use in port. If you have chips left over from the casino, bought through your onboard account, cash them out at the cashier's desk as you will be given the currency the ship uses. This can save you having to withdraw money using either the onboard ATM at guest relations or from a cashpoint in port, all of which will probably incur an inflated charge.

# Life Onboard

### Attend the Port Lectures
While these talks are designed primarily to sell the ship's excursions, they also offer up useful information on the popular things to do in port and they often give away money-saving vouchers to use ashore, as well as spa giveaways.

### Birthdays, Anniversaries and Milestones
Inform guest relations, either prior to your cruise or once onboard, if anyone in your party is celebrating a special birthday, anniversary, a business or personal achievement, a graduation or a wedding proposal, as the ship will usually organise a free cake at dinner and decorate your cabin door. If you want to arrange a cocktail party or candlelit meal as part of the celebrations, the ship's crew will be more than happy to help put your plans in place.

### Buy in Advance
Several cruise lines offer package deals on dining and spa services if purchased before you sail. These are definitely worth looking into, as certain lines give as much as a 25% discount.

### Casino Rewards
The casino will often have spot prizes and giveaways for those using their facilities, including t-shirts, designer handbags or even a free cruise.

### Coffee Stations
Instead of buying hot drinks from an onboard bar or cafe, most ships have complimentary tea and coffee stations in their 24-hour buffet restaurant. Bring an insulated mug from home to keep your drinks warmer for longer and so you can fill up as required, plus it's much better for the environment. For specialty coffees, it might be worth buying a package, especially if you are going to indulge frequently. If you are very picky about your coffee, you can always bring your own.

### Duty-free
Keep an eye out for the 20% discount on cigarettes and alcohol on the first day of your cruise, especially as the deal is not usually repeated.

### Shore Excursions

Consider exploring on your own while in port rather than booking a tour through the ship as cruise lines typically apply a 30-40% mark-up. This is particularly worthwhile if you dock in a city where the main attractions are close by. Going independently also allows you to set your own schedule and soak up the atmosphere at your own pace.

### Free Drinks

There are usually quite a few events onboard that give out free drinks. Certain cruise lines give out a glass of champagne when you first embark, followed closely by a tipple or two at the Captain's Welcome Party. Keep an eye on the daily programme for events that offer a complimentary libation. The spa, jewellery shops, casino and art gallery will often host promotional days with drinks and a free raffle.

### Future Cruise Programme

Most ships will try to tempt you to book your next trip before you've even disembarked, with offers of discounted fares, reduced deposits, onboard credit, no-penalty cancellation, free parking, free internet and free upgrades. Some also let you pay a reduced deposit which can be put towards any cruise which sails within a set period of time. The validity depends on the cruise line, but can typically be applied within a one to three year period. These are often excellent ways of saving money on future cruises as it is unlikely you'll get as many perks through a travel agent. Some cruise lines allow you to cancel these bookings without penalty, so you really have nothing to lose, and if you prefer, the cruise line will even transfer your booking to your travel agent to take advantage of any extras they might offer.

### Gift Cards

There are several companies offering gift cards, including *giftcardspread.com* and *giftcardgranny.com*, at a fraction of their face value, meaning they can be a great way of saving extra money on a cruise booking. Most companies offer a 100% lifetime guarantee never to expire or lose value.

### Gift Certificates

If you've just got married or are about to celebrate a special milestone, cruise line gift certificates (both physical or electronic) are the perfect present

# Life Onboard

to ask for. They can be applied directly to the purchase of a cruise or to onboard services (if you already have one booked), such as one of the specialty restaurants, tour excursions or spa treatments.

## Gratuities
Seabourn, Regent Seven Seas, Silversea Cruises, SeaDream Yacht Club and P&O now include tips in their cruise fares, while others automatically add tips to your onboard account each day. If you wish to adjust the amount or want to pay in cash, visit guest relations and ask them to amend it accordingly.

## Internet
Several cruise lines will offer free time online if you sign up for their internet package. These deals are usually only available on the first day of your cruise, but it's worth keeping an eye on the daily planner for any other special offers during your voyage.

## Juices
Juices are free at breakfast but often cost afterwards. Bring an insulated mug from home so you can fill up at the beverage station in the mornings.

## Laundry
Each stateroom has a laundry list and bag to use if you wish to use the laundry or pressing service. Some lines, including Carnival, Disney, Fred. Olsen, Oceania, P&O, Princess, and Silversea, have self-service laundry facilities across their fleet, while Marella (*Celebration*) and Saga (*Sapphire & Pearl 11*) only offer them on specific ships. The self-service facilities are equipped with washers, dryers, ironing boards and irons, and have detergent for purchase. The washers and dryers are usually coin-operated so try to keep some change handy. On some sailings, special promotions can be offered in the last week of your cruise such as 'fill a bag' - your steward will leave a large paper bag in your cabin, and for a set price, the laundry room will wash all the items you can fit in the bag. Your cabin's shower cubicle will probably have a retractable clothesline for drying smalls so you won't have to use the laundry room just to dry your swimsuit.

> **Don't Ask:**
> Why is this raw! (said to the waiter after ordering steak tartare)

***A Clean Deal:*** *Azamara, Crystal (Serenity & Symphony), Cunard, Regent Seven Sea, Seabourn and Viking Cruises all offer complimentary washing machines, dryers, irons and detergent.*

***A Not So Clean Deal:*** *Celebrity, Costa, Holland America, MSC, Norwegian and Royal Caribbean do not have self-service laundry facilities.*

**Loyalty Programs**

An estimated two-thirds of passengers each year are repeat cruisers, and these loyal stalwarts are rewarded by the cruise line's loyalty tier scheme. There is a whole breadth of inducements, including priority check-in, upgrades, lapel pins, laundry services, onboard discount vouchers, cocktail party invites, priority tender tickets, complimentary nights, and access to an exclusive club for the length of the cruise.

Signing up as a new member is generally a simple process, as you are automatically enrolled on the completion of your first cruise and points are then accrued with every night spent on board. The more you cruise with one line, the higher your loyalty tier and the better the reward. Simply apply your loyalty rewards number when you book your next cruise.

**Lunch**

If you're a fussy eater or on a tight budget, pop back to the ship during a port day and enjoy a free lunch, as opposed to paying for something ashore.

**Mobile Phone**

You'll save yourself a fortune by turning data roaming off on your phone and making use of free Wi-Fi when in port.

**Onboard Credit**

When it comes to onboard credit, the motto is 'use it or lose it'. The guest relation's staff will not offer this perk as cash, so passengers often tend to buy useless and overpriced souvenirs just to use up their credit, however, these is a way to redeem this credit for cash: insert your cruise card into one of the slot machines and load whatever is left of your onboard credit, then simply cash out the funds with the casino cashier. Make sure you do this while at sea as the casino will close once you near a port.

# Life Onboard

**Onboard Shops**
Before you buy anything onboard, check your ship's daily planner for the next scheduled sale. Waiting a few extra days to buy your souvenirs could save you a fortune. It isn't unusual for a 'Blow Out' sale to be held before the end of the cruise, offering substantial savings.

**Photographs**
Don't be tempted into buying every picture the onboard photography team takes, as they will quickly add up. Try to use your own camera or mobile phone, asking fellow passengers to capture a special moment for you if you want to be in the picture. Then, use a website like *freeprints.com* and have up to 500 of your photographs printed for free when you get home.

**Picnic**
Before going ashore for an excursion or just to explore a port, fill up on breakfast items from the buffet: make a few rolls and bring some nibbles like fruit, muffins and biscuits for the road. Shore outings can mean long days and it isn't always possible to buy a snack when you want one, especially if you have children with you. Fill up an insulated mug if you need to take mediation en-route or just in case you get thirsty.

**Seasickness**
If you feel slightly under the weather, Guest Relations or the medical centre will usually provide complimentary seasickness medication.

**Shopping Programme**
Gem sales and high-end jewellery are massive industries in the Caribbean, and most of the larger cruise ships host a shopping scheme led by specialist consultants who work for independent American companies rather than the cruise line. These companies pay considerable premiums to secure contracts at sea, allowing them to implement their shopping program onboard the ship.

Throughout the cruise, the consultants will give lectures disguised as port talks that recommend where you should shop. The high standards that are claimed cannot be tested, nor can their reputation, and while the consultant will have you believe that every dealer has been carefully checked to ensure they meet certain standards, the bottom line is that the shop has paid for the privilege of making the 'approved' list. The consultants will offer scare tactics to tourists about the dangers of shopping elsewhere and of getting ripped off, and will repeatedly use phrases like 'guarantee', 'high end' and 'best prices', but as always there is usually a drawback. If a deal seems too good to be true, then it probably is.

Forewarned is forearmed and while the Caribbean does offer fantastic gems and prices, don't feel intimidated by the onboard shopping consultants into only looking in the shops that they have recommended. Shop around and if you do want to invest in a costly purchase, make sure it comes with an international guarantee.

Wherever you shop, you must learn to haggle. In many countries and cultures, bartering is a way of life, and you'll be pleasantly surprised at what a vendor will actually accept. It is extremely difficult to haggle for something if the shopkeeper knows you or your partner desperately wants an item, so put on your best poker face and play nonchalant. Once you've looked at an object, put it back on the display shelf and feign a lack of interest. The vendor's eyes will have seen dollar signs the minute you picked the item up, and they will start by offering a highly inflated price, which will quickly spiral down to more realistic levels. In fact, you could even try walking towards the exit, as it is very unlikely that you will make it to the door without a further onslaught of bargaining. Once you are happy with the price, be gracious and accept with a smile.

***Be Aware:*** *Many guests feel comforted by the 30-day return guarantee if purchasing jewellery on the ship, but the small print often states that you must contact a third-party agent to claim a refund. Once you're home and a problem arises with your purchase, you'll find that neither the company that hosts the shopping program or the cruise line will help.*

**Souvenirs**
The prices you pay in the shops onboard the ship for souvenirs are usually inflated, the cruise line taking advantage of having a captive audience, but if you wait and buy your holiday keepsakes ashore, you stand to save a small fortune.

**Spa Orientation**
Your first day onboard can be bewildering to say the least, and every department is aimed at coveting your business during your cruise, whether

that be selling drinks packages, reservations at specialty restaurants, casino lessons or wine tasting seminars. The spa and wellness centre offer a tour of their facilities which ends with a facial or massage demonstration. Stick your hand up quickly and volunteer to be the 'demo' person to receive a free treatment while your fellow passengers look on in envy. Raffle tickets are also often given out on arrival and prizes given out at the end of the induction.

**Spa Promotions**
If you fancy being pampered with the latest in massage therapies but don't want to pay full price then wait until the ship is in port. With most of the passengers disembarking the ship en masse, the beauty salon, spa and hairdresser will generally be empty and so will offer up to 50% off bookings. You can go ashore, but by disembarking just a few hours later or returning a couple of hours earlier to accommodate for your appointment time, you'll still be able to take advantage of the special offers.

**Specialty Restaurants**
Specialty restaurants usually incur a surcharge, but you can often find off-peak deals, including 2-for-1, half-price menus, or a free appetiser or dessert. These special rates often apply on the first night of a cruise when most passengers are getting their bearings or if the ship includes an overnight stop in port. Some cruise lines offer a dining bundle on the first day that could save you a lot of money over the course of the cruise if you plan to eat at the specialty restaurants frequently.

**Toiletries and Incidentals**
If you find you've left your sunscreen at home or that you didn't pack spare batteries or memory cards for your camera, hold off on buying replacements until you're in port as ship prices are generally extremely high in comparison to what you'll find ashore.

**Travel Reward Points**
Collecting travel reward points can offer loads of bonuses and free trips. Make sure you apply for an appropriate credit card before you board the ship and simply register it to your onboard account on embarkation so your final cruise bill will be charged to it. During your cruise, buy as much casino credit as you can afford, don't gamble with any of it, and simply cash it out before the

end of your holiday. Once home, use the cash to pay your credit card bill immediately, so you don't incur any interest charges. In doing this, you will have racked up hundreds of free rewards on your credit card for spending absolutely nothing.

**Voucher Codes (**_vouchercodes.co.uk_**)**
More than 5000 codes are offered each day on the Voucher Codes website, including money-off vouchers and promotional codes to use on cruises, excursions, hotels, restaurants and airport car parking. Even better, the company guarantees every single one of them works.

**Water**
Buying bottled water from the ship can be expensive. Most lines allow you to bring aboard water purchased from a port of call where it is often much cheaper.

**Wine**
Cruise lines make a large profit on alcohol and apply a strict policy preventing guests from bringing locally purchased alcohol onboard to drink during the cruise. If you do try to bring some onboard, it will be confiscated and given back on the last day of your holiday. That being said, some lines will allow you to bring one or two bottles of wine (750ml) or champagne onto the ship at the beginning of the voyage - drinking it in the restaurant will incur a corkage charge, but you can enjoy it in your cabin for free. The exception is Costa, who doesn't allow any alcohol to be brought on board at any time.

Ordering wine by the glass is, as usual, far more expensive than ordering by the bottle, and because your waiter will happily cork and keep your wine for your next meal, there's little reason not to buy by the bottle. You can even ask for it from a different restaurant - just request it the next time you want wine with your meal and your waiter will find it for you.

# Onboard Apps

The app market has exploded in the last few years and there are quite literally hundreds that can enhance your cruise experience and entertain you. Split into two categories, the first is for the shutterbug enthusiast. It's been said that a photograph is worth a thousand words and these apps will help you to enhance your photography and video skills and help capture that perfect moment. The second section is there purely to help you catch your breath, chill and relax.

### Pixlr
Create incredible photos with over two million combinations of effects, overlays, and filters. Remove blemishes and red-eye, smooth skin, or whiten teeth with simple tools for fantastic results. Turn your picture into a pencil drawing, an ink sketch, or a poster, add text and share your masterpiece on your favourite social networks.

### PicsKit – Free Photo Art Effects Editor
An all-in-one photo editor enabling you to create fabulous designs with full-featured tools including 100+ filter effects, a collage and grid maker, colour splash, dispersion effects, and pixel effect dispersion.

### Trips by Lonely Planet
Upload your photos and videos, have them turned into visual stories with maps and time and place data, then share your travel experiences with friends and loved ones.

### Flipagram
Create amazing videos using your own selfies and photos, and even add your favourite music to the end result. Create slideshows, transitions, and apply filters, and effects to your masterpiece, before sharing it with your friends.

### Instagram
Offers a simple way to capture and share your favourite holiday memories. Edit your photos and videos with filters and creative tools and combine multiple clips into one video before connecting with your friends and followers.

### TouchNote
Design and send physical cards of your travel photos straight from your phone to anywhere in the world. Pick your favourite snap, personalise it with photo filters, travel stickers, customisable stamps and a personal message, and it will be printed and sent off on your behalf.

## Postagram
Personalise, print and send any photo you take while away to friends and family anywhere in the world for just $.99.

## FreePrints
Get up to 500 free 6x4 photo prints every year with no subscription or commitment. Just select the photos you want to print from your phone, Facebook or Instagram, choose your paper, and your free prints will be delivered to your door within days, for just the price of delivery.

## PressReader by Newspaper Direct
Stay connected with the stories you love with unlimited access to thousands of magazines and newspapers from around the world. Catch a story the minute it hits the newsstands and set automatic downloads so you never miss an issue.

## City Papers
Access more than 3000 English-language newspapers worldwide, read the local paper in the country you're visiting and keep your finger on the pulse even whilst away (Android users use World Newspapers).

## Fishes: Greater Caribbean
This resource helps identify 1,693 species of fish, with the help of more than 8,200 colour photos. Search using common generic names, location and fish features (shape, colour, pattern). Each species has its own page with information, including its form, colour, size, habitat and depth-range.

## Star Walk
Tilt your smartphone or iPad skywards and see which stars, satellites, and constellations you're looking at. Just tap on the screen to unveil the names of the stars and grab a screenshot to email or share on social media.

## Cruise Tycoon
If you've ever wanted to run your own cruise company, this game gives you the tools to buy ships, hire a captain and set a sailing schedule. Train your crew, increase passenger satisfaction and expand your empire.

## Ship Visits

In the past it was possible to board a vessel temporarily if you knew someone who was sailing, but due to increased security onboard, friends and relatives are no longer allowed to visit the ship unless they are on the passenger manifest. Some ships allow wedding personnel and guests for an onboard ceremony and lunch, but of course, they must disembark before the ship sails.

## Port Calls

Cruise ships usually arrive in port first thing in the morning, and the vessel has to wait to be cleared by port officials. Passengers who have pre-booked one of the ship's shore excursions will be asked to meet up in one of the public areas and are usually the first people allowed off, together with suite guests and anyone with a priority pass. People with special needs can enjoy ports of call, but a companion or caregiver should accompany them. How you choose to explore is up to you, and while your first option might have been a shore excursion, if your cruise line doesn't cater for the disabled, you'll be left to make alternative arrangements. explore by yourself.

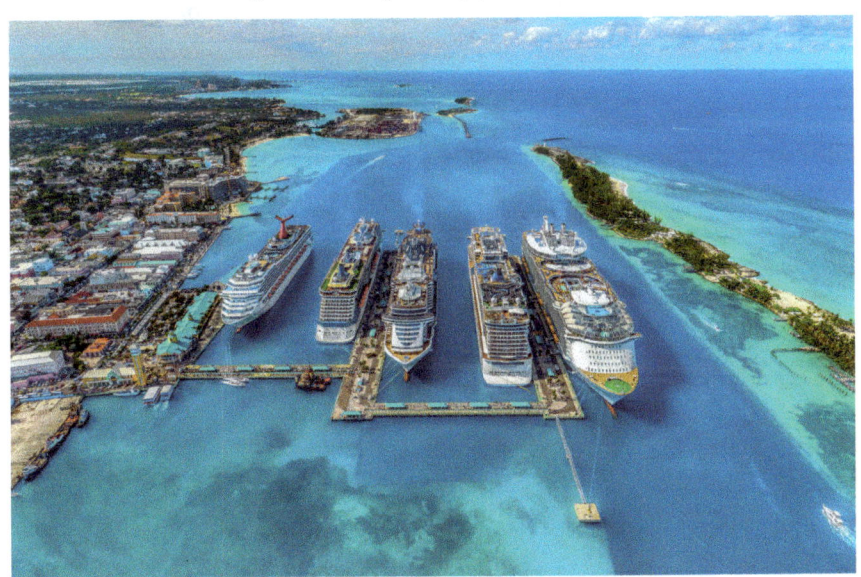

*Credit: Nassau, Bahamas - Fernando Jorge, Unsplash*

# The Autonomous Cruiser

Sometimes your ship will dock minutes from the town centre and its amenities, other times you might find yourself in an industrial port, where more often than not, walking is not allowed, and if that is the case, the port authority will lay on a free shuttle to take you to the port gates. Every effort is made by the cruise lines to supply wheelchair-accessible shuttle buses in every port, but unfortunately, it isn't always possible as it is dependent on the destination, location of the berth, how many other ships are in port on the same day and the availability of adapted vehicles. The majority of ports have a host of taxis waiting at the quayside or by the port exit, but there is no guarantee there will be any that are wheelchair-accessible. Most will be able to carry a collapsible chair in the boot (sometimes for a charge), but you'll be required to transfer into the taxi unassisted. If there are no suitable cabs, go to Guest Relations and ask if they can secure an accessible vehicle for you.

***Transport Tip:*** *If using public transport, always buy a return train or bus ticket so you won't have to queue again on the way back.*

If you pre-booked an excursion with an independent tour operator, they will be waiting on the pier for you with a sign bearing your name. If, on the other hand, you did not reserve anything before arriving in port, don't despair as there are usually dozens of vendors standing near the pier or at the port exit offering tours around the area.

***Excursion Warning:*** *Certain ports like Civitavecchia are more than an hour away from the main attractions of Rome, and Warnemunde is nearly three hours away from Berlin so if you are at all worried about the time constraints of independent travel it is best to book an excursion through your ship or a reputable company. Travelling under your own steam can be risky with public transport especially as punctuality is not a strong point of the train service to and from Rome.*

***Tour Tip:*** *If you have a hearing impairment, ask your tour guide to use a transmitter microphone, which will allow you to listen to the narrative over radio waves via your hearing aid's receiver.*

## Port Disembarkation

Staff will be able to provide wheelchair or arm assistance from the top to the bottom of the gangway, but only when and where it's safe to do so. Apart from tendering restrictions, there will also be a few occasions when a wheelchair or scooter user may not be able to disembark the vessel because of tidal variance. Ships use a variety of gangway configurations to cope with tidal conditions, some of which are not suitable for those with mobility impairments.

Certain ports of call have a substantial tidal variance, resulting in a significant height difference between the quay and the gun-port doors, making the gangway too steep for the safe passage of wheelchairs or mobility scooters. The ship's daily planner will have restrictive tidal times displayed for a particular port, and announcements are usually made advising passengers of the times to avoid when embarking or disembarking the vessel. In certain circumstances, it might mean a wheelchair or scooter user cannot alight the ship at all.

Whichever port you dock at, there will be a significant number of souvenir shops and stalls selling everything from postcards and novelty t-shirts to local sauces, either on the quayside or in the terminal. Just remember that any alcohol purchased in the terminal's duty-free shop will be confiscated when you re-board the vessel and won't be given back to you until the last night of the cruise.

**Insect Bite Risks:** *Insect bites and stings are common when travelling, especially mosquito bites, which are responsible for spreading malaria, dengue, chikungunya and Zika, to name just a few. Don't think they are confined to exotic countries, the dengue virus has, in recent years, been reported in France, Madeira, Portugal and Spain. DEET, an insect repellent that is used in several products, is said to be the most effective in preventing bites, but if you are allergic to the formula or overwhelmed by the strong smell, Sawyer Permethrin is an alternative that creates a mosquito barrier and actually kills ticks, mosquitoes, chiggers, mites and more than 55 other kinds of insects on contact. Unlike DEET it is odourless and won't stain or damage your clothing or any plastics. For those that prefer plant-based products, you might try 'Mosi-Guard' which contains lemon eucalyptus oil. Wrist and ankle bands soaked in an insecticide can provide protection for days. If you are prone to being bitten, wear clothing that covers as much of your body as possible and spray yourself all over with insecticide, not forgetting any exposed areas like your wrists, ankles and feet. Bites tend to blister and can be itchy, but they usually go away in a few days if you can resist the itch - apply something like Eurax to help ease the itching for up to ten hours. Most bites are not all that serious, but travellers should take extra care as they could suffer an allergic reaction or the area could become infected; if in doubt see a doctor.*

***Transport Tip:*** *Negotiate and agree on a price before you get in a taxi and make sure it is for everyone and not per person. If you require a round-trip transfer don't pay for both journeys upfront, but pay for each separately.*

***Time Watch:*** *The most important thing to take with you is your ship's daily planner as it will advertise the times you are in port, the 'all-aboard' time and the port agent's contact details.*

Unless your ship specifically requests it, never take your passport ashore but instead carry a photocopy. Some people also keep a photograph on their phone in case of an emergency. Minimise the amount of jewellery you wear, as all ports carry the risk of pickpockets and wearing something obviously expensive can make you a target.

***Taboo:*** *Government guidelines at most ports worldwide prohibit you from bringing plants, fruit or any non-packaged foods either off or onto the ship.*

For passengers with autism, port days are excellent opportunities to remain on the ship and take advantage of the lack of people onboard, offering you the chance to fully enjoy some of the usually crowded parts of the ship. If you do venture ashore, the best tours are free walking tours that usually leave the town's tourist office at a set time each day. They are not usually overcrowded, and you have the option of leaving at any time. Be aware of the tell-tale signs of sensory overload so you can stop the activities for the day in favour of a cooling down period and quiet time.

Hot climates can lead to heat exhaustion, the body's inability to cool itself, which isn't usually serious, but can lead to sun or heat stroke, both of which can, at worst, prove fatal if not properly or promptly treated. Overheating the body leads to fluid loss through sweating and can cause headaches, nausea, faintness and clammy skin. Dark urine is a sure sign that you are dehydrated, so make sure to drink plenty of water and avoid alcohol and direct sunlight.

When cruising to Norway, the Arctic and Antarctic, it is important to take exposure precautions if going outside for a long period, especially against hypothermia, the body's inability to produce enough energy to heat itself. Elderly, frail and wheelchair-bound passengers are especially susceptible, because they tend to have impaired mobility or might not be able to communicate exactly how they physically feel, so it is important to retain as much inner core heat as possible by dressing correctly. The head, neck, sides of the chest, armpits and groin need extra protection as they tend to lose heat more quickly than other parts of the body. Layering is a very effective way of protecting the body against the cold as warm air becomes trapped between the layers and acts as insulation. Your feet, hands, nose and cheeks are vulnerable to frostnip, the early sign of frostbite, so it is essential to wear insulated gloves and waterproof footwear and cover the head and neck to prevent heat loss because of extreme cold exposure. If symptoms do occur, such as shivering, confusion or numbness of the hands or feet, move inside or take sheltered cover, remove any wet clothing, stamp your feet and move your arms in circles to create heat, and drink a warm sugary non-alcoholic beverage.

# Tendering Protocol

With more and more super-liners on the high seas than ever before, it isn't always possible for your ship to berth in a port of call, sometimes because of the sheer weight of port traffic and often because the vessel is simply too big. In these instances, the ship will anchor just offshore and small boats, typically carrying 100 people at a time, will transport passengers free of charge to the quayside. These boats are referred to as tenders, and it's usually the ship's lifeboats that make the short journey across to the shore, though on occasion the cruise lines are required to use the port's local shuttle boats.

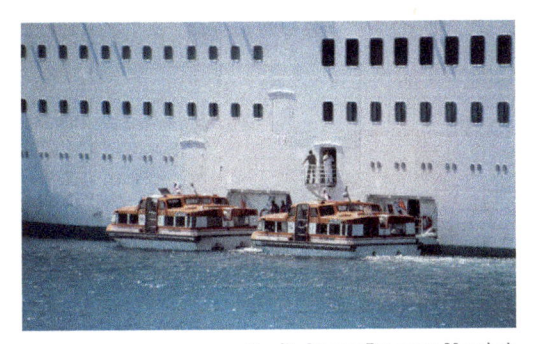

*Credit: Jeremy Bezanger, Unsplash*

***Cruise Tip:*** *Appropriate non-slip footwear should be worn for accessing the tender.*

Due to the sheer number of passengers onboard any chosen vessel, a ticket system will be put in place for those wanting to get off the ship early. Information on the times and procedures will be printed in your daily cruise planner. Some cruise lines issue Priority Tender Tickets as perks to specific guests, often those in suites and members of their Loyalty Club. If you are entitled to one, your tickets will be delivered to your cabin the night before the ship docks in port.

**Cruise Tip:** *If you have booked an independent excursion in a tender port, allow plenty of time to disembark and meet the tour operator.*

Once the majority of guests have gone ashore and tender congestion has dissipated, an announcement will be made over the ship's tannoy system declaring 'open tender', meaning passengers no longer require a ticket to disembark and can get off at their leisure. Vacating a ship can take as long as three hours depending on how many passengers are onboard, how many tender boats are in operation, the length of the journey to the quayside and the conditions of the sea.

**Cruise Tip:** *Book an excursion through your ship to avoid the tender queues as it'll give you priority disembarkation.*

There is no ticket system in operation for returning to the ship. You simply go back to where you alighted earlier, show your cruise card and wait for the next available tender. There will almost always be a queue, but if you don't like crowds, it might be wise to avoid particularly busy periods such as lunchtime, when those on a budget rush back for the free buffet. Also, seeing as most guests like to maximise their time ashore, it's common for the tender service to be congested an hour before the back-on-board time. If you want to avoid a queue altogether, you can try to catch the last tender, but do so at your own risk!

## Don't Miss the Ship

With all there is to do in some ports it can be easy to lose track of time but it is important that you know what time you have to be back on board your vessel as the ship will not wait for you. On arrival in port, announcements will be made informing you when the ship has cleared customs and what the 'back onboard' time is. The time will also be printed in your ship's daily planner and on signs at the gangway. Tender ports will also clearly state what time the last tender leaves.

# Life Onboard

***Cruise Tip:*** *Take a photograph of the 'back onboard' time on your mobile phone or camera and set an alarm on your phone to act as a reminder.*

You should always set your watch or mobile phone to 'ship time' as it is not always the same as the local time in port. Not doing so is the number one reason people miss the ship and it is simply not possible for the captain to wait for latecomers. You should also take note of exactly which port you are docked at or you could run into trouble. One couple went exploring in Stockholm and caught a taxi back to the port, except they were taken to the wrong one (the city is spread across 14 islands with three different ports). It took 40 minutes and an expensive cab fare to get them back to the ship, and with only minutes to spare.

> **Don't Ask:**
> The photographer took my picture, how will I know which one is mine?

***Medication Alert:*** *Always carry enough medication for your time ashore.*

There are numerous reasons why the ship can't wait for latecomers, and while the captain has the last word, their decision is not based on a whim. They have to take into consideration extra port charges, fees for harbour workers, payment for additional security and the costs of burning more fuel to make up for lost time. If there are two or three ships in port and your ship's scheduled slot time is missed, the captain will have to wait for the pilot to allocate another. There are even more considerations as to whether to wait for late passengers, including tidal times for both the departure and the arrival at the next port, impending weather conditions and if another vessel coming into the harbour requires the berth. Finally, waiting will also mean the shops and casino will have to remain closed for longer, adding up to even more lost revenue.

If someone is thought to be missing after the 'back onboard' time, several announcements will be made to make sure the guest isn't onboard, as on occasion, cruise cards don't register when they're swiped coming back onboard. If there is no response, a crew member will be dispatched to check the passenger's cabin. Once the decision is made to sail, the ship's crew will often remove the guest's essential items – passport, medication, or money – and leave them with the port agent.

Although there is a 30-minute gap between the onboard time and departure, don't assume you will be allowed back on the ship just because you make it back before the ship has actually left. The crew will invariably have lifted the gangway and released ropes, and it's not easy to reverse the process. Also, once the 'back onboard' time has passed, port security will usually close the gates, making the quay inaccessible.

In the unlikely event you do miss the ship, go to the cruise terminal and make contact with the port agent, who will be in constant contact with the vessel. Items such as your passport or medications might have been handed over to a ground representative just before sailing, so you will need to retrieve them. The agent will help work out the logistics of either getting you back to the ship at the next port or arranging transport back to your home country, and can assist in booking a hotel, an onward ferry, taxi or flight. The cruise line's customer service department, your travel agent or insurance company might also be able to help with onward plans. The cruise line is not financially liable if you miss the vessel, so getting to the next port of call or travelling home will be at your own expense. As such, don't get off the ship without a debit or credit card, as you can't know how much a flight, overnight accommodation or a lengthy taxi ride might cost.

*Cruise Essential*: *Make sure you know where your ship is docking next.*

If you haven't got the required identification papers, you can't contact the ship or cruise line and can't speak the local language, you will need to contact the local embassy who might be able to help you catch up with your ship. If you come to the conclusion that the trip is a washout and decide to go home, you'll have to make arrangements with the cruise line to have your luggage forwarded, which might incur another hefty fee.

# Port Apps

*With so many apps available it's difficult to know which are actually useful and which are gimmicky, so here's a selection of some of the best to help you make the most of your time in port.*

**Safer Travel Caroline's Rainbow Foundation**
This free app does not rely on international roaming to work and offers maps and essential information for over 350 travel destinations around the globe,

and even advises you of places to avoid. Travellers can access emergency numbers for their location, find out where hospitals are, locate the nearest embassy, or even find the closest tourist office.

## World Clock – Time Zones
Organise your favourite cities onto one page so that you can easily find out the correct local time and the most relevant time zone information for every city in the world. Choose from five clock designs and the format you want your clocks to run on.

## Weather Pro
Weather reports for well over two million locations, giving you access to cloud formations, atmospheric pressure, wind speed and humidity.

## Dark Sky
Accurate down-to-the-minute forecasts of hyperlocal weather information enabling you to pinpoint exactly when the rain will start or stop, right where you're standing. The app includes a full 24-hour forecast, a detailed seven-day forecast, current conditions, multiple saved locations, historical data, and weather maps.

## LinGo
A fun way to learn essential foreign phrases. There is also a tip calculator and currency converter, while the premium version offers audio lessons and a live translator, helping you to converse in 180 languages.

## iTranslate Voice & Text Translator
Just talk into your phone and this app will immediately reply in any of 90 languages. This app is excellent for translating everyday conversations, traffic signs, maps, and local news. You can even send translations via email, SMS, Twitter or Facebook.

## Google Translate
This service provides a quick translation for 103 languages you might come across on your travels. Hold your camera up to any text, like a sign or a menu, and Google will translate it for you instantly. Two-way conversation is available in 32 languages.

## Google Maps

Navigate over 220 countries and territories, with hundreds of millions of businesses and places shown on the map. Get real-time GPS navigation, traffic and transit information, and explore local neighbourhoods by knowing where to eat, drink or locate cash in a foreign port. You can even browse some places in first person to see if they're wheelchair-accessible.

## Maplets

Maplets is the perfect complement to Google Maps, with maps of national parks, state parks, the metro, subway systems, bike routes, rail trails, ski resorts, college campuses, zoos, and theme parks.

## Sygic Travel Maps

Build your own day-to-day itinerary with an easy-to-use trip planner. See estimated travel times and walking distances. The perfect companion for any tourist looking for the best attractions, such as cafés, restaurants, museums, parks, beaches, waterfalls, caves or even bird observatories. The most popular places come with descriptions, photos, opening hours, and admission fees.

## XE Currency

Features a currency converter with live rates (when connected to the internet) for every country, and which stores the rates for when you can't access the internet. Transfer money in 65 currencies to over 170 countries, receive notifications on your transfers, and keep an eye on up to ten currencies of your choice.

## ATM Locator/Cash Machine Finder

This extremely reliable app scans multiple current databases to instantly locate the nearest ATM in any foreign location.

## Mastercard Nearby

This powerful app lets you search for more than two million ATMs in 200+ countries. You can set different filters, including the name of your financial institution, no surcharges, no access fee, chip-enabled, drive-through, or 24-hour service. You can also get a list of local retailers that offer cashback.

## Life Onboard

### Find Near Me
Are you looking for the closest hotel, cinema, petrol station, café or taxi rank? This app works worldwide, with results that will include the facility's rating, website, address, phone number, images, its distance from your current location, user reviews, working hours and price levels.

### Musement
Book tickets in over 1000 cities across 70 countries for any sporting event, museum, attraction, or experience, instantly and securely. Build itineraries, save your favourite activities and source the best, most authentic local experiences.

### TripAdvisor
Get practically all the information you could possibly need on any port, from the most popular things to see and the best places to eat, to the top bars to visit and the most swish spas to pamper yourself. With thousands of reviews, locations and photos, you can search and book tours, attractions and experiences at any port in the world.

### Viator Tours & Activities
This app enables you to book 200,000+ amazing tours, activities, travel experiences, tour guides and private sightseeing trips around the world. Get vouchers, mobile tickets, exclusive deals and instant booking confirmation. Read millions of reviews and photos, watch videos of the top activities and get a sneak peek before you go.

### Cool Cousin
Discover incredible places with reliable city guides who are passionate about their native lands and happy to share their insider tips. Get travel advice from trusted locals who share your interests and will help you find the things you want to do, not just what the guidebooks recommend.

### Culture Trip
Discover unique cultural experiences from design, photography and street art experiences, to ethnic food tours, underground history, and sightseeing from local experts in 450+ destinations. This app lets you explore and discover the best things to do wherever you are.

# The Autonomous Cruiser

**Wefi**
A massive network of hundreds of millions of hotspots that helps you find and connect to the best Wi-Fi hotspot anywhere across the globe.

**Triposo**
This app works offline and delivers recommendations for three million points of interest across 50,000 destinations, covering hotels, transport, activities, food, nightlife, sights and attractions. You'll also find it has a currency converter, phrasebooks, weather forecasts and extensive information about local wildlife, festivals, food and culture.

**Port Shopping Guide**
Available on both Celebrity and Royal Caribbean, this handy port shopping app covers every store in every port. It comes with descriptions, insider deals and an interactive map, so you know where to get the best brand-name deals, sought-after jewels and unique souvenirs.

**Open Table**
Discover, explore, book and manage restaurant bookings instantly, anywhere in the world. You can search with dozens of filters, including neighbourhood, cuisine, price and rating, so you can narrow your search to find the perfect eatery from their 52,000+ restaurants. Sneak a look at menus, photos and reviews, and find a jewel near you.

## Travel Scams

One way to ruin a great holiday is to have your wallet or mobile phone stolen while in port. Despite this, a lot of holiday travellers don't seem to be as vigilant abroad as when they are at home. Scammers are continually devising new and varied ways to make money from unsuspecting tourists, but their schemes usually fall into any of three categories: overcharging for goods, deceiving or coercing you into paying for a service you don't want, and outright theft. You might read this and think you could never be suckered in by an obvious ploy, but you'd be shocked at how many tourists fall victim to even the most common scams.

The main criterion for a safe and happy day out is to be observant and take stock of your surroundings. Never engage in conversations with strangers and don't accept an invitation to go to their house for tea, a bar for a drink or to their brother's shop. Don't let your guard down when it comes to protecting your possessions just because you're on holiday.

## ATM Scams

Be extremely careful in tourist-heavy areas when using an ATM as your money could be whipped out of your hand almost as soon as it is dispensed. Thieves may also watch as you key in your PIN, steal your card and empty your account before you can contact your bank. Thieves may not necessarily take your card by force, instead someone might tap you on the shoulder to ask a seemingly innocent question or offer to help you as you try to find the language setting, using the distraction to slip your card or cash away without you even realising. Try to use ATMs inside a bank whenever possible and always cover the keypad when you enter your PIN. If someone near an ATM looks suspicious, find another machine or come back later.

You should also do your best to make sure any ATM you use hasn't been tampered with. Some scammers rig the machine so that it swallows your card and will retrieve it once you've stormed off into the bank, and some will attach an almost invisible device that will read off your card details without you even knowing. First off, watch someone else take money out of the machine first and make sure they get their card back before starting your transaction, then when it's your turn, feel around the card feeder to make sure there's no easily removed device that shouldn't be there

**ATM Con:** *Hidden cameras might be recording your PIN, so always cover the keypad with your other hand.*

## Baby Scam

Someone, often a lone female, carrying a baby in a blanket will approach you and without warning will throw the child into your arms or drop the baby in front of you. Accomplices will then grab your valuables amid the confusion. After the thieves run away, you'll quickly discover that the baby is just a doll or some other inanimate object.

## Bag/Luggage Scam

Be careful if a pretty girl asks you to look after her shopping bags while she uses the coffee shop toilet as she may be part of a scam. While 'in the toilet' a stranger will approach the girl's table and take her bags. This is a distraction technique, and it usually sees you, the mark, give chase. Meanwhile, another member of the scam team has lifted all your personal belongings that you have left unattended on your table.

### Bar/Café Scam
Single male travellers are a common target of scammers, using attractive young women to entice them to a local drinking hole or café. TheySll order several drinks, but by the time the exorbitant bill comes, the women have long gone.

### Broken Camera
A 'tourist' may ask you to take their photo at a busy sightseeing location, and as you return the camera, which will almost always be worthless, they'll mishandle it and ultimately drop it. Causing a scene, they'll blame you, saying you were at fault and demand the money to pay for the damage.

### Closed Attraction
Your taxi driver may suddenly inform you that the tourist attraction you want to visit is closed for renovation or a religious holiday, or it isn't worth your time. Instead, they may offer an attractive alternative, but it will invariably be more expensive, and the driver will receive a kickback for taking you there.

### Cruise Ship Auctions
Not all ships have their own art gallery, but most of the super-liners do, with auctioneers that work for a land-based auction house that rent the space from the cruise line. These companies pay considerable premiums to secure contracts with the cruise lines that allow them to run their art auctions onboard the ship.

What you might think is investment-grade, collectable art, is often actually industrial inkjet printed copies, euphemistically called *giclée*. Because the auctions take place at sea, it is difficult to research a piece of art or check that the auctioneer is actually licensed. Since the sales are conducted on a respectable cruise line, passengers are lulled into a false sense of security and don't consider that the artwork might be misrepresented, and since the sales are conducted in international waters, they are exempt from any consumer protection or fraud laws.

The artwork is usually displayed before a big event, and once it comes up for sale, a successful bidder will find that they haven't actually purchased the one which was on display, but instead a similar piece that they'll later find out is only worth a fraction of the purchase price. Furthermore, the winning bidder won't even be able to carry the artwork off the ship; it will be shipped from the company's warehouse in the States at huge expense. All this would be a painful lesson in itself, but the rub isn't over, as Customs and Excise are likely to seize the package en-route, requiring the payment of exorbitant fees for them to release it.

***Did You Know:*** *Because of outlandish prices and hard-sell tactics, onboard art auctions are the second-largest source of complaints from cruise guests, after spas.*

The problem stems from the point registration. Flyers are mailed to every cabin offering free champagne and lithographs just for attending the auction, and those that want the freebie are presented with a registration form that has to be signed in order to participate. The back of this form is an overcrowded lengthy screed of terms and conditions that few bother to read before signing, meaning once you've made a bid after getting caught up in all the excitement, you'll have very little recourse against any excess charges.

'Shill bidders', a term for stooges who bid on an auction to inflate its price, are often used, and it's also common practice for a buyer to be stung with additional fees. Surprise costs like appraisal fees, added sales tax, shipping, handling and insurance bills, and the price of framing, all add to your original bid, so you end up paying a lot more than you expected or offered.

If you search the internet, you will find it littered with articles implying that these auctions are little more than high-end scams, and that the auction houses use deceptive ruses to part you from your money. Several auction companies have been outed for shady practices, and the huge amount of passenger complaints is in part why some cruise lines have removed the auctions at sea completely.

## Crying Child
A lone, seemingly distraught child may approach you and says they are lost. The parent will suddenly appear and thank you, meanwhile, the child will be lifting your wallet or purse as you're distracted.

## Dual Menus
Bars and restaurants flaunt low prices on menu boards outside their establishment in an effort to lure tourists in, but when the bill arrives, it may

cost far more than you had anticipated. There is little point arguing as they will produce a menu reflecting the inflated prices and insist you pay. Some eateries don't display any prices at all, leaving the staff to charge whatever they want. A variation of this scam is being offered the 'dish of the day' which is not on any menu and, once again, you will be stung because you didn't ask for the price before ordering.

**Fake Drowning**
Whilst on the beach you might spot someone who appears to be in trouble in the water. Your instincts will kick in, and you'll run to help the person in distress, only to come back to find your possessions, which you left unattended, have disappeared.

**Fake Police**
Some of the most popular cruise ports are rife with drugs, with locals that will openly offer them for sale. A common scam will simulate this, during which people appearing to be local police will approach you, flashing their fake badges. They may insist you hand over your passport and wallet then and there, or they might ask you to walk with them to the police station so they can verify who they are. Never hand over your passport or wallet; tell them it's on the ship and that they will have to escort you through security at the terminal. Most of the time, they'll disappear.

**Fake Tickets**
Taxi drivers may offer to sell you attraction tickets at a discounted price, or they'll tell you they have a partner with an excursion desk on the roadside. Beware, as the tickets may be fake, and by the time the venue has refused you entry the taxi driver will be long gone.

**Fake Wi-Fi Hotspots**
Wi-Fi is freely available in most busy ports, but some of those free connections can be high-risk when it comes to protecting your identity. Hackers set up unsecured hotspots in public locations, and once you're connected, your personal information, passwords, online accounts, and other sensitive information will be transmitted back to the hackerWs computer. Always use a café, coffee shop or cruise terminal connection to ensure it is an official hotspot. It might cost you a cup of coffee, but it's a small price to pay for digital privacy.

# Life Onboard

**Free Souvenirs**

This scam is gradually widening its net to include most countries, but is currently most prominent in Egypt. A trader may approach you and place something in their hand or tie something in a double knot around your wrist, telling you it's a gift. They'll then demand money and will cause a scene if you refuse, in the hope you'll hand over some cash just to get rid of them.

**Gold Ring Scam**

Often found on the streets of Paris and Lisbon, scammers hang out near places like the Eiffel Tower and the Monument to the Discoveries and pretend to find a 'valuable' gold ring. They'll offer to sell it to you for a ridiculously low price, but it is in fact worthless.

**Group Photo Opportunity**

A local will offer to take a group shot in a busy tourist location, and while you are busy organising yourselves, the local has made tracks with your expensive mobile phone or camera. If you want a photo memory of your group, ask a local business owner or someone you recognise from the ship - there are hundreds of them in port.

**Map Scam**

A seemingly smart-looking couple will ask for directions as they are 'lost' and while distracting you with the map, other members of the con will snatch your wallet or bag.

**Medical Emergency**

Don't give out details of your trip on Facebook or other social media platforms. Doing so alerts scammers to the fact that you will be away, something your friends would also know. The hacker will then gain access to your email account and send pleading messages to your friends or relatives requesting funds be wired to you for some desperate reason while you're abroad, with reasons varying from being mugged to a medical emergency. Before you travel, tell your network of friends and family never to wire you money abroad, and that if there were a need for emergency funds, you'll ring them first. Better yet, agree on a codeword or phrase that you'll include in an email.

### Milk Powder

In some countries, including India, you'll see lots of people begging in the streets, but sometimes instead of asking for money, they'll plead for items like milk powder for their babies. You'll perhaps even follow them to a local shop where you can purchase an overpriced product and hand it over. Once you have left, the milk powder will be given back, and the vendor will split the profit with the 'beggar'.

### Mopeds

Always keep your handbag on your person, and don't place it or your shopping bags on a chair next to you if you decide to sit down, as moped riders whisk through the street and may swipe your possessions. They'll be long gone before you even realise what has happened.

### Pickpockets

While cruise lines highlight Rome, Barcelona, and Venice as well-known hotspots, pickpockets are at work in all major cities. Often working in teams, one member will create a distraction while a second acts as a lookout and a third member relieves you of your wallet, purse or backpack, with the latter being the number one target for thieves.

Don't carry mobile phones or wallets in the back pocket of jeans; it only takes a second for someone to lift it while you're distracted and you won't even feel it. Also, try to avoid hanging your handbag on the back of your seat or under a table as it makes it far more susceptible to theft. If you do have to put your bag under the table, then place a table leg through the handle. Finally, don't wear unnecessary jewellery in ports of call and don't carry large amounts of money. If wearing a money belt, keep a few notes somewhere else so you're not wiped clean if you experience a pickpocket first hand.

### Spilt liquid

A common scam in Europe, someone may 'accidentally' spill something on your clothing or bump you from behind. It may seem innocent, but it's just another disruptive tactic to divert your focus towards the spill and away from your personal belongings. While helping clean up the mess, the scammer may pick your pockets, or someone else may steal your bags. Avoid this scam by declining any help and go to the nearest bathroom (with bags in hand) and clean the stain yourself.

## Life Onboard

**Taxis**

Notorious for ripping off tourists worldwide, taxis are your biggest threat when it comes to relieving you of your money with overpriced fares. Too many passengers refuse to heed the advice of agreeing to a fee before they get in the vehicle, or to clarify whether the agreed price is per person or for the entire party. Cabbies have been known to rig meters, swap bills with counterfeits, take much longer routes, charge a higher fixed fare, or take a detour to a tourist shop where they are paid a commission.

Another fairly common scam, when paying a fare with a note, the driver will drop it and make a switch to a bill of lower value. They will then argue that you have underpaid them and may not let you out until you shell out even more cash. Keep your cash in your hand until they get out the correct change and then pass it over, or verbally clarify how much you're giving them as you hand over the money.

It is not uncommon for cabbies near train stations and port terminals to notify passengers that the meter is broken or the rate is cheaper without the meter. However, if the meter isn't used, passengers can be held responsible for outrageous taxi fees. Insist the driver turns the meter on, or negotiate the rate before driving away from the curb. If the driver refuses, get out and choose a different taxi.

Watch your luggage or shopping bags if loaded into the boot to make sure nothing is misplaced. Also, some drivers might refuse to return them unless you pay a much higher price than the actual fare. If this happens, tell them your wallet is in your luggage.

To avoid most (if not all) problems, only take official services whenever possible, agree on a price for your whole party before you get in the taxi, and try to have the exact fare for the journey.

**Three-card Monte**

You'll often see people on the street playing a game like find the Jack, three-card Monte or hiding a ball in a cup. It'll seem as though other tourists around you are guessing correctly and winning money. You might decide to play and may even win the first time, but further attempts will see you lose time and time again. This is one of the oldest travel scams on the streets of Europe, and the 'tourists' who win are actually accomplices and part of the con.

### Timeshares
Be wary of stalls offering free excursions to luxury resorts. When you get there you'll be subject to a hard sell by a timeshare salesperson, who'll get extremely rude if you refuse to attend the session.

### Toilet Scams
Scammers sometimes position themselves outside a restroom, insisting you must pay to use the facilities. Once you've paid, two things can happen: you might be met by the official attendant in the bathroom and told you have to pay again, or you may find out the toilets were free to use anyway. It's hard to argue if you really need to go!

### Tumbling Tourist
A well-dressed elderly tourist will fall in front of you, and while offering your assistance, you'll be relieved of your valuables without even realising. There are several variations of this scam, like someone dropping their coins in the street or having their bag stolen in front of you. Your natural instinct will be to comfort or help the 'victim', during which you'll no doubt be distracted and more vulnerable to theft.

### Turkey Drop
A scammer will 'accidentally' drop money on the floor in front of you and keep walking seemingly unaware of their loss while a co-conspirator either waits for you to pick the money up or picks it up themselves and offers to split it with you. The scammer will then come running back, challenge you and accuse you of stealing the money, and while the confrontation is in full throes, your own wallet or phone will be stolen.

## Technology at Sea

It wasn't that long ago when a holiday meant you left all the problems and stresses of everyday life at home and a cruise ship offered a serene and tranquil atmosphere where you could kick back and get away from it all. Several years on, technology has changed this drastically.

According to Ofcom, 94% of the British adult population personally own or use a mobile phone, and so it stands to reason that going away

## Life Onboard

now means most people take their phones with them. The good news is, with new technologies, using your phone abroad has become a lot easier, more convenient, and in some cases, far cheaper. Internet access at sea has become the norm as cruise lines have bowed to public demand and today nearly every ocean-going vessel provides the service. With millions of pounds being invested in satellite communications, shipboard mobile services are also improving, but it is still a slow and expensive method of staying in touch with loved ones.

If you plan to use your mobile at sea, it's important to note that the ship's network, which is relatively expensive to use, will be turned on once you sail away from the embarkation port. If you have roaming enabled your device will connect automatically and could seriously put a dent in your pocket. Telenor Maritime, 90112, 90118, Nor-18, INMARSAT or Cellular at Sea are just some of the International Marine Roaming services, and the high costs of making and receiving calls and texts on this network will be added to your mobile bill, not your onboard account.

Once you're within about 12 miles of land and approaching port the ship's network will be switched off, and the local land-based mobile phone service will become available. These are often cheaper (or even free) dependent on your home provider's tariff. Most service providers offer cruise ship plans with lower rates than maritime roaming charges, so it's a good idea to contact your mobile phone provider before your holiday and check whether you can swap over to a better pricing plan for your trip.

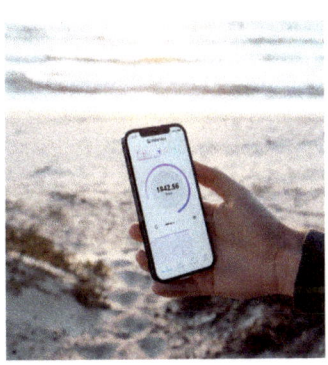

*Credit: Frederik Lipfert, Unsplash*

**Cruise Essential:** *Make sure you turn off data roaming before leaving every port.*

**Brexit Warning**: *The UK formally left the UK on 31 January 2020 and an 11 month transition period was put in place to decide the terms of the withdrawal deal. The guarantee of free roaming for UK mobile users has now ended with mobile companies able to apply charges if they want to. Check with your provider as to exactly what is included in your tariff and the rates that will apply. If you want to make calls abroad, you also need to check with your provider that International*

# The Autonomous Cruiser

*Roaming is enabled on your contract. To protect the public from being charged excessive rates from mobile companies who do implement fees, the UK government has introduced a law to cap the charges at £45 a month.*

**Mobile Plans:** *Three Mobile customers on an Advanced Plan can use their monthly allowance of texts, calls, and data at no extra cost in 71 destinations worldwide, including the USA, Australia and Singapore.*

Most cruise lines now offer an internet service aboard their ships, but they can vary greatly in quality and price across lines: some will charge by the minute, some by megabyte and others will offer up package deals of varying size. Whichever way you connect will undoubtedly add a hefty surcharge to your overall holiday cost - it's up to you as to whether the price is worth it. The availability of internet connectivity also varies across each ship. Some have bow-to-stern access, while others might only provide hotspots in a few public areas. On smaller lines, you might be restricted to using the ship's internet café.

It is often best to limit your internet usage where you can and avoid downloading large files at sea if you're trying to save money. A trick to lower your costs if you pay by the minute is to compose your messages offline so that once you connect to the internet, you only have to push send instead of wasting precious minutes typing. Streaming can also be very expensive as it consumes a lot of data; you can avoid the charges by downloading your movies directly to your devices before your holiday so you can watch them offline.

If you do want to keep in regular touch with family back home or if you need to make frequent use of the internet for work, it may be worth investing in a package deal as it could work out cheaper in the long run. It's best exploring your options when you first embark as cruise lines tend to offer their best deals, often the 'early bird' package, on embarkation day only.

Turn your mobile roaming off or switch to 'airplane mode' while at sea (i.e. when an International Maritime service is your only option) or in ports where you can't roam for free. Doing so will help you avoid hefty fees, as most smartphones will run app updates, automatic software updates and push notifications in the background that all use your cellular data, even if you are not actively using your device.

**Cruise Essential:** *Once you have set your phone to 'airplane mode' you will have to manually update the time on your phone if the ship's clocks change.*

> Skype, Facetime, WhatsApp, Facebook Messenger, Viber, Google Duo, Signal Private Messenger, Telegram and Google Hangouts are all very useful for making cheap or even free phone calls to anywhere in the world while on holiday. The trick to reducing your costs is to limit your use to when you can connect to free Wi-Fi in port. Just download the app(s) that you want to use, open an account, and you'll be ready to go, though you'll need to make sure all your friends and family that you might want to contact also have accounts. It really couldn't be easier.

The most common complaint after price is that the onboard internet connection can be agonisingly slow, meaning websites often freeze and phone calls regularly disconnect mid-conversation. The connection is dependent on factors like location, weather and general level of traffic, so avoid trying to connect during peak times as the fewer people that are on it, the faster your internet speeds. The best times are usually early mornings, late nights, at mealtimes or while in port.

A lot of passengers head straight to the nearest internet café or Wi-Fi hotspot as soon as they get ashore. If you are unfamiliar with the port, a good bet is to follow the stream of crew, who seem to know where all the local hotspots are in the destinations they visit.

Free Wi-Fi is available just about everywhere, especially if you plan ahead and know where to look. Big chains are often a good bet, with the likes of McDonald's, Burger King and Costa Coffee all offering complimentary internet. Also, Starbucks has recently partnered with Google to bring free and unlimited Wi-Fi access to each of their locations. Airports, airline priority clubs, cruise terminals, libraries and hotels usually have complimentary connections too, with some railway and bus stations also offering a free service. In fact, an increasing number of train operating companies are providing onboard Wi-Fi facilities - National Rail has the full list on their website.

Cyber Cafes (*cybercaptive.com*) and Cyber Cafe (*cybercafe.com*) are the largest internet-based information providers for the Internet and Cyber Café market. They offer an excellent list of the pitstops available for the towns, cities, islands or countries you are visiting. Smaller enterprises constantly open and close, so although the site is continually updated, some information might fall through the cracks.

One thing to remember when using public Wi-Fi networks is that they aren't always the most secure. In fact, you can seriously place your online security at risk if you're careless. Unfortunately, nothing is private on open Wi-Fi, no matter where you are, though you can offer some level of protection by going to your 'sharing settings' and disabling them, or by turning off 'network discovery' on your device.

The most effective way to stay safe on public Wi-Fi is to install a Virtual Private Network (VPN) client on your devices. It will encrypt the data travelling back and forth from your laptop or phone to the internet and hook you up to a secure server, making your online information much more secure. If you are on a long cruise, meaning you will be connecting to lots of different public networks, a good VPN is a worthwhile investment. The only downsides are that it can be a little costly and it will slow your connection down a bit.

**Cyber Tip:** *Before leaving home, make sure your gadgets all have the latest security software updates, and don't download or install anything new over an open network unless you absolutely have to.*

**Battery Saver:** *To help preserve your phone battery: turn your screen brightness down, implement the 'low power' mode in your battery settings, disable auto app updates, disable background app refresh, switch off fitness tracking, and turn Bluetooth off if you're not using any accessories. If you often use your phone for extended periods, it might be worth investing in a portable power bank.*

### In-cabin Telephone

Mobile phones with international capability may not work while at sea, but ship-to-shore communication will still be available 24 hours a day to all guests through their stateroom phones, meaning you can make and receive calls whilst onboard without the need for a mobile phone. Friends or family ringing into the ship will have to pay for the call with a credit card, but there is no charge for waiting or dialling time, and the fees will not be applied until the caller connects to the ship.

## Phone Apps

*Keeping in touch with loved ones while you're away has become the norm in this advanced technological age, and it's now easier and cheaper than ever.*

# Life Onboard

**Signal – Private Messenger**
This app allows users to send texts, pictures and video messages without SMS and MMS fees, and make phone calls without incurring long-distance phone charges. Developers, donations and grants support the app, so there are no adverts or trackers.

**Telegram**
Telegram is the most secure messaging app on the market, connecting people around the world. Synced across all your devices, Telegram has no limits on the type or size of media you use, leaving you without the worry of running out of disk space, plus, everything is backed up and stored on their own cloud service.

**WhatsApp**
Phone and text your friends and family for free even if they're in another country, avoiding international SMS and calling charges. WhatsApp uses your phone's internet connection, whether through your mobile network or through a Wi-Fi connection to communicate.

*Finding a hotspot can be challenging, especially in more remote areas, so here are a few of the best apps to help you get connected.*

**Free Wi-Fi**
Quickly locate over 120 million verified public Wi-Fi hotspots worldwide, with passwords and reviews of the locations.

**Wi-Fi Map**
Discover 100 million hotspots all over the world and get directions to them instantly. Plus, you can download the maps so you can use them later without an internet connection.

**JiWire**
Locate over 150,000 confirmed public Wi-Fi hotspots in 136 countries through multiple search options.

*Here are a few small apps that can save you time, stress and money if your device is lost or stolen.*

**Find My** (*iOS*)
If you misplace any of your Apple products (Mac, iPhone, iPad, or iPod Touch, etc.), this handy app will let you use any other Apple gadget to find it and protect your data. Once you locate your missing device online, you can remotely lock it, play a sound alert, display a message on the screen, or erase the data on it altogether.

**Google Find My Device** (*Android*)
Instantly find a lost, stolen or missing Android phone, tablet or watch, whether it belongs to you, your spouse or your child. If the missing or stolen device is moved, its position is updated instantaneously with real-time location updates on the app's map.

# Safety & Security

Cruise lines and their crew are committed to maintaining a safe and secure environment aboard their ships to ensure passengers can enjoy their holidays to the fullest without having to worry. Cruising is one of the most reliable forms of travel, with accidents a rare occurrence across the entire industry - and they want to keep it that way.

Cruise ships undergo rigorous safety procedures and have to follow a significant number of rules and regulations to protect both the passengers and crew on board. All ship personnel, passengers and even luggage must pass through several meticulous security checkpoints before being able to board the vessel. Trained security staff are found on every cruise ship and CCTV cameras are located in all public areas.

The onboard policies and procedures are all designed to give the guest the confidence that their safety remains the top priority and include:

- Responsible service of alcohol - security staff will deal firmly with all alcohol-related issues, including underage drinking, with the possibility of those involved being disembarked.
- Zero-tolerance to illicit substances - the cruise line reserves the right to search you, your luggage and cabin, and they will deny boarding or disembark any guest in possession of an illegal substance.

> **Don't Ask:**
> Why are the ruins in such bad condition? (talking about the Acropolis)

# Life Onboard

- Zero-tolerance to behaviour that affects the safety or enjoyment of other passengers - security staff will deal firmly with the culprits, which could result in those concerned being removed from the ship.

## Cabin Safety

- All cabins are non-smoking.
- Irons are strictly prohibited.
- Electrical items should not be left plugged in while unattended.
- Candles, naked flames or other burning material in either your stateroom or on your balcony is strictly prohibited.
- Do not use power extenders with surge protectors.
- Do not tamper with smoke detectors or sprinkler heads.
- Do not hang clothing out on the balcony.
- Do not cover or place items on top of light fittings.
- Muster station safety instructions are on the back of every cabin door.
- A safety video is broadcast 24/7 on the in-cabin television.

## Personal Safety

- Do not sit or stand on your ship's railings.
- Never hold the frames of open doors as the sudden movement of the ship can cause the door to slam.
- Always hold the handrails while moving about the ship, especially when the vessel is pitching or rolling.
- Do not tamper with the deadlights (steel plates over portholes). If there is cause to close them during your voyage, your steward will reopen them when the captain gives the okay.
- Use extreme caution when walking on open decks in bad weather or if the area becomes wet due to swimmers or cleaning procedures.
- Remain aware of any raised thresholds on the vessel, particularly around fire doors, exterior doors, the bathroom entrance in your cabin and the public areas of the ship.
- Never place your hands between a lift's closing doors.
- Do not leave valuables unattended in public areas.
- Place valuables which you don't regularly use in your cabin's safe.
- Lock your cabin door at night.

### Children's Safety

- Never attempt to raise or lower the top bunk bed yourself. Ask your steward instead.
- Young children should not sleep or play on top bunks.
- Ladders must only be used to access bunks.
- Never leave your child unattended, especially around the pool areas and on a cabin balcony.

### Pool Safety

- Use extreme caution around the pool areas, which can be slippery.
- Keep in mind that most cruise lines do not employ a lifeguard.
- Jumping or diving into any pool is strictly prohibited.
- Alcohol is forbidden in the pool and hot tubs.
- Do not attempt to access pools or hot tubs that have been netted off.
- Call a member of staff if you see anyone in trouble.

### Ship's Security

- Keep your cruise card on you at all times.
- You are required to show your cruise card at the gangway every time you leave or return to the ship.
- You are required to place your bags and parcels through the ship's x-ray machine each time you board the vessel throughout your cruise. You may also have to open them if asked by security.
- Do not agree to bring anything onboard the ship for a stranger.
- It is strictly prohibited to enter any crew area on the ship, even if invited by a member of the ship's staff. The only exception is an escorted Galley or Bridge tour.

### Personal Safety Ashore

- Travel in numbers and stay in open public spaces.
- Be aware of your surroundings, especially at night.
- Do not wear expensive jewellery.

# Life Onboard

- Be cautious in the care of your handbag, mobile phone, camera and other valuables.
- Respect the dress code of the country you are visiting.
- If possible, use an ATM inside a bank rather than on the street.
- Use discretion when handling cash publicly.
- Do not accept rides from unofficial taxis. Make sure to look for certification and proper licenses.
- Do not leave drinks unattended when in bars and restaurants.
- Do not provide personal information to strangers.
- Keep clear of gathering crowds, rallies or demonstrations.

**Medical Safety**

- Cruise lines screen anyone who has visited or travelled through Liberia, Sierra Leone or Guinea within 21 days of a cruise departure.
- Cruise lines screen any guests who have come through an area or had physical contact with a person suspected of having Ebola.
- Cruise lines screen any guests who have come through an area or had physical contact with a person suspected of having coronavirus.
- All passengers, crew members and ship visitors must complete a mandatory health screening questionnaire upon embarkation. If deemed necessary, guests may be asked to submit to further screening before boarding.
- Hand sanitisers are available and clearly visible throughout the vessel - it is important to make use of them and to wash your hands frequently.
- Any situation where medical assistance is required should be reported to the medical centre or Guest Relations.

**Smoking**

Cigars, cigarettes, e-cigarettes and pipe smoking are only permitted in designated areas on board, and ashtrays are provided accordingly. Smoking is strictly prohibited in all staterooms and on most cruise ships' private balconies, with the exception of AIDA, Fred. Olsen, Costa and Hapag-Lloyd. Some of the American ships have indoor smoking lounges and designated areas within the casino and nightclubs. Cigarette ends, cigars or matches should not be thrown over the side of the vessel as they can be drawn back into a ship and cause a fire. While some cruise lines will impose heavy fines for such infractions, others are not so lenient and will disembark any culprit. More information on smoking onboard is available in 'Up in Smoke'.

If you should discover a fire, raise the alarm by activating one of the red fire alarms located throughout the ship and advise a member of the crew as quickly as possible. In the event of a fire or other emergency, the Officer of the Watch will call for the First Stage Response — a group of key personnel who will investigate the incident. No action is required by passengers.

**Emergency Drills**
These are deemed compulsory under maritime law and everyone, without exception, must attend them on the day of embarkation.

**Pirate Drills**
Piracy in some waters, particularly near East Africa, is still a huge threat to passenger liners, but while yachts and merchant vessels have been held hostage in the past, a successful pirate attack on a cruise ship has never occurred. In addition to standard ongoing security measures, an additional drill is led before any cruise ship enters unfriendly infested waters, particularly the Arabian Sea and the Gulf of Aden. The drill requires guests to close and lock their balcony door and sit on the floor outside their cabin door after the alarm sounds. Sitting to the side of the cabin door with a wall directly behind you is the safest place, and the handrails can be used in case the ship has to veer sharply away from pirate ships.

Larger ships have the advantage of speed, and though they may come into contact with a pirate boat armed with grappling hooks and rope ladders, it is doubtful that the ship will be infiltrated due to the height of the Promenade deck. Privately contracted armed security officers have been used on smaller vessels, but they are there more to reassure passengers than because of an imminent danger of attack. The onus of safeguarding up to 2000 people is taken seriously, so it is safer to put these extra procedures in place than become complacent.

Measures, usually in force for seven to ten days, require that all surplus external lighting on the ship is extinguished from dusk to dawn and the vessel only uses its navigational lights at night. Curtains are drawn, outdoor bars and swimming pools are closed and balcony use and deck parties are suspended during the blackout period.

Fire hoses, water cannons, sonic projectors, and barbed wire are the most common defence against unwanted intruders, and on British ships, armed guards using night vision goggles will patrol the decks around the clock. Several countries, including the UK, the USA, France and Germany, have strengthened security for cruise and cargo ships around the prevalent areas and work together to keep everyone safe. Typically, ships sail in a convoy of other vessels with protection at both ends, which has proved to be a very effective countermeasure. Navies from various nations, together with NATO and the European Union, have all shared in the patrolling duties.

## Man Overboard

Three long blasts on the ship's whistle indicates that a person has gone overboard. If you see anyone jump, fall, or be pushed overboard, throw a lifebuoy or anything that floats over the side of the ship and inform the nearest crew member by shouting 'man overboard'. If there are no crew members nearby, call reception from any onboard phone as quickly as possible.

## General Emergency Alarm

The General Emergency Alarm is sounded by seven short blasts and one long blast of the alarm and ship's whistle. If you have not had a warning that a crew exercise

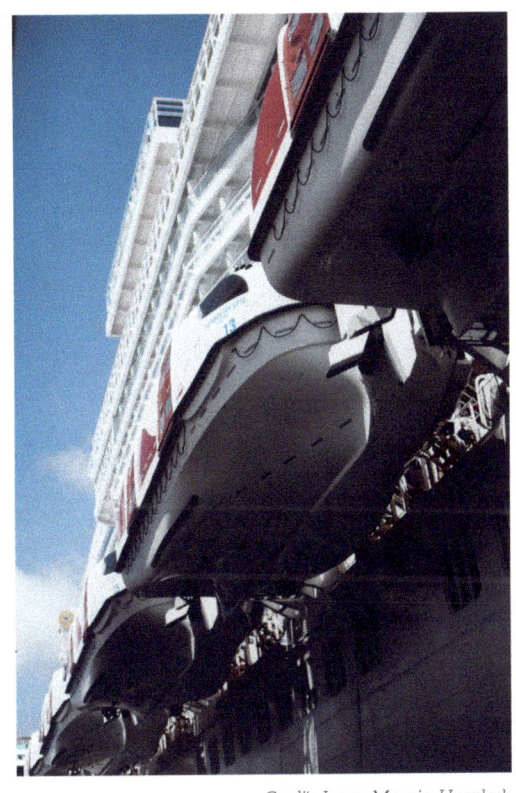

*Credit: Jenny Marvin, Unsplash*

is taking place, you must go straight to your cabin and collect your lifejacket, warm clothing, sensible footwear, essential medication and cruise card, and proceed directly to your tender/muster station. Your assigned station is on your cruise card and the safety notice behind your cabin door.

When carrying your lifejacket, do your best to stop the straps from trailing on the floor. Low location strip lighting will automatically switch on in the event of an emergency. If visibility is badly affected so that it becomes hard to see exit signage, it might help to crawl, and by following the lighting strips you will be led to an exit. The use of lifts is strictly prohibited during an emergency, as in the event of a power failure you may become trapped.

A member of the ship's staff will be dispatched to anyone with mobility difficulties who have informed the crew before boarding. Any children in the youth clubs will automatically be taken to their muster station to meet up with their parents or guardians. Finally, once you reach your muster station, listen for further instructions - they will either come across the public address system or from the officers at your station.

**Abandon Ship**

In the unlikely event that you need to abandon ship, do your best not to panic. You will be directed to your muster station and told to await further instruction. The lifeboats are capable of being loaded, launched and manoeuvred away from a ship within 30 minutes of the captain's order, far less time than it takes for a cruise ship to sink.

# Disembarkation

Planning for the end of your holiday before you've even set sail is certainly not fun, but it is necessary; a little planning can take away the stress of disembarkation. As a first step, it's always best to review all disembarkation instructions issued by your cruise line, even if you are a seasoned cruiser, in case of changes to standard procedures.

*Brief Note:* Guests can review the Cruise Director's disembarkation briefing on their stateroom television.

Some cruise lines allow a late checkout for a modest fee, but it needs to be arranged in advance. For example, on their European sailings, Celebrity Cruises charge a fee that will allow you to stay on board until 90 minutes before the ship sails, giving you an extra half day's access to all the ship's facilities, including the pool, gym, bars and even lunch. You can also use the showers in the spa to freshen up before leaving.

During your cruise, you will have been asked to fill in a form detailing your onward travel plans so that those with early flights or coach travel can be given an earlier disembarkation time. If the instructions you receive don't suit your exit plans, simply go to Guest Relations and ask for an alternative time. If you're catching an onward flight, you can use the ship's Internet Centre to check-in online and print off your boarding card.

The ship will issue number or colour-coded luggage labels to all passengers which correspond to the time your luggage will be available to pick up from the terminal. Make sure that you write your name and mobile number on the labels in case they get lost. Some cruise lines no longer issue new luggage labels for disembarkation, instead expecting you to reuse the ones you came aboard with, but if you do need more, ask your steward or collect them from Guest Relations.

**Luggage Essential:** *All your cases should have the same colour or number-coded labels.*

**The Night Before**
You have two options when disembarking: you can opt for the 'Early Bird Express', or you can leave your cruise line to deal with your luggage. Choosing Early Bird Express (also 'self-assist' or 'walk-off') means you'll be among the first to alight the ship almost as soon as it has cleared customs, but you'll have to carry your luggage off the ship yourself. This is obviously quite physically demanding as it could involve stairs, the gangway and a long walk to the terminal and so is the wrong option for some passengers. You should also be aware there will be no porters or trolleys available to help if you choose this option.

If you opt for the ship to take care of your luggage you'll be required to place any bags outside your cabin the night before you disembark by a designated time (typically between ten pm and midnight), and while you are sleeping, they will be collected and made ready to be sent ashore the next morning upon arrival. Using this complimentary service is very convenient but will mean you'll have to wait until your designated time, often later in the morning, until you can disembark. Once off the ship, your luggage should be waiting for you in the arrivals hall. Once you're packed and ready to put your luggage outside the door, doublecheck that you've left out the clothes you want to travel home in, and put all your medication, travel documents, glasses, keys and any other essential items in your hand luggage. Finally, if you have an onward flight, remember the 100 ml liquid restriction and ensure all liquids, creams, lotions, gels, pastes, perfumes, contact lens solution and toiletries over the allowance are packed in your suitcase.

# The Autonomous Cruiser

***Don't Forget:*** *Any duty-free alcohol purchased or confiscated on the cruise will either be delivered to your stateroom or will need to be collected from a designated area.*

***Don't Forget:*** *Make sure you buy any last-minute prints from the Photo Gallery as it won't be open in the morning, and if you've ordered a DVD of your cruise, make sure you pick it up before the Gallery closes.*

There are a few ways to reward exceptional members of the crew that went above and beyond to make your holiday extra special. Of course, you can give them tips directly, but do so on your last night as it is unlikely you will find them during the chaos of debarkation. Also, take the time to fill out a Crew Recognition Card, usually obtained from Guest Relations - it's simple to do and makes a big difference to the staff who could earn a privilege or even a promotion.

If paying off your onboard balance with cash, you will need to settle your final account at Guest Relations before retiring for the night, and your final invoice will be delivered to your cabin in the early hours of the morning. If you disagree with any of the charges you will need to go to Guest Relations in the morning and talk it through with one of the receptionists; you cannot argue any discrepancies once you've left the ship. If you don't intend to pay off your bill with cash and you registered your credit or debit card at the beginning of the cruise, there is nothing further to do as your card will be charged automatically the morning you disembark.

***Bought too much?*** *If you've run out of luggage space, don't rush down to the onboard shop and buy a holdall to carry all of your souvenirs. Instead, go to one of the onboard shops and ask them to keep a cardboard box for you after they next refill their stock. It's free and often just as effective.*

***Packing Tip:*** *Use your free shower cap to cover up dirty shoes before you pack them.*

Nearly 80% of travellers opt for black or brown cases, meaning yours might be hard to identify amongst the other 2000 in the luggage hall unless they stand out. Wrap something distinctive around your baggage handles, like coloured or patterned duct tape, neon ribbon or fabric, so they are easily distinguishable. It will make finding it in the luggage hall much easier, and it'll be less likely to be lost or stolen.

# Life Onboard

***Luggage Tip:*** *Take a photo of all your luggage before you place it outside your cabin as it could make it easier for the ground staff to locate if it does get lost. It also acts as proof of its condition should you need to make an insurance claim for any damaged items.*

Don't steal the fluffy bathrobes or the cabin umbrella that's been hanging in your wardrobe, as they are only put in your cabin for you to enjoy while you are on board. Robes are usually available to purchase from an onboard shop, and if you think you've had the last laugh by sneaking it off the ship, you won't be laughing as loudly when you see an added charge on your credit card bill that the cruise line has applied for the missing item.

**Morning of Departure**

On the morning of your return home, breakfast will be available in select locations, with specific timings that will differ from a regular sea or port day. Room service is usually not an option on debarkation day. If you don't need to be anywhere in a hurry, take your time over breakfast or settle into a comfy chair and let the crowds die down. You probably won't be able to get off earlier than your allocated time, but you can get off later. Typically, you will be required to vacate your cabin by 7.30 am. Make sure you empty the safe and leave its door open, grab your hand luggage and make your way to one of the designated waiting areas. Guests requiring wheelchair assistance should proceed to their designated waiting areas in one of the public lounges at their specified time slot, where a porter will arrive to help them off the ship. Guests staying in suites will have a dedicated lounge away from the chaos. It's a great place to gather your thoughts if you are not among the first groups leaving the ship.

Do not wait in the stairwells or by reception, as doing so could massively slow down the disembarkation process - several thousand people are all trying to leave the ship from a limited number of exit points, so it's important to avoid any delays. Time slots are allocated to ensure

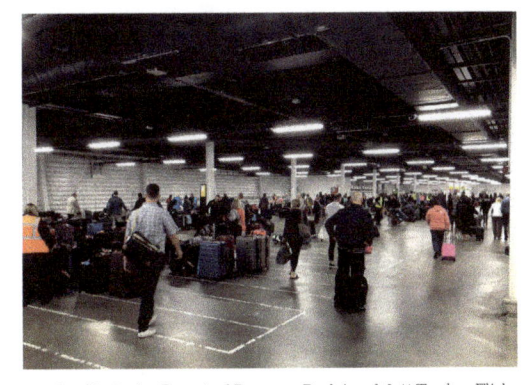

*Credit: Cruise Terminal Baggage Reclaim - Matt Taylor, Flickr*

the mass exodus of the vessel is staggered in order to keep lines moving, and so areas inside and outside of the ship are not overly congested.

*Early Bird Tip:* *The staff aren't usually policing the deck numbers as passengers stream off, but there will be incredibly long lines if you try and sneak off early. If you do disembark before your allocated time slot, you could find yourself waiting in the terminal for your luggage for a long time, as there is a possibility it might not have been offloaded yet.*

Depending on your disembarkation port and your nationality, you may be required to fill in a customs declaration form and go through passport control in the terminal. Some passengers might even be required to meet with immigration officials onboard for a face-to-face interview. At a lot of British ports, you might not necessarily see customs, but that doesn't mean they are not there. They are typically out in force if your ship has been to Gibraltar, the Canary Islands or the Caribbean, as guests often stock up on cheap duty-free items. Cases are usually x-rayed and inspected by sniffer dogs before passengers disembark.

Your cruise card will be scanned one more time before heading towards the baggage holding area where your luggage will be in a bay with the same number or colour-code you were issued. Trolleys are usually available, but you can make it easier on yourself by opting for a porter. For the cost of a tip they'll take your bags all the way through the terminal for you, and they usually have a dedicated express line through customs, allowing them to get back and help more guests as quickly as possible, but also meaning you may get through the terminal more quickly.

*Luggage Essential*: *Make sure you check your luggage labels carefully before you leave the terminal to make sure you have the right bags, as other guests may have the same make, model and colour cases as you. If you inadvertently take another passenger's case home, any costs incurred in having the bags returned to their owner will be at your own expense.*

**Transport Back Home**
Guests who drove to the port for embarkation can head straight to the car park upon leaving the terminal. If you take advantage of a porter they will walk your luggage across to your car and help you load it. Guests who have

purchased transfers should proceed to the buses outside the terminal with their luggage for transportation to the airport.

A lot of cruise lines offer excursions on disembarkation day for guests who have time to stay in the area (e.g. those with late flights, those that live locally, etc.) and some tours will even end with a drop off at the airport. If you do take advantage of this option, make sure your luggage is on the same coach as you before you leave the cruise port.

**Guest Satisfaction Forms**
Digital surveys have replaced the majority of paper end-of-cruise guest satisfaction questionnaires. It's important that you complete them, as your comments will be taken very seriously by the cruise line's top brass and will have a genuine impact on future cruises. The burden on staff to achieve near-perfect ratings each cruise is incredibly high, with anything less than an 'excellent' for each question considered somewhat of a failure, and can sometimes result in a crew member losing their job.

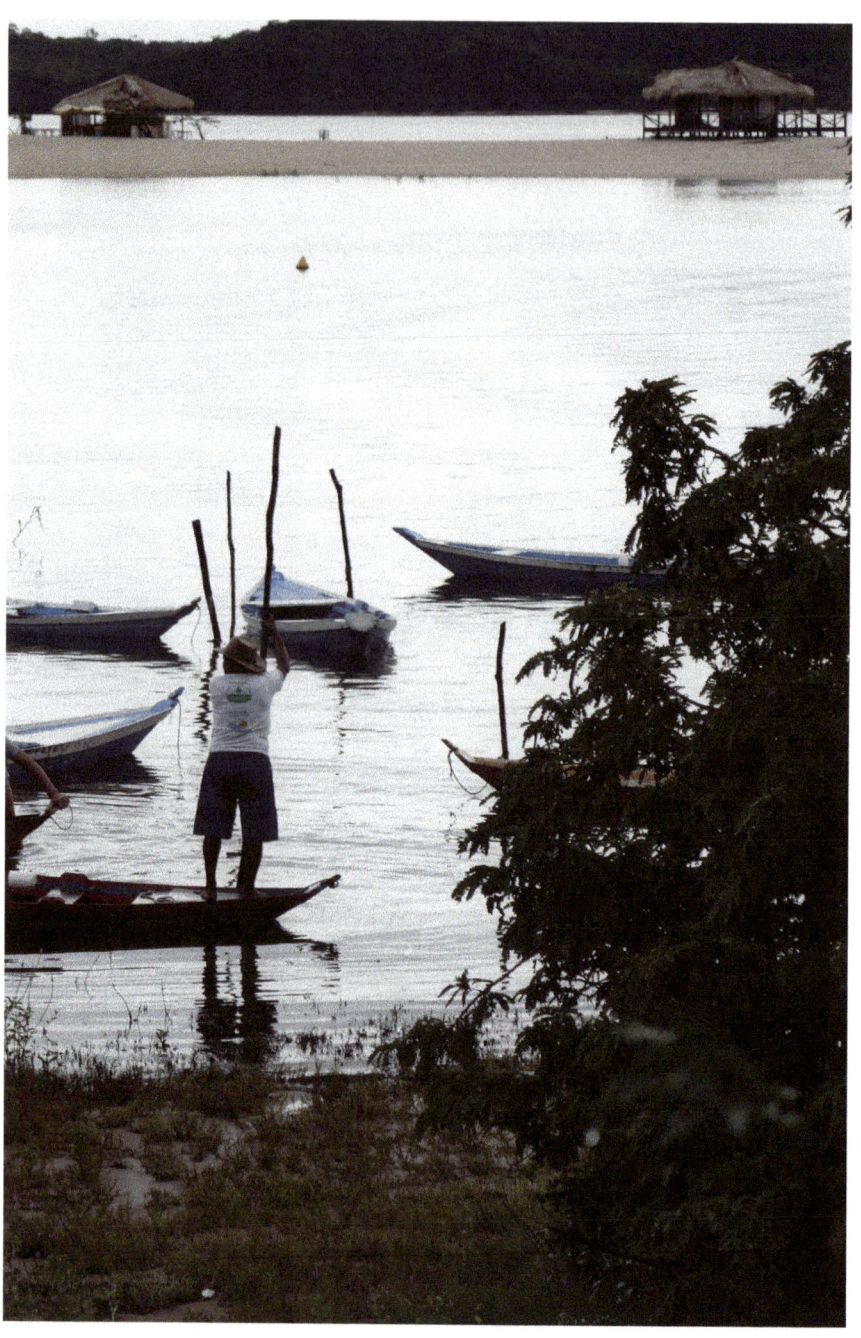

Credit: St Lucia

# Directory

## UK Cruise Ports

Sailing from the UK offers a wide range of top destinations and removes the cost of a long-haul flight and the inconvenience of an airport, and over recent years, a huge number of cruise lines have chosen to 'home port' in cities across the UK. As the biggest cruise port in the UK and thus a gateway to some of the world's most beautiful destinations, Southampton is the choice for many of the major cruise brands, including Royal Caribbean, Azamara, Princess, Celebrity, and P&O who have been sailing from Southampton since the 1850s.

The good news for less-southern Brits is, unlike the past, Southampton is no longer the only realistic option when it comes to cruising from the UK. For example, Fred. Olsen specialise in providing no-fly cruises with a focus on broadening the range of regional programs and sailings they offer from around the British Isle including Dover, Liverpool, Newcastle and Rosyth. Wherever you live in the United Kingdom, you should be able to find an escape route that suits you.

You should be able to find a company that offers accessible taxis near most UK cruise ports - if you have trouble finding one, check out the wheelchair taxi directory at *wheelchairtaxis.co.uk*.

A UK taxi comparison site, minicabit enables you to connect and compare quotes from over 800 taxi companies that will take you to and from any cruise port across the UK. For more information on what companies offer accessible vehicles, visit *minicabit.com*.

Train Genius provides a countrywide service to all UK National Rail destinations. Whilst trains may not stop directly at the port of your choice, you will find that there is usually a train station just a short distance away in a local taxi. Being independently impartial, you are guaranteed to be offered the train tickets that suit your needs at the best price, sometimes with as much as an 80% saving. For more information, visit *traingenius.com*.

# The Autonomous Cruiser

Park on My Drive is a service which connects you with people that are offering the use of their driveway parking spaces, often less than a mile away from your chosen port. To check locations available dates and prices, visit *parkonmydrive.com*.

**GPS Tip:** *Satellite navigation systems vary in how accurately they pinpoint a given postcode. Once you're near to your destination port, ignore your satnav and follow the relevant signage.*

## Bristol, England – Port of Call/Turnaround
*Bristol Cruise Terminal, Avonmouth Dock, Bristol, BS11 9DB*
*Bristol Cruise Terminal, Royal Portbury Dock, Bristol, BS20 7XQ*

**Recent cruise operators:** *Cruise & Maritime Voyages.*

Located at the River Avon's mouth, this industrial port is only six miles from Bristol and not far from junction 18 of the M5, or the A4 (Portway), with access via the main port entrance at West Town Police Gate. The Port Authority does not allow passengers to walk from the port entrance to the cruise terminal, so all guests must arrive via some form of transport.

Bristol Port is made up of two docks, either side of the River Avon, a junction apart on the M5 motorway. Generally speaking, Avonmouth handles most embarkations as the berth and terminal are dedicated to cruise ships, but with the increase in sea traffic, Royal Portbury has been put into service - and for the immediate future, the terminal, a temporary structure in the way of a marquee, has been opened for the cruise season.

Bristol Airport is thirteen miles away or you have a choice of local railway stations, with Bristol Temple Meads only seven miles away or Bristol Parkway just ten miles away, both of which have taxi ranks. Ask your taxi driver to take you to the Cruise Terminal off the A4 Portway, Avonmouth Docks. There is a branch line service to Avonmouth station, but it is three miles from the terminal and walking inside the dock is not permitted. There is no taxi rank at Avonmouth Station so you must pre-book one if you choose to use this route. Returning from your cruise, there is a taxi rank to the right as you exit the terminal.

Car parking is available close to the cruise terminal but must be pre-booked with your tour operator or travel agent. Ensure your parking permit is clearly displayed on your windscreen prior to your arrival and follow the signs to the drop-off area so you can unload your luggage before heading to the car park which is a short distance away.

A Taxis of Bristol offer wheelchair-accessible cars that will transport guests to their destinations across Bristol. With ramped access as standard, their drivers offer transfers to and from Avonmouth, or day tours to see the local sights. To secure your booking, email *info@bristoltaxihire.co.uk* or phone 0117 378 1212.

The Avonmouth Cruise Terminal is convenient for those living in the West, the Midlands and Wales, though the facilities are rather primitive and only include a seated waiting area, café and public toilets. The single storey building does have ramped access and temporary disabled toilets.

Royal Portbury is not far from Junction 19 of the M5 and is signposted all the way to the dock. The drop off/pick up area and taxi rank will be by the Marquee Terminal, which has toilet facilities for able and disabled passengers. A local café from the village sets up a pop-up stall on cruise days in each terminal.

> **Don't Ask:**
> What language is this in? (tour to the ballet)

## Belfast, Northern Ireland – Port of Call/Turnaround
*Belfast Harbour, Grotto Wharf, Northern Road, Belfast, BT3 9AP*

**Recent cruise operators:** *Fred. Olsen, Cruise & Maritime Voyages, Princess Cruises, Cunard, Seabourn, Ponant, Celebrity, AIDA, Azamara, Carnival, Royal Caribbean, Crystal, Holland America, MSC, Oceania, MSC, P&O, Regent, Saga.*

Located on the River Lagan, Belfast is Northern Ireland's principal maritime gateway and the country's capital. Only five minutes from the city centre and close to the M2, the port is easily accessible. Two airports serve the city, George Best Belfast (within the city) and Belfast International, 15 miles to the west.

Having invested in new gangways and luggage scanners, Belfast Harbour is now marketing itself as an embarkation port, offering locals the chance to join their cruise directly instead of having to fly to Southampton or another regional port.

Two docks service passenger ships: Stormont, used by larger ships, and Pollock Wharf, used for berthing smaller vessels and where passengers are

# The Autonomous Cruiser

welcomed with musical performances. Both docks have wheelchair-accessible toilet facilities quayside.

Cruise Harbour has opened the first dedicated cruise terminal to cater for Belfast's growing cruise trade. The upgraded quayside facility now includes a Visitor Information Centre, staffed by Visit Belfast's travel advisors and utilises the latest digital and audio-visual technology to showcase Belfast and Northern Ireland's biggest attractions, including the Giant's Causeway, Hillsborough Castle, Mount Stewart and Titanic Belfast. The Visit Belfast Welcome Centre provides all necessary assistance for tourists, including information, bureau de change advice, schedule changes, booking services, a box office (special events and tours), gift shop, left luggage and free internet. Opening hours are often extended to accommodate the visit of a cruise ship.

A tourist information desk is available at the quayside, staffed by multilingual travel advisors who supply maps, brochures, discount vouchers, a daily event listing and a shuttle bus timetable.

Just three miles from the city centre, accessible shuttle buses run regularly between the harbour and Donegall Square North. The shuttles are low-floor with kneeling facilities and ramped access, and they provide a dedicated space for one wheelchair user and five other priority seats for disabled passengers. Some cruise companies choose to provide these as a complimentary service, but some do charge.

Belfast Cabs offer wheelchair-accessible vehicles for transfers to and from Belfast, as well as day tours to see the local sights. To secure a booking, email *info@belfastcabs.com* or phone 0744 601 4761.

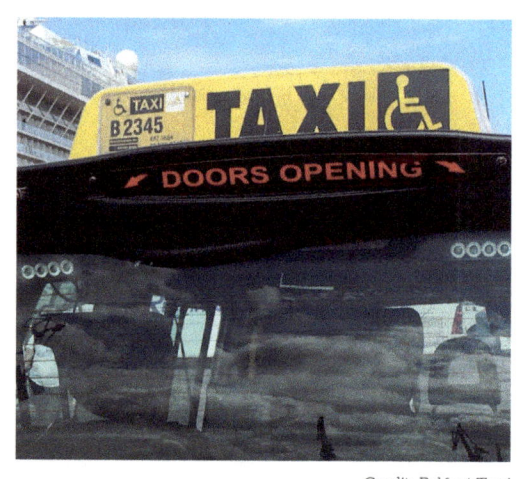

*Credit: Belfast Taxi*

# Directory

## Cardiff, South Wales – Port of Call/Turnaround
*Port of Cardiff, Queen Alexandra House, Cargo Road, Cardiff, CF10 4LQ*

**Recent cruise operators:** *Cruise & Maritime Voyages, Saga, Phoenix Reisen.*

Located on the north side of the Severn Estuary, connected to the rail network, and within easy reach of the M4 motorway, the new and developing Port of Cardiff has three approved berths for small cruise ships (Queen Alexandra Dock, Roath Dock and Roath Basin) and is only minutes away from the city centre by car, coach or water taxi.

Cardiff Airport is 13 miles away and taxis are readily available for onward travel. Cardiff Central Station is less than two miles away from the port entrance and has direct links to London, the Midlands and the southern coast of England. Taxis are available to meet arriving trains, but at present, the local buses do not service the port.

There are two entrances to the port, the West Gate, located near the BBC Studios in the Bay, and the East Gate, located off Rover Way. Cruise passengers need to enter the port via the East Gate to comply with port security. Because the cruise terminal is within a secure facility, passengers are not permitted to walk within the area, but free shuttle buses are provided.

A temporary accessible marquee is on site for transit passengers. Disabled and public toilets are available on the quayside. A complimentary wheelchair-accessible shuttle bus transfers passengers into town.

Cardiff is a popular port of call, especially on cruises around the British Isles, but in recent years it has also been used as a turnaround home port, enabling local passengers to start and end their cruises without having to fly or travel to the more popular ports of Southampton, Dover or Liverpool.

There are convenient and secure parking facilities within the port area, but parking must be pre-booked with your tour operator or travel agent. Once at the port, drop off your luggage before driving to the adjacent parking facility.

There is an accessible, temporary marquee in place for embarking guests, that houses check-in facilities, disabled and public toilets and a pop-up coffee shop. There is also disabled access to the vessel.

Capital Cabs are Cardiff's wheelchair access specialists as well as carrying a fleet of larger than average cabs to suit one to eight people. Boasting the lowest taxi meter charges in Cardiff, they offer short runs in the city, airport and train station transfers and a courier and parcel delivery service. Book

# The Autonomous Cruiser

online at *capitalcabs.co.uk*, through their app (available on Android and iOS) or by phoning 02920 777 777.

## Cork (Cobh), Ireland – Port of Call/Turnaround
*Port of Cork, Cobh Heritage Centre, Lower Road, P24 CY67*

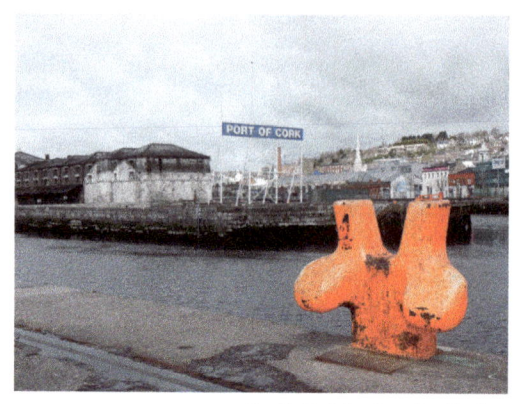

Credit: Christian Maeder, Pixabay

**Recent cruise operators:** *Cruise & Maritime Voyages, Norwegian, Celebrity, Princess, Royal Caribbean, Silver Spirit, MSC.*

Ireland's second largest seaport after Dublin, The Port of Cork serves as the main port for the country's southern coast and houses Ireland's only dedicated cruise ship berth in Cobh. Most ships dock at the Cobh Cruise Terminal, however, they can also use Ringaskiddy Deepwater Quay and the City Quays.

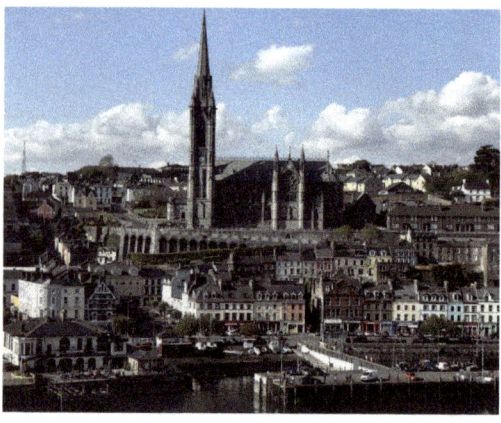

Credit: Port town of Cobh

Cruise ship passengers disembark directly from the quayside alongside Victorian Railway Station, which serves as the gateway to Cork's city centre, 20 km away - trains leave on the half hour and travel time is approximately 26 minutes. The Cobh Heritage Centre is located inside the station, as is a café, shops and disabled toilets.

# Directory

Located within 100 m of the quay, the town of Cobh is renowned for its maritime past and attracts a vast amount of attention as the last port of call for the ill-fated Titanic. There are also a variety of pubs, restaurants and cafes within walking distance of the quay.

Marketing organisation CorkCruise was formed to promote Cork as a cruise destination and their team provide a very special welcome to visiting cruise ships. On arrival, representatives greet each guest with a friendly smile and offer advice and tourist information. If time permits, a display of traditional Irish dancing is presented in the ship's theatre and an emotional farewell sees your ship slip off its mooring to the sounds of a local brass or pipe band playing on the quayside.

Although there is presently no cruise terminal, there are plans to build one at Port Cobh's Deepwater Quay, but no finishing date has been given as of yet. In the interim, there is a marquee on the quayside which is being used as the check-in point.

Waterfront Car Park is a free long-term parking facility adjacent to the quayside, known as the Five Foot Way, and overlooked by the police station. Once parked, it is a short walk along the waterside path to all the attractions and amenities that Cobh has to offer.

A Cabs Cobh provides affordable fixed fare taxis with wheelchair-accessible vehicles that will transfer you on short trips, as well as laying on day tours to see the local sights. To secure a booking, call 021 481 4000.

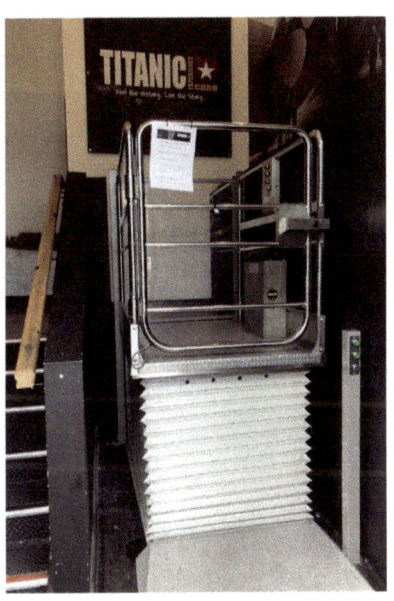

Credit: Experience Cobh

## Dover, England – Port of Call/Turnaround
*The Port of Dover, Harbour House, Marine Parade, Dover, Kent CT17 9DQ*

**Recent cruise operators:** Crystal Cruises, Holland America, Princess, Seabourn, Disney, Fred. Olsen, Saga, Royal Caribbean, Regent Seven Seas.

# The Autonomous Cruiser

Located 76 miles to the south-east of London, Dover's two state-of-the-art port terminals offer some of the most modern facilities in the UK, and for all those that want to see the famous White Cliffs, you will have a magnificent view as you set sail.

If you travel by car it's an easy journey down the A2 or A20, with clear signage to Dover Cruise Terminal, which has a dedicated car park with over 1,000 car parking spaces and undercover parking facilities - for bookings, email *carparking@doverport.co.uk* or phone 0844 504 1771. Due to the size of the onsite parking compound, a bus service is provided to facilitate transit to the terminal building.

A train from London Charing Cross, London St Pancras or London Victoria will take just under two hours, alighting at Dover Priory Station, only minutes away from the cruise terminal.

Tourist Information is located on Old Town Gaol Street and is open Monday to Friday from 9 am-5.30 pm and on Saturdays from 10 am-4 pm. In July and August, it's open daily from 9 am-5 pm.

The three terminal buildings that serve Dover each offer modern facilities that are fully accessible and include fast check-in, a spacious departure lounge, cafe bars, disabled and public restrooms, wheelchair ramps and walkways, a currency exchange, free internet and baggage handlers. The two main terminal buildings have a taxi rank outside.

Cruise Terminal 1 was originally built in 1914 as Dover Marine Railway Station but the building has since been renovated as a state-of-the-art cruise terminal. For those interested in the port – reflecting its heritage as a royal gateway over the centuries – information boards tell its fascinating story.

Cruise Terminal 2 is the largest of the terminals and was purpose built in 2000 along the lines of an airport terminal. It is sleek and modern, with every inch representative of a 21$^{st}$ century cruise terminal. From the first-floor departure lounge passengers can experience unimpeded, spectacular views of the harbour, the world-renowned White Cliffs and Dover Castle.

Cruise Terminal 3 has an adjacent berth ideal for smaller ships and port of call visits. At the far end of Admiralty Pier, Cruise Terminal 3 provides berthing for cruise ships up to 180 m in size. Passengers travelling out of this terminal check-in at a specially designed, dedicated gazebo space.

Wheelchair Taxis provides 24/7 accessible transport for disabled guests with integral ramps as standard on all their vehicles. To secure your booking, email *enquiries@licensedlondontaxi.co.uk* or phone 07519 055 741.

# DIRECTORY

## Dublin, Ireland – Port of Call/Turnaround
*Terminal 7, Tolka Quay Road, Dublin, N53 21 12/W6 12 33*

**Recent cruise operators:** *Celebrity, Princess, Seabourn, Windstar, Ponant, Noble Caledonia, Silversea Expeditions, Crystal, Regent Seven Seas, Hapag Lloyd, Oceania Cruises, Sea Cloud, Scenic Luxury Cruises & Tours, Cruise & Maritime Voyages.*

Situated off the east coast of Ireland near the Irish Sea, Dublin is home to Ireland's largest port and is the country's capital city. Primarily a busy cargo facility, it is dominated by containers and cranes, though cruise ship appearances are becoming a regular sight. During the 2018 season, Celebrity Cruises became the first major cruise company to use Dublin as a homeport and more cruise lines have since followed suit.

Dublin Airport is conveniently located eight miles north of the city centre and has excellent links to most major cities in the UK and continental Europe. Dublin is positioned at the heart of Ireland's road and rail network, making getting to the terminal by car or train incredibly easy. Dublin Tunnel is situated on the perimeter of the port and provides quick access to the M50 & M1 motorways, the main routes to the North and South of Ireland. Car Parking is available at the cruise terminal by contacting Dublin Port in advance, either via their website *dublinport.ie* or by phoning 01 887 6000.

Passengers arriving by small ship will arrive in the heart of the city at the quayside of the River Liffey, at North Wall Quay Extension, close to the East Link Bridge. Transport to town is usually provided by the cruise line, but a frequent service from the cruise port to the city centre is also provided by bus line 53, or alternatively it's less than a ten-minute taxi ride. Luas tram/light rail system is adjacent to East Link Bridge (next door to 3Arena) and has a direct route to the city centre. Tram stations' ramps, low floors and wide spaces mean that wheelchair users can easily board. For those more energetic, it's about a two-mile walk along the river.

Larger vessels berth in Alexandra Quay (Ocean Pier 33), only minutes from the city centre. If your cruise line doesn't provide a shuttle bus, there is a city bus service near the terminal, as well as taxis. Due to heavy port traffic in the area, walking isn't advised.

If your itinerary has Dublin down as a tender port, the disembarkation will be in Dún Laoghaire Harbour, a small suburban town located eight miles from Dublin's city centre. A free shuttle service is usually provided from the port to Dun Laoghaire's railway station from which you can easily catch a cab into the city (located on Marine Road). There is also a Dublin rapid transit system (DART) station near the pier which runs every 15 minutes and will get you into the city centre in about 20 minutes. Passengers have the option of leaving the train at three stations, Pearse Street, Tara Street and Connolly Station, all of which are accessible. DART trains feature generous space for wheelchairs, but not every station on the line is wheelchair-accessible. Search for your station online via Irish Rail and check its accessibility.

To facilitate the growth of homeporting from Dublin, the port commissioned a unique, fully equipped 30,000 square foot Evolution building, with dedicated check-in facilities, porter assistance and disabled and public toilets. The cruise lines provide tea, coffee and water for their passengers inside. Just a short distance away is Circle K, a 24-hour convenience store chain offering a variety of products for people on the go, including rolls, sandwiches, coffee and free internet. The Gateway Restaurant is located above the forecourt and a lift is available for guests who are mobility challenged.

Wheelchair Xpress offers accessible transfers to and from Dublin, as well as day tours to see the local sights. Their wheelchair taxi is the only one of its type in Dublin, safely accommodating two wheelchairs and six people. To secure a booking, email their office at *wheelchairxpresstaxis@gmail.com* or phone on +00 353 876 271 363.

The Alexandra Basin Redevelopment project is due for completion in 2023, which will transform the port's infrastructure by lengthening the berths and deepening the basin, allowing larger-sized cruise ships to dock there.

## Dundee, Scotland – Port of Call/Turnaround
*The Port of Dundee, East Camperdown Street, Dundee City DD1 3LG*

**Recent cruise operators:** *Cruise & Maritime Voyages, Princess, Silver Wind, Azamara, Crystal.*

Located on the north bank of the River Tay estuary, on the east coast of Scotland, midway between Aberdeen and the central belt, the Port of Dundee, a UNESCO City of Design, is conveniently close to City Quay and the rejuvenated Dundee Waterfront.

A free shuttle service is available from the port to the city centre and to the nearby shopping community of Broughty Ferry. The city's new V&A Dundee is proving to be a big hit with tourists and its ever-changing temporary exhibitions mean there is always something new to see. Next door is the RRS *Discovery*, Captain Scott's old ship, a highlight to those who love maritime history. Forth Ports Ltd works very closely with Dundee City Council, who provide tourism students and Sea Cadets at the port to offer assistance and tourist information when required.

Dundee Airport (DND) is located just two miles southwest of the Scottish city and has easy links to the surrounding towns and cities of St Andrews, Perth, Montrose and Forfar. Dundee Railway Station is 1.5 miles from the terminal and taxis are readily available for the short journey.

Dundee has been a popular port of call for some time, especially on cruises around the British Isles, but in recent years it has also been used as a turnaround homeport, enabling passengers to start and end their cruises without having to travel the distance to Southampton, Dover or Liverpool.

Forth Ports (Dundee) offer car parking located within the port area but it must be pre-booked with your tour operator or travel agent. On arrival at the port, drop your luggage off at the cruise terminal before heading towards the car park. Ensure your parking permit is clearly visible in the windscreen of your vehicle.

All embarking guests should be aware that the Dundee Cruise Terminal is located within a secure port facility, so you must follow the signs for the 'Cruise Traffic' area of East Camperdown Street.

Forth Ports is currently investing in an update to the terminal facilities which are currently housed in a shed, but there are disabled toilets next to a marquee which is used as the passenger waiting area. Baggage handlers are provided at the discretion of the cruise line (CMV always does).

Tele Taxis offers accessible taxi transfers to and from Dundee, as well as day tours to see the local sights. Bookings can be secured by emailing *teletaxi@btconnect.com* or by phoning 01382 825 825.

## Edinburgh (Leith, Newhaven, Rosyth, South Queensferry), Scotland
*Leith – Port of Call/Turnaround*
*Cruise Port Terminal, 100 Ocean Drive West, Leith, EH6 6JJ*

**Recent cruise operators:** *Fred. Olsen, Cunard, Princess, MSC, Sea Cloud, Silversea Expeditions, Azamara, Windstar.*

# The Autonomous Cruiser

Home to the Royal Yacht *Britannia*, Leith is located on the Firth of Forth's southern shore and is only three miles from the centre of Scotland's capital city, Edinburgh.

The cruise terminal has easy access to major motorways in Scotland, including the A1, Edinburgh bypass, the M8 and the M9, and parking is adjacent to the cruise terminal. Train networks are well connected to Edinburgh Waverley Station and are only a short taxi ride away from the port. Edinburgh Airport is only a 30-minute taxi ride.

The modern terminal has good passenger facilities, including check-in desks, a reception, waiting area, baggage area and handlers, security personnel, scanners, internet and disabled toilets. There is also outside seating and a smoking area.

> **Don't Ask:**
> Is the island completely surrounded by water?

The CruiseForth Welcome Team will be in the terminal to provide detailed advice on the town's accessibility. The shore excursion buses are located in the car park outside the terminal building and some cruise lines run shuttle services into Edinburgh.

The Ocean Terminal Shopping Centre, a five-minute walk away, offers a modern leisure and retail complex including shops, banking facilities, restaurants, cafes and car parking. It is also the access point for the Royal Yacht *Britannia*. A short walk away in Leith itself are celebrity chef restaurants, historic pubs, art studios and highland-dress outfitters.

Edinburgh supports the National Key Scheme (NKS), which offers disabled people access to public toilets across the city.

Getting around from Leith is easy with the Lothian Hop-On-Hop-Off bus service (Majestic Route) stopping at the terminal door. A variety of local buses take passengers to different parts of the city, including the railway station and the airport. All Lothian buses are wheelchair-accessible and passengers with restricted mobility have found the service to be competitively priced and an easy way to see the city. Taxis, most of which are wheelchair-accessible, will be waiting on the quayside, just beyond the cruise terminal, the majority of which accept credit cards.

Central Taxis proudly state that all 465 of their vehicles are wheelchair-accessible, with accessible ramps as standard and drivers that are specially trained to interact with all disabled passengers. The company offers accessible transfers to and from Leith, as well as day tours to see the local sights. Bookings can be secured by emailing *customer.services@taxis-edinburgh.co.uk* or by phoning 0131 229 2468.

Leith can only accommodate smaller ships so larger vessels drop anchor at Newhaven and tender guests ashore to Newhaven Pier.

## Newhaven – Port of Call

***Recent Cruise Operators:*** Viking, Norwegian, Seabourn, Hapag Lloyd, Silversea, Celebrity, Royal Caribbean, Oceania.

One of two tender ports serving Edinburgh, Newhaven Harbour is adjacent to the port of Leith and handles guests from larger ships that cannot get under the Forth Rail Bridge or through the lock gates. Forth Ports have invested in a pontoon which can handle up to four tenders at one time and connects to the quayside by a ramp. Assistance is provided to wheelchair users if required and CruiseForth Welcome Volunteers will be present on the quayside to provide more detailed information on the area's accessibility.

The shore excursion buses leave from a parking area adjacent to the pontoon. Care should be taken on the uneven ground of the car park at this historic port. Disabled toilets are provided in a building on the quayside.

A free shuttle service is provided by the port authorities to take guests on the five-minute journey to the Ocean Terminal Shopping Centre, from which the Old Port area of Leith can be accessed. Most of the shuttles are wheelchair-accessible.

Getting around from Newhaven is easy, with the Lothian Hop-On-Hop-Off bus service (Majestic Route) located approximately 100 yards away. All tour buses are fully accessible with low floor ramped access and two wheelchair spaces. A variety of local buses take passengers to different parts of the city, including the railway station and the airport. All Lothian buses are wheelchair-accessible, but there is only one space on each bus and mobility scooters are not permitted. The buses can be lowered to the ground and have retractable ramps that come out to give step-free access. Passengers with impaired mobility have found the service to be an easy way to get around the city.

Edinburgh's two main black cab firms are wheelchair-accessible, with over 900 taxis between them. Taxis are located 100 yards from the pontoon, many of which are wheelchair-accessible and accept credit cards. If you want to ensure you have an accessible taxi waiting, contact Central Taxis by emailing *customer.services@taxis-edinburgh.co.uk* or by phoning 0131 229 2468. The company offers accessible transfers to and from Newhaven, as well as day tours to see the local sights.

## Rosyth – Port of Call/Turnaround
*The Port of Rosyth, Exmouth Building, Rosyth, Fife, KY11 2XP*

**Recent cruise operators:** Fred. Olsen, Cruise & Maritime Voyages, Azamara Club Cruises, Voyages to Antiquity, Windstar Cruises, Viking, Oceania.

Known as the gateway to Fife and just 13 miles from Edinburgh, Rosyth is centrally located on the north bank of the Firth of Forth, just to the west of the three impressive bridges that join North and South Queensferry. Of the three, The Forth Bridge, a magnificent railway viaduct, is now a UNESCO World Heritage Site. The Forth Road Bridge is now restricted as a bus, taxi, cyclist and pedestrian route, and the recently completed Queensferry Crossing connects Rosyth with the arterial motorway infrastructure, allowing easy travel for all vehicles in all directions. Rosyth Cruise Terminal is approximately 25 minutes away by taxi from Edinburgh Airport.

Parking at the port is extremely limited for visitors, but it's usually possible to bring your car close to the terminal building to drop off and collect guests. Rosyth does have a dedicated car park next for embarking passengers, but you'll need to speak to your cruise operator about parking availability for the duration of your cruise.

Passengers in transit pass through a marquee and are greeted by the CruiseForth Welcome Team who provide tourist information and point guests with pre-booked tours in the direction of their coaches. They also offer a courtesy bus for the 3-mile journey to Dunfermline, the ancient capital of Scotland, birthplace of Andrew Carnegie and burial place of Robert the Bruce. The courtesy bus does not have a wheelchair ramp, but local taxis, some of which may be accessible, are available at the terminal building. If your taxi driver doesn't take credit cards they will happily drive you to a local ATM. The Shopmobility operator in Dunfermline permits the use of their equipment on production of your cruise card.

Disembarking passengers collect their luggage in a marquee before continuing on their homeward journey. Embarking passengers check in their luggage at the cruise terminal and proceed to a 250-seat lounge which offers tea and coffee facilities, disabled and public restrooms and free internet. Once processed, passengers are transferred in low-level buses down to the ship for boarding. Baggage handlers are available if required.

There is currently no public transport service at the port, but cruise lines often provide a shuttle bus to Inverkeithing Railway Station, a busy depot on the East Coast Main Line that is 25 minutes from Edinburgh Waverley Station, however, the shuttle bus does not guarantee a wheelchair ramp. The station is also served by London and North Eastern Railway (London to Aberdeen) and Virgin Cross Country (Aberdeen to Plymouth).

Wheelchair-accessible cars with ramps fitted as standard are available from Central Taxis. Bookings can be secured by emailing *customer.services@taxis-edinburgh.co.uk* or by phoning 0131 229 2468.

## South Queensferry – Port of Call

***Recent cruise operators:*** *Princess, Holland America, Crystal, MSC, Royal Caribbean.*

One of two tender ports serving Edinburgh, South Queensferry handles guests from the larger cruise ships that cannot get under the Forth Rail Bridge or access the lock gates at Leith and transfers them into South Queensferry, whose anchorage sits in the shadows of the UNESCO World Heritage Forth Bridge, under which tenders pass on the journey to Hawes Pier.

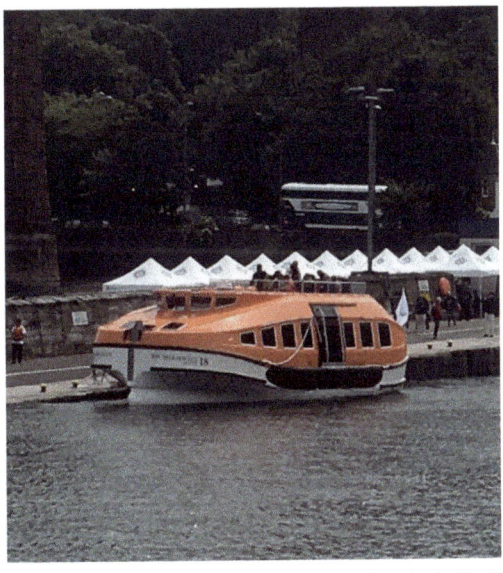

*Credit: South Queensferry Hawes tender – Cruise Forth*

The arrival point is around nine miles from Edinburgh city centre. Excursion buses are parked on the nearby promenade, where they depart north or south by accessing the nearby M90 and the Queensferry Crossing. The distance to the buses depends on the tide, with around 200 yards walk on a gentle incline during low tides, and a 100-yard walk on a gentle incline during high tides. Toilets are available at the head of the pier but there are no disabled facilities.

South Queensferry itself is a popular town for day visitors, with cobbled streets and traditional houses, pubs and restaurants overlooking the bridges. The CruiseForth Welcome Team will be available on the pier and are only too willing to offer assistance and tourist information on the options available to you on your day's visit. They can also provide a list of outlets that offer free internet.

Getting around from South Queensferry is made easy by the 99X Cruiselink Service which runs directly from the head of the pier to St Andrew Square in central Edinburgh (*journey time around 35 minutes depending on traffic*). The service is operated by Lothian Buses and is wheelchair-accessible.

A regular train service from Dalmeny Station takes passengers into Edinburgh in 15 minutes, but access to the station is by way of a set of 120 steps or an 800-yard walk up a steep incline. There are ramps to both platforms and for train access.

Taxis are also available at the head of the pier. Wheelchair-accessible cars, with ramps fitted as standard, are available from Central Taxis. Bookings can be secured by emailing customer.services@taxis-edinburgh.co.uk or by phoning 0131 229 2468.

## Greenock, Glasgow, Scotland – Port of Call/Turnaround
*Greenock Ocean Terminal, Patrick Street, Greenock, PA16 8UU*

**Recent cruise operators:** *Fred. Olsen, Cruise & Maritime Voyages, P&O, Cunard, MSC Azamara, Princess, Royal Caribbean, Crystal, Disney, Saga.*

Located at the entrance to the sheltered and scenic Clyde estuary on Scotland's Atlantic coast, Greenock's Ocean Terminal is now one of Scotland's best natural deep-water cruise facilities, with convenient access to rail, air and motorway networks. Just a five-minute walk from the main town, the port is easily accessible for travellers from Glasgow, Edinburgh and the surrounding Scottish towns.

Greenock is the gateway to some of Scotland's most breath-taking scenery and a host of exciting excursions and attractions, including the architectural, cultural and shopping delights of Scotland's largest city, Glasgow, just 35 minutes away.

Greenock is served by two international airports, Glasgow Airport and Glasgow Prestwick International Airport. The easiest way to get from

Glasgow Airport is from Paisley St James Station to Greenock West; a direct train departs hourly and takes about 25 minutes. There is no direct train from Glasgow Prestwick International Airport, you have to travel to Greenock West via Paisley Gilmour Street, a journey of about 85 minutes.

There are two train stations that can take you from the port to Glasgow Central Station, in the city centre, both just a short drive away from the terminal - Greenock West and Greenock Central have trains to the Scottish city running every 20 minutes, with a journey time of approximately 40 minutes. For the return journey, take the train, which runs every 30 minutes, to Greenock West.

For passengers embarking, Greenock provides car parking on site but it must be pre-booked through your booking agent. Once at the port, offload your baggage at the terminal before heading to the car park where you can catch a short shuttle ride back to the cruise terminal after dropping off your car. If friends are seeing you off, Cathcart Street West car park offers free parking for up to three hours, but a free parking disc, available from most shops in the town centre, must be displayed.

The port has a modern, accessible terminal building with excellent facilities, including tourist information areas, disabled and public restrooms, a currency exchange, internet connectivity and several vendors. The terminal is also ideally sited close to a supermarket and shopping mall.

After docking, tourists are typically greeted by traditional bagpipers, dressed in their distinctive tartan uniforms, while the Inverclyde Tourist Group provide volunteers to assist with local information, maps, and complimentary two-hour coach tours of the local area. Three different tours are offered at varying times throughout the day, but spaces are limited so make sure you book your place with one of the volunteers as soon as you disembark. The complimentary tours are only served by small minibuses and, unfortunately, are not wheelchair-friendly.

Inverclyde Taxis has a dedicated concierge at Ocean Terminal on hand to assist when you disembark that will offer up independent tours of some of the highlights of Scotland. They provide wheelchair-accessible vehicles that can accommodate passengers with a range of special needs and which incorporate ramps as standard. An induction loop is incorporated in the intercom system of all their accessible taxis for hearing aid users. Bookings can be made by emailing *enquiries@inverclydetaxis.co.uk*, downloading their app before leaving home or by calling 01475 734563.

## Harwich, England – Port of Call/Turnaround
*Harwich International Port, Parkeston Quay, Harwich, Essex, CO12 4SR*

**Recent Cruise Operators:** Cruise & Maritime Voyages, Fred. Olsen, Costa Cruises.

Harwich International Port is located on the River Stour's south bank on England's east coast. The original port of the *Mayflower*, Harwich has given the town a historic significance - if you have time to spare you could opt for a guided tour.

In the past, Harwich has acted as a major turnaround port for round-trip departures from the UK. Being a deep-water harbour, some of the biggest ships can dock here, but the last few years have seen a decline in the cruise operators that use the facility because of the lack of modern cruise passenger facilities.

The purpose-built accessible cruise terminal includes a departure lounge with seating for 300, disabled and public restrooms, a 24-hour tourist information point, free internet and the Quayside Café. The Visitor's Centre is open seasonally (May-September). The adjacent ferry terminal hosts another eatery, vending machines, a currency exchange machine, a cash machine, a railway ticket counter and more restrooms, including unisex disabled toilets. All walkways leading to cruise ships are wheelchair-friendly.

Trains take an hour from London's Liverpool Street into Harwich International train station, which is conveniently right next to the ferry and cruise terminals. If you are driving to the port then you can access the port's secure car park via the M11, M25 or A14, all of which have links to the A120 eastbound and are signposted for Harwich International Port. Four of London's major airports, Heathrow, Gatwick, Luton and Stansted, are under a two-hour drive. Taxis are readily available outside the terminal.

Parking can be pre-booked with Harwich Cruise Parking, who offer enough space for 600 vehicles. Follow the signage to your designated car park where a courtesy bus is provided to make the five-minute transfer to the cruise terminal. Trained staff are available to assist you and provide a wheelchair if needed.

Wheelchair Taxis provides 24/7 accessible transport for disabled guests with integral ramps as standard on all their vehicles. To secure your booking, email *enquiries@licensedlondontaxi.co.uk* or phone 07519 055 741.

# Directory

## Hull, England – Port of Call/Turnaround
*Port of Hull, King George Dock, Hedon Road, Humberside, HU9 5PR*

***Recent cruise operators:*** *Cruise & Maritime Voyages.*

> **Don't Ask:**
> *How high above sea level are we? (asked while floating on the sea)*

The only passenger port on the Humber River, the Port of Hull is often very busy with ferries and commercial shipping, but less so with cruise ships; Cruise & Maritime Voyages was one of the few cruise companies to use Hull as a homeport. The port has excellent road and rail links from most UK locations and Humberside Airport is 23 miles to the south, the equivalent of a 40-minute taxi ride.

Hull Station can be found within the Hull Paragon Interchange, the integrated rail and bus station in the city centre. Step free access is provided from the station entrance to all platforms and the staff will provide assistance throughout the station and with boarding and alighting the train, but it needs to be pre-booked by contacting the Assisted Travel Team on 0800 107 2149. A regular bus service is available from Hull Paragon Railway Station to tackle the four-mile journey to the dock - the bus takes about 15 minutes but only takes you to the port entrance, which is quite a long walk from the cruise terminal. The nearest taxi rank is outside the station.

Those travelling by car should follow the clear signage to King George Dock and enter at the Northern Gateway. On arrival, staff will direct you to the luggage drop off area before you head to your designated car park, from which it is a short shuttle ride back to the terminal. Parking must be pre-booked with your tour operator and you are asked to make sure the provided permit is clearly visible in your windscreen. There is no disabled parking close to the terminal building and all passengers are required to travel by shuttle to the check-in area, but the shuttle is wheelchair-accessible.

There is no dedicated terminal, instead cruise ship passengers use a temporary marquee with limited facilities, but accessible toilets are available in the ferry terminal. In September 2017 plans were drawn up for the construction of a new cruise ship terminal and riverside berth at Sammy's Point, which could be operational by 2024.

Wheelchair-accessible transport is available from 50 Cars, who provide transfers to and from Hull, as well as day tours to see the local sights. They operate a text/call back system that provides you with their vehicle's details and

# The Autonomous Cruiser

lets you know that your car is outside the terminal. To secure your booking, email *info@hulltaxisltd.co.uk* or phone 01482 505050 or 01482 505052.

## Leith (Scotland)
See Edinburgh

## Liverpool, England – Port of Call/Turnaround
*Liverpool Cruise Terminal, Pier Head, Princess Parade, Liverpool, L3 1DL*

***Recent cruise operators:*** *Fred. Olsen, Cruise & Maritime Voyages, Princess, Celebrity, Oceania, Disney, AIDA, Seabourn, Viking, Cunard, Saga, Ponant.*

Liverpool Cruise Terminal is situated at Pier Head and is one of the few ports in the world where cruise ships dock right in the heart of the city. Centrally located in the Irish Sea, the port is perfectly sited for itineraries around Britain and is an excellent starting point for transatlantic, North European and Baltic Cruises.

The city's John Lennon Airport is only nine miles away, while Manchester Airport is a longer journey at 40 miles. Lime Street Station is only a five-minute taxi ride away from the port and has routes to and from Manchester, London, Scotland and the rest of the UK. If coming by car, leave the M6 at junction 21a and take the M62 towards Liverpool city centre. Follow the brown signs on the arterial routes for Liverpool and/or Waterfront until you reach the Liver Building, from which the cruise terminal is easily identifiable.

Pre-booking is required for embarking passengers who require car parking. Cruise and Passenger Services are the main providers and bookings can be secured by emailing *info@candps.com* or by phoning 0345 071 3939. Once at the port you will be directed to the secure parking facility.

For embarking travellers, the drop off point is located in front of baggage reclaim. Due to limited space in front of baggage reclaim, the port is unable to provide a pick-up point on site. The closest short-term parking is adjacent to the Liver Building on St Nicholas Place, which also houses the nearest taxi rank. Mini buses and adapted vehicles are provided to cruisers with reduced mobility from the car park when travelling to baggage reclaim.

A small accessible terminal is housed in a single storey, modular building which has wheelchair-accessible toilets and refreshment facilities. Due to its size, it is not advisable to arrive before your allocated check-in time, as both embarkation and disembarkation takes place in the same shared space. Guests who do arrive early are not permitted to enter the building until disembarkation and luggage reclaim has been completed. The distance from the passenger lounge to the quayside is about 150 m but there are adapted vehicles for passengers with reduced mobility to the ship's gangway. If you have time to kill, explore the many restaurants, cafes and bars located directly adjacent to the cruise terminal on Pier Head. Alternatively, Albert Dock is only a 10-minute walk and boasts numerous places to eat and drink. There is a Taxi Rank adjacent to the Cruise Terminal on St Nicholas Place.

For those visiting the port for the day please note that the link-span bridges connecting the quayside to the shore-side can be steep at low tide.

A new cruise terminal has now been given planning permission with the proposed facility set for completion in 2023. The anticipated transformation will see their current terminal services moved to the Princes Jetty at Princes Parade, which will have the capacity to handle around 3600 passengers, three times larger than the existing terminal. The new facilities will include passport control, a waiting lounge, a baggage hall, public restrooms, a cafe, a restaurant, a dedicated taxi rank, coach and vehicle pick-up areas and terminal car parking for up to 300 cars. The new facility will be completely DDA compliant and ease of access for those with mobility issues has been built into the design.

Hackney Direct welcomes wheelchair users - in fact, their whole fleet is accessible and comes fitted with folding ramps for easy access. Offering transfers to and from Liverpool or bespoke tours of the city, bookings can be secured by emailing *info@hackneydirect.com* or by phoning 0151 645 8080.

### Newcastle, England – Port of Call/Turnaround
*International Passenger Terminal, North Shields, Tyne & Wear, NE29 6EE*

***Recent cruise operators:*** *Fred. Olsen, Cruise & Maritime Voyages, Marella Cruises, AIDA, Disney, Norwegian.*

The Newcastle International Passengers Cruise Terminal, also known as The Port of Tyne, is located in North Shields, adjacent to the Royal Quays Marina; it helps locals avoid the inconvenience of having to fly or travel the distance to the southern UK ports of Dover, Harwich and Southampton.

With great connectivity by road, rail and air, the port offers superb facilities for both turnaround calls and day visits. Sailing from Newcastle will save you almost a full day at sea compared to the more southerly options if booked on a Baltic cruise. The closest airport, Newcastle International, is just 14 miles from the port - a 35-minute taxi ride or an effortless journey via the A1 if driving. The city centre's coach station has good links to all parts of the country.

Newcastle Central Station is eight miles away, and if this is a port call your cruise line might lay on a shuttle to take you from the terminal to the station, with shuttle tickets available through the shore excursion desk the night before docking. The nearest Metro from Newcastle Central Station is Percy Main Station, a 20-minute walk and then a further 20-minute walk to the terminal (the cruise terminal is in Zone C).

The Port of Tyne offers secure car parking for passengers just a few minutes' walk from the International Passenger Terminal, but the service must be pre-booked through your tour operator. On entering the car park you'll get a ticket which must be taken with you and not left in the car. Arriving back from your cruise, baggage will be in a reclaim point within the car park for those with parked cars.

Recently refurbished, the terminal is fully accessible and has excellent pre-boarding facilities, including six check-in desks, lounge seating for 700, luggage facilities, tourist information and a currency exchange. The terminal also boasts shops, a café, a bar, disabled toilets, internet access and ATM machines for both euros and sterling. A beautiful refurbished waterfront offers excellent shops, eateries and amenities. There is a dedicated taxi rank in front of the terminal and a special minibus service is available to help wheelchair users, or those with reduced mobility, and their companions board the ship.

Budget Taxis have a large selection of wheelchair-accessible vehicles prepared to accommodate all passengers' needs, but to avoid disappointment bookings should be pre-booked by emailing *info@nodataxis.co.uk* or phoning 0191 298 5050. Their sister company, Noda Taxis Newcastle, also offers wheelchair-accessible transport with ramped access for taxi transfers to and from Newcastle or for day tours to see the local sights. To secure a reservation, pre-book by emailing *info@nodataxis.co.uk* or phoning 0191 222 1888.

## Newhaven, Scotland
See Edinburgh

# Directory

## Oban, Scotland – Port of Call

***Recent cruise operators:*** *Silver Cloud, Seabourn, Hebridean Princess, Holland America, Azamara, Cruise & Maritime Voyages, Quark Expeditions, Ponant, Prinsendam Cruises, Voyages to Antiquity, Windstar, Princess.*

The coastal town of Oban ('little bay' in Gaelic, Scotland's ancient Celtic language) is a popular and vibrant destination and is regarded as the seafood capital of Scotland. Oban is well connected to the central belt of Scotland and is only two and a half hours' drive through stunning countryside from Glasgow.

The North Pier pontoons offer accessible embarkation and disembarkation directly into the town centre for those arriving by tender. The Oban Town Ambassadors do their best to meet and greet every cruise ship passenger, offering maps and plenty of suggestions of things to see and do in the local area. Oban's Visitor Information iCentre, is also conveniently located just off the North Pier at the Columba Hotel and can help independent cruise ship passengers plan their visit to Oban. Open daily, the VisitScotland counter staff sell a selection of gifts, books and souvenirs, as well as tour tickets for walking tours, boat trips and other activities.

Disabled toilets are within the harbour office on the North Pier and are open to all cruise ship visitors. Though there are no ATMs at the pier, you are actually tendered into the centre of town where the nearest cash machine can be found on George Street at the Nationwide Building Society, a two-minute walk from the landing area. Currency exchange transactions can be done at the Post Office within a Tesco's supermarket just a ten-minute walk from the pier.

West Coast Motors offers bus services throughout Oban and beyond and all their buses are wheelchair-accessible with low floors and ramps for easy access, though each bus only has space for one wheelchair. The company sometimes lays on a coach on certain routes, but these are also accessible by a lift. The company allows class two mobility scooters up to a maximum size of 39.3 inches (1000mm) long and 23.6 inches (600mm) wide, with a maximum turning circle of 47.2 inches (1200mm) on all their vehicles. Service dogs are welcome onboard and bus drivers are instructed to stop for customers with a white cane and state their service number and destination.

With a fleet of over 800 taxis, Glasgow Taxis are the largest supplier of licensed taxis in Glasgow, and the largest in the UK outside of London.

Impressively, their entire fleet is wheelchair-accessible and offers transfers to and from Oban, as well as day tours to see the local sights. To secure a booking, email their office at *office@glasgowtaxis.co.uk* or phone on 0141 429 7070.

## Poole, England – Port of Call/Turnaround
*The Port of Poole, New Harbour Road, Poole, Dorset, BH15 4AJ*

**Recent cruise operators:** Cruise & Maritime Voyages, Fred. Olsen, Grand Circle Line.

Poole Harbour is the largest natural harbour in Europe and is widely recognised for its spectacular beauty and exciting tourism sites, including the Jurassic Coast World Heritage Site. The port has seen an increase in small cruise ships in recent years, but with the recent completion of the deep-water South Quay, the port can now also welcome larger ships. The port houses a modern, accessible terminal, equipped with a departure lounge, disabled and public washrooms, bureau de change, cash machines, internet access and a café.

The port has a central position on the South Coast and is easily accessible from London, the Midlands and the West Country, and offers convenient road and rail access. Poole is linked to London by the A31, M27 and M3, the A350 runs north to Bristol and the A35 to Dorchester and Exeter. Once nearby, drivers are advised to head into the town centre and then follow signs for the port - access is via two bridges which are open at different times, but advice is given on the variable message signs situated along the approach roads as to which one is open.

Bournemouth International Airport is just a 30-minute drive from the cruise terminal. Poole Railway Station is located in the town centre and is just 1.5 miles from the port and access is via the main port entrance at New Quay Road. Taxis are readily available around the station.

After dropping your luggage at the terminal, you will be directed to the nearby parking facility which offers the options of both short- and long-term stays. The port operates the car park themselves and has a pay and display machine which accepts either cash or credit cards. You need to display the ticket in your car whilst you are away and pay on your return.

Disabled Transport Services have eight specialist wheelchair-adapted taxis, offering door-to-door transport for users of all types of wheelchairs, including electric chairs and scooters, and for those with limited

# Directory

mobility. Bookings can be secured by phoning 01202 480111 or by emailing *info@wheelchairtaxisbournemouth.co.uk*.

## Portsmouth, England – Port of Call/Turnaround
*Portsmouth International Port, George Byng Way, Portsmouth, PO2 8SP*

**Recent cruise operators:** *Saga, Noble Caledonia, Cruise & Maritime Voyages, Ponant, Sea Cloud, Crystal, Fred. Olsen, Viking, Celestyal, Hapag-Lloyd, Lindblad Expeditions, Phoenix Reisen, Quark Expeditions, Silversea.*

Situated near the historic Naval Dockyard on the south coast of England, Portsmouth International Port is only one mile north of the city and offers superb facilities as both a turnaround port and for day visits.

The port itself is easily accessible by plane, train and car. Southampton Airport (20 miles), London's Heathrow (64 miles) and Gatwick (76 miles) are all within driving distance of the port. Both Portsmouth Harbour and Portsmouth & Southsea train stations are linked from London Waterloo and Cardiff, and from either station it's just a short ride by taxi, or free bus service in the summer months, to the terminal.

Just an hour and a half from London, Portsmouth enjoys enviable access by road, with the A3 connecting Portsmouth and London, and the nearby M27/A27 that brings the rest of Britain within reach. Once you're nearby, follow the clearly marked signs to reach the port and its multistorey parking facility, located just a few minutes' walk from the main terminal building. There is a long-term car parking facility servicing the port which must be pre-booked through Cruise Passenger Services. If you are picking up or dropping off passengers there are 20-minute parking bays directly outside the terminal.

A special minibus service is available to help wheelchair users, or those with reduced mobility, and their companions board the ship. Assistance is also available for those travelling by car, with designated spaces for guests with disabilities.

The award-winning passenger terminal is spacious and offers comfortable seating in contemporary surroundings, with check-in desks, internet access and a Travelex currency exchange, with snacks and drinks provided by the World Marche café or Costa coffee lounge. There is an ATM on the ground floor on the side of the Travelex Bureau which offers both euros and sterling, and an Amigo shop for any last-minute purchases. A dedicated taxi tank can be found outside the terminal.

A member of the Sunflower Lanyard Scheme, Portsmouth International Port has staff specially trained to recognise a wearer as having a hidden disability and can offer additional help if needed. Disabled toilets are located throughout the port. The terminal has recently installed a new toilet/changing room for people with complex needs on the ground floor; this 'Space to Change' facility includes a peninsula toilet, an adult-sized height-adjustable changing bench and ceiling-tracking hoist, plus there is extra space for mobility equipment and caregivers. The toilet is accessible by radar key, or you can ask for access at the security desk if you don't have the key with you.

The terminal is easily accessible by wheelchair users and has two large customer lifts, providing access to the 1st floor. There is seating marked for disabled and elderly passengers in the terminal and all food outlets on both floors are accessible to wheelchair users.

Paragon Taxis offers accessible vehicles for long distance transfers to and from Portsmouth. Each vehicle can take one wheelchair and up to six passengers. They also offer bespoke trips to the local tourist hotspots, such as Stonehenge, Windsor Castle, Winchester and the New Forest. Bookings can be secured by emailing *info@paragontaxis.co.uk* or by phoning 0771 409 0273 or 0787 019 8968.

The Route4U app is easy to download and offers maps and routes for the city that have been specially tailored for wheelchair users and those with impaired mobility.

## Rosyth, Scotland
See Edinburgh

## South Queensferry, Scotland
See Edinburgh

## Swansea – Port of Call/Turnaround
*The Port of Swansea, Head King's Dock, Port Tennant, Swansea SA1 1QR*

**Recent cruise operators:** *Phoenix Reisen.*

Swansea has been transformed in recent years, from its industrial past of coal mines and iron works, to its current bustling city centre and waterfront. This modernisation has also extended to its cruise port which is just a few miles

# DIRECTORY

from the city centre, the Gower Peninsular and other local tourist attractions. There are two approved berths for cruise ship calls, and shuttle buses to town may be laid on by your cruise ship operator. Public bus stops are available on the peripheral roads the port and taxis can access the cruise terminal for collections and drop-offs. An accessible temporary marquee is used for embarking guests and houses facilities such as a seated waiting area, security and baggage screening, baggage assistance, public and disabled toilets and a pop-up café for refreshments.

Swansea airport is sited nine miles from the port, a journey of around 26 minutes in light traffic. The port is less than three miles by dual carriageway to Junction 42 of the M4 and offers secure car parking within the port compound that needs to be pre-booked through your cruise line operator.

The port also has direct links to the national rail network - Swansea station is less than ten minutes from the cruise terminal, with easy connections to most of Britain, including London, Bristol, Manchester, Swindon and Cardiff, and regional services that run to Carmarthen, Pembroke Dock, Llanelli and Shrewsbury. The station has four platforms, all with step-free access, and has an adjacent taxi rank.

As one of Wales' most popular waterfront cities, Swansea is a great cruise call with several local attractions, activities and shopping on its doorstep. The staff exude a real Welsh welcome to guests in transit and typically greet passengers with traditional harp music at the quayside and an opportunity to sample some of their fabulous local wares. The staff are also on hand for those needing visitor information or itinerary planning and will help passengers enjoy the best the city has to offer.

Data Cabs is proud that 70% of their 102-vehicle fleet is wheelchair-accessible and available for short or long distance transfers to and from the Port of Swansea. Each vehicle can take one wheelchair and up to six passengers, with a number of vehicles that can accommodate two wheelchairs. They also offer a bespoke service around the local sights. Bookings can be secured by emailing *steve@datacabs.com* or by phoning 01792 474747 or 01792 545454.

# The Autonomous Cruiser

**Tilbury, England – Port of Call/Turnaround**
*The London Cruise Terminal, Tilbury, Essex, RM18 7NG*

**Recent cruise operators:** *Cruise & Maritime Voyages, Fred. Olsen.*

The Port of Tilbury (aka Tilbury Docks) is located just 25 miles east of central London at the head of the River Thames. As London's only deep-water cruise facility, it is home to the London Cruise Terminal, which Cruise & Maritime Voyages previously made their home. The area is a cheerless mix of freight depots and commercial docks, and the terminal is much the same - a single-storey listed building occupying a flat site. It is wheelchair-accessible and offers a passenger lounge and a kiosk selling hot and cold drinks and snacks. A wider selection of food and drink is available from the ASDA right next to the port.

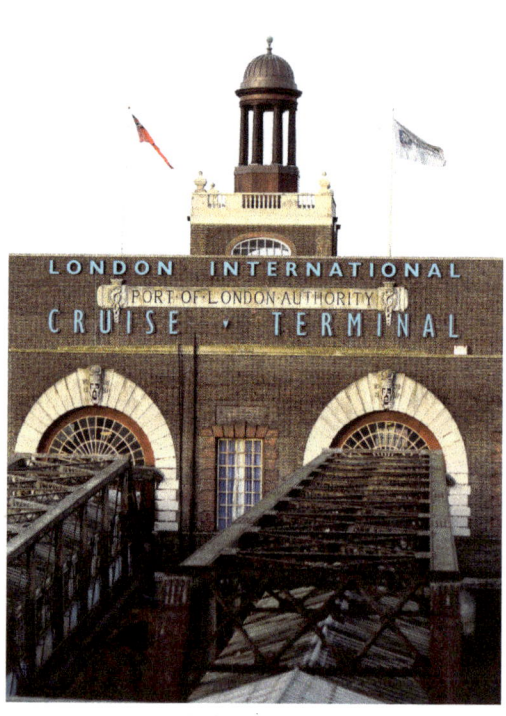

*Credit: Tilbury Docks - Jerry Clack, Flickr*

Allowing for good traffic, the journey from Heathrow or London City Airport runs about 90 minutes. There are regular trains to Tilbury Town on the main London Fenchurch to Southend line and taxis are available from the station to make the mile's journey to the cruise terminal. Alternatively, free shuttle buses meet the trains and take you to the Tilbury to Gravesend ferry which is situated right next to the terminal building. Special coaches are frequently laid on from Victoria Coach Station to tie in with the cruising schedule.

The Port of Tilbury offers secure passenger car parking within the port compound that needs to be pre-booked through your cruise operator. Please note, you will need to drop your luggage off at the terminal first if embarking

# Directory

as the car parking facilities are at least two miles away. Once parked up you will need to take the short shuttle bus journey back to the cruise terminal.

Wheelchair Taxis provide 24/7 accessible transport for disabled guests, with integral ramps as standard on all their vehicles. To secure your booking, email *enquiries@licensedlondontaxi.co.uk* or phone 07519 055 741.

## Cruising from Southampton

**Western Docks**
**City Cruise Terminal – Berth 101, via Dock Gates 8, 10 or 20, Solent Road, Western Docks, Southampton, SO15 1AJ** (Dock Gate 8 is closed for the annual Southampton Boat Show every August and September).
**Mayflower Cruise Terminal – Berths 102/104/106, via Dock Gates 10 or 20, Herbert Walker Avenue, Western Docks, Southampton, SO15 1HJ**

**Eastern Docks**
**QE2 Terminal – Berth 38/39, via Dock Gate 4, Test Road, Eastern Docks, Southampton, SO14 3GG** (Enter the port through Dock Gate 4 and at the first roundabout, take the 2nd exit and proceed along Test Road for approximately one mile where you will find the terminal on your right).

**Ocean Cruise Terminal - Berth 46/47 – via Dock Gate 4, Cunard Road, Eastern Docks, Southampton, SO14 3QN** (Enter the port through Dock Gate 4 and at the first roundabout, take the 3rd exit, proceed 100 yards and turn left - the terminal will be in full view ahead of you).

*Recent cruise operators:* AIDA, P&O, Princess, Cunard, Royal Caribbean, Celebrity, MSC, Carnival, Fred. Olsen, Marella, Norwegian, Oceania, Regent Seven Seas, Saga.

As the cruising capital of the UK, Southampton sees some of the finest cruise

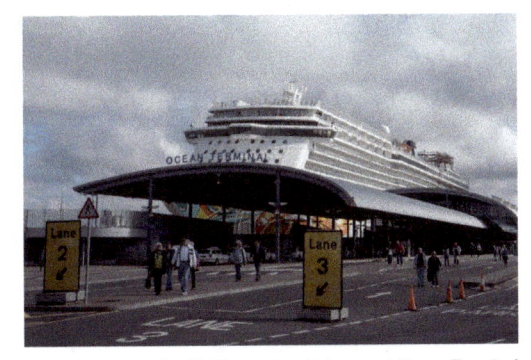

Credit: Norwegian Getaway at Ocean Terminal Southampton - Richard Vaillancourt, Flickr

# The Autonomous Cruiser

lines sailing from four terminals strung along two miles of waterfront: The Mayflower Cruise Terminal, QE11 Cruise Terminal, Ocean Cruise Terminal and City Cruise Terminal. The port continues to grow, with Royal Caribbean recently signing a deal securing the City Cruise Terminal as their official UK cruise departure port until 2023. If you're not sure what cruise terminal your ship is going to dock in, visit *southamptonvts.co.uk* to check the schedule.

Southampton is now the UK's principal cruise port and one of the most popular embarkation points in Europe because of its fabulous road links and the regional airport just a spitting distance away. These different transport options can make it difficult to assess which will be the quickest, easiest or cheapest route to take when getting to your cruise ship terminal.

## Cruise Terminals

### City Cruise Terminal

A full redevelopment of the building was completed by the RCCL Corporation, who have since made the City Cruise Terminal Royal Caribbean's official UK homeport for roundtrip itineraries. The renovations include paperless check-in at one of 50 service desks, digital signage (wayfinders), Wi-Fi, a new security area and full accessibility throughout the building. A large departure lounge offers ample seating, a fully licensed bar and cafe serving refreshments and sandwiches, disabled and public toilets and complimentary magazines. There is, however, no ATM in the building.

Facilities in the arrivals area include disabled and public toilets, vending machines offering a limited range of drinks and snacks, a range of complimentary magazines and a guide and map of Southampton. Ceanos operate an outside catering kiosk with a large covered seating area and offer refreshments, snacks and hot food. Adjacent to the Isle Of Wight Ferries terminal, and just a three minute car ride via Herbert Walker Avenue, Mayflower Park is an excellent vantage point to watch ships sail away. A dedicated taxi rank is adjacent to the terminal.

### Mayflower Cruise Terminal

The accessible terminal has a sizable departure lounge with plenty of seating, a vending machine, Wi-Fi, complimentary magazines and disabled and public toilets. Please note, there is no ATM at the terminal. Ceanos, a fully licensed cafe, operates both within the departure and arrivals lounges, offering a selection of refreshments, snacks and fresh handmade sandwiches.

# Directory

The Arrivals Hall offers visitors a chance to watch ships sail out of Southampton from the viewing gallery, which opens an hour before the departure time; visitors will need photo ID to obtain a security pass to access the viewing gallery. The Arrivals Hall houses accessible and public toilets, a selection of refreshment options, and a taxi rank just outside - the terminal is 1.5 miles from the dock gates, so anyone wanting to go into town is best off catching a taxi.

## QE2 Terminal

Home to Cunard ships, the fully accessible terminal underwent a huge refurbishment in 2016 which included the installation of a state-of-the-art ship-to-shore walkway. The departure lounge, located on the first floor, has ample seating, disabled and public toilets and complimentary magazines. Please note, there is no ATM in the terminal. Café Ceanos is fully licensed and offers refreshments, as well as hot and cold snacks.

The arrivals lounge has comfortable seating, disabled and public toilets, a vending machine and complimentary magazines. The lounge is open to the public who want to see friends and family off, but the viewing gallery is not open to visitors. Disembarking guests can have tea, coffee, cold drinks, cakes, snacks and crisps during the company's opening times. There is a dedicated taxi rank outside the Arrivals Hall.

## Ocean Cruise Terminal

One of Southampton's newest and busiest cruise terminals, the fully accessible Art Deco building leads you into a ground floor reception area with seating for nearly 150 people. There is a water cooler located next to three vending machines which offer refreshments and snacks, and there are complimentary magazines, including a map and guide of Southampton, available. Disabled and public toilets are available in both the reception area and the departure lounge upstairs.

An escalator, stairs or a lift are available to take you up to the first-floor departure lounge, with staff on hand to point you in the right direction. About 40 service desks make up check-in, with the first four or five desks sectioned off and dedicated to priority check-in. There is ample seating and Wi-Fi in the terminal, but no ATM. Ceanos operate within the upstairs departure lounge and offer a selection of teas and coffees, cold drinks, beers, wines, spirits, crisps, cakes and snacks. In addition, there is a selection of hot food and fresh handmade sandwiches and another complimentary magazine rack. Both the coach and train station are about a mile from dock gate 10 and there is a dedicated taxi rank outside the terminal.

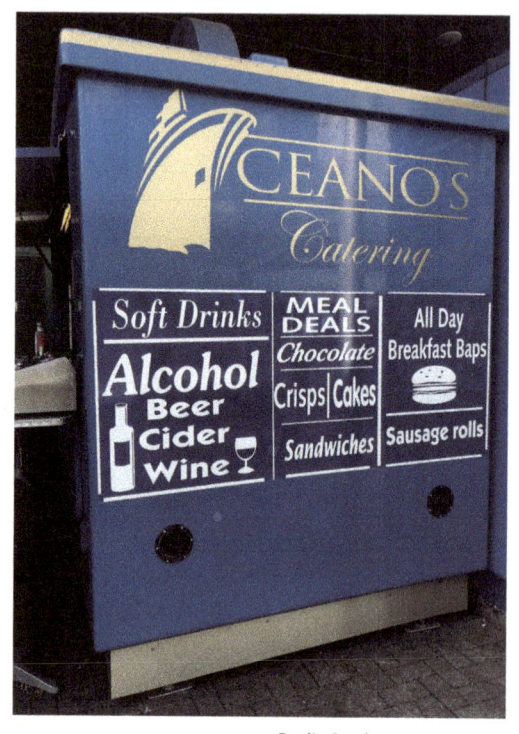

*Credit: Southampton Catering*

**Smokers Essential:** *The terminals are non-smoking throughout but there are designated smoking areas outside the four terminal buildings. Remember to use the bins provided, as littering in the UK has an £80 on the spot fine.*

The aim of the information below is to give you an overall picture as to what transport is available to get to Southampton from several major cities throughout the UK, but remember that flight, train and coach timings are dependent on public demand and the dates of travel, so it is possible that the details listed might be slightly different for your travel plans.

### Domestic Flights
The excellent transport links between Southampton's airport and port make it a tempting departure point for cruisers from all across the UK. Located on

# Directory

the outskirts of the city, just five miles from the port, and within easy reach of the M27 and M3, the airport is easily the leading 'fast track' airport in central-southern England. It is the destination of a host of domestic flights, making it incredibly easy to fly to from all across the UK. Several low-cost airlines, including Eastern Airlines, operate domestic routes to and from Southampton Airport. The easiest way to find cheap flights is to use a comparison site like Directline Flights - *directline-flights.co.uk*.

The airport is on one level, making wheelchair access easy, and there is a lift in the departure lounge for accessing the restaurants and bars on the first floor. Accessible bathrooms are located on the main concourse and within the departure lounge itself. The airport has an Access Partnership with Guide Dogs and airport staff have received specialised training enabling them to assist travellers with visual impairments.

Airport facilities include plenty of cafes and bars, a large branch of WH Smiths and free wireless broadband throughout the airport. If you don't have personal access to a wireless connection, pay-as-you-go computer terminals are available near the 'help point' and on the top floor of the departure lounge. Checkercars has a taxi desk located on the main concourse within the airport terminal and offers accessible vehicles for wheelchair users. Pre-booking is recommended, as it is for your return journey as the possibility of several ships disembarking at the same time could mean long queues. To secure a booking, email *southampton@checkercars.com* or phone 02380 651 110. The airport is also home to its own train station (Southampton Airport Parkway Station) which can get you to Southampton Central Station in under ten minutes.

If you are flying into Southampton the night before your cruise you can stay at one of a wealth of hotels conveniently placed between the airport and cruise terminal, all within 15 minutes of the port, with the majority linked to the port by a shuttle bus. There are also good options when it comes to wheelchair-accessible hotels in the area, perfect for pre and post cruise stays including Novotel Southampton, Ibis Southampton Centre, Ibis Budget Southampton, Holiday Inn Southampton, Moxy Southampton, Leonardo Royal Southampton Grand Harbour, Premier Inn at West Quay Harbour Parade, and Jurys Inn Southampton.

Despite Southampton Airport's close proximity to the port, most fly-cruise passengers fly into Heathrow (70 miles) or Gatwick Airport (90 miles), neither of which are particularly close by car. There are, however, direct trains from Gatwick Airport to Southampton Central train station, but not

# The Autonomous Cruiser

from Heathrow. Your cheapest options are to either book a transfer package through your cruise agent or book the direct service through National Express. You should be aware, though, that the National Express bus depot is in Southampton's town centre and not at the port, so you will still need to catch a taxi to your cruise terminal.

## Driving

Travelling by car to the cruise port is the obvious option for many holidaymakers as it can offer a faster and easier route than other modes of transport. From the North, London and the Home Counties, the M3, M27 and A34 provide fast, direct road links into Southampton city centre. The A36 is the major route from the West Country, Bristol and Wales. From the East, follow the A27/M27 and exit at Junction 8.

***GPS Tip:*** *Postcode accuracy on satellite navigation systems is variable. Once you're near your destination, follow the relevant signage.*

It is important to check which berth your cruise ship is berthed at before you leave home - go to Associated British Ports (ABP) website *southamptonvts.co.uk* and click on Live Information/Shipping Movements and Cruise Ship Schedule.

### Motorway Directions from the North, East & London regions
*Route One*

Travelling on the M3 southbound, follow signs for Southampton. Merge onto the M27 and follow the signs for the M27 West. Leave the M27 at Junction 3 and at the roundabout take the 1st exit signed M271 toward Southampton/The Docks. At the next roundabout (Redbridge), take the 1st exit onto the A33 which will lead you along a dual carriageway heading into Southampton to the relevant Dock Gate assigned for your cruise. This route will bring you in via Dock Gate 20 or Dock Gate 10 for the Mayflower Terminal, or Dock Gate 10 or 8 for the City Cruise Terminal.

*Route One Alternative*

From the end of the M3 at junction 14 follow A33 signs for Southampton & The Docks. This route will bring you out close to the Eastern Docks and Dock Gate 4, where the Ocean Cruise Terminal & QEII Terminal are situated. For

# Directory

the Western Docks, proceed to City Cruise Terminal via Dock Gate 8 or to Mayflower Terminal via Dock Gate 10.

### *Motorway Directions from the West*
From the A31 Poole and Bournemouth areas follow the road through the New Forest to join the M27. Leave the M27 at junction 3 and at the roundabout take the 3rd exit signed M271 toward Southampton/The Docks. At the next roundabout (Redbridge), take the 1st exit onto the A33 which will lead you along a dual carriageway heading into Southampton to the relevant Dock Gate assigned for your cruise. For the Western Docks, proceed to City Cruise Terminal via Dock Gate 8 or to Mayflower Terminal via Dock Gate 10. For the Eastern Docks, remain on this road and follow the signs for Dock Gate 4, where the Ocean Terminal & QEII Terminal are situated.

## Southampton Car Park Services
For those that opt to drive to the port, there are good options when it comes to secure car parking services.

**WePark4u** (*wepark4u.co.uk*)
A leading airport, cruise ship and port parking comparison site, this company knows all the best parking services at all major UK air and seaports and are 'Park Mark' accredited.

**ABParking** (*abparking.co.uk*)
Each of ABParking's car parks is a dedicated facility located directly adjacent to your cruise terminal and in full view of your ship. They also have a dedicated Blue Badge car park which must be booked in advance. ABParking has been awarded the prestigious 'Park Mark Safer Parking Award', giving you peace of mind that you have left your vehicle in a safe and secure area.

**Cruise & Passenger Services** (*CPS*) (*cruiseparking.co.uk*)
CPS provides safe, secure, long-term parking at Southampton's terminals. They are 'Park Mark' accredited and an ABTA partner. Located right on the docks alongside the cruise terminals to avoid wasted transfer time, CPS are the approved Carnival parking service provider and are available to assist should your arrival at the terminal be delayed for any reason. Parking is also available for passengers sailing with Cunard, P&O Cruises, Princess and Silver Sea.

The company also offers a range of additional services, including fuel top-up, SureStart and Valet Service.

**Parking for Cruise Ships** (*parkingforcruiseships.co.uk*)
A highly competitive company based at Southampton docks offering a safe and reliable service for their customers. The staff are efficient and friendly, even taking photos of your car and logging the mileage to give their customers total peace of mind that their vehicle is secure. They also offer a fuel top-up service, a loyalty scheme and are 'Park Mark' accredited.

**Parking4Cruises** (*parking4cruises.co.uk*)
Parking with Parking4Cruises takes away the worry about where to park safely while you're having an amazing time on your cruise. All cars are checked into their secure, CCTV monitored compound which is protected by steel entry barriers. Their Meet & Greet team will be waiting at the short-term car park for you when you arrive and at the end of your cruise. A car valeting service is offered.

**EzeParking** (*ezeparking.co.uk*)
EzeParking is the longest running meet and greet parking service at Southampton Cruise Ship Port and they guarantee to beat any comparable quote by at least 15%. They remain the only parking operator at Southampton to collect your car and return it to you right outside the terminal entrance doors if you are a Blue Badge Holder. They are 'Park Mark' accredited and offer a car valeting service.

> The Park Mark® Safer Parking Award is given to parking facilities that have achieved the requirements of a risk assessment conducted by the Police and the British Parking Association. The Safer Parking Scheme is an initiative from the Association of Chief Police Officers (ACPO), Police Scotland and the Police Service of Northern Ireland, aimed at reducing crime and the fear of crime in parking areas.

**Petrol Filling Stations**
Texaco Queensway SSTN – 13-15 Queensway, SO14 3BL
Texaco Co-Operative – Millbrook Road, SO15 0JZ
Shell Roselands Service Station – Redbridge Road, SO15 0LT

# DIRECTORY

**Electric Car Charging**
Ecotricity – West Quay Road, SO15 1GY

## Rail Travel

There are easy routes to Southampton station from most major cities in the UK, with either Great Western Railway, London Midland, Virgin, Cross Country or TransPennine Express. Route planning is made a lot easier by the fact that all train operator's information, whether fare prices, train times or ticketing details, are available on the one website (*nationalrail.co.uk)*.

*Ticket Tip:* Use either *ticketclever.com* (UK credit cards) or *raileurope.co.uk* (International credit cards) for all your ticket needs. They both only charge the traveller the official fare, with no booking fees added on top.

There are several train stations in Southampton, with the most pertinent to cruise passengers being Southampton Central, located on Blechynden Terrace, SO15 1AL. The station is fairly basic, housing a ticket office, toilets and basic refreshment facilities. That being said, the station is fully accessible, with a height adjusted ticket counter and an induction loop system. All South Western Railway ticket machines are accessible and can sell tickets with a Disabled Persons Railcard discount. Wheelchair-friendly toilets are located in the waiting rooms on platforms one and four and are operated by a RADAR key which is available on request from station staff.

### Disabled Persons Railcard

If you travel the train networks regularly it might be worth investing in this special travel card, which costs £20 a year. The benefits include ⅓ off adult rail fares on the National Rail network in Great Britain, and the discount also applies to your travel companion. There are no time restrictions on the railcard, so you can use it for travel at any time of the day. Visit disabledpersons-railcard.co.uk for more details.

### Royal Association of Disability and Rehabilitation (RADAR)

The RADAR Key Scheme or National Key Scheme (NKS) offers disabled people independent access to more than 10,000 locked public toilets around the UK. You can find them in shopping malls, pubs, cafes, department stores, bus and train stations and many other locations throughout the country. Official keys can be purchased from Blue Badge Co (*bluebadgecompany.co.uk*) or by calling them on 020 7250 3222 or by email at *radar@radar.org.uk*.

If you're travelling from London and want a train to take the strain, use the direct South Western Railway service from London Waterloo or the Southern train service from London Victoria. If Paddington Station is an easier option, travel with First Great Western, but you will have to go via Reading. The journey from London to Southampton Central Station takes about an hour and taxis are readily available outside the station to take you the short distance to the cruise terminal.

There are a limited number of wheelchair spaces on each train so you should book your space through National Rail in advance. Some trains cannot accept electric scooters because their weight may exceed the accessible ramp's safe working load. If travelling with South Western Railway, you will need to go to their website *southwesternrailway.com* and complete a Scooter Card application form, allowing up to ten working days for it to be processed.

***Mobility Tip:*** *There is a combined weight restriction of 300 kg for mobility aids (e.g. wheelchairs or mobility scooters) and passengers on train ramps.*

For those with mobility challenges you need only contact one train company and they will organise assistance for your whole journey and ensure the train and stations that you want to use are wheelchair-accessible and that they will provide a ramp on and off your train. You can book assistance by phone or online with the rail company directly or centrally with the Assisted Travel team online at *disabledpersons-railcard.co.uk/travel-assistance* or by phone on 0800 022 3720 or 08000 223 720.

If you require luggage assistance at Southampton Station, an Assisted Travel Service is available. To make a booking, call a member of the team at

Southampton Station Assisted Travel on 0800 5282 100 or 0800 6920 792. You should be aware that the railways impose restrictions on the size and number of luggage items - for more information, go to national.rail.co.uk.

The WheelMate app (*available for iPhone and Android users*) is free and provides a dynamic overview of your nearest wheelchair-friendly accessible toilets and parking spaces. WheelMate currently has more than 35,000 locations across 45 countries, with more being added every day.

## Coach Travel

Southampton Coach Station is located on Harbour Parade, SO15 1BA. Facilities include an automated ticket machine, waiting facilities, coffee shop, charging points, cash point, payphones and disabled and public toilets. There is a 20 pence fee to use the toilets that requires exact change. The nearby coffee shop is not inclined to offer change unless you purchase something. Disabled customers should seek out a member of staff to open the barrier, as the charges do not apply to wheelchair users.

*Toilet Hint:* Cross over to the City Bus Station and use their toilets for free.

The coach station is exclusive to National Express - nationalexpress.com, the largest British coach operator, with a nationwide network of more than 1200 destinations and offering nonstop travel to Southampton from Nottingham, Bristol, Brighton, Winchester, Portsmouth, Basingstoke, Fareham, Bournemouth and Stansted. There are also direct buses from London Victoria Station, Gatwick Airport, Heathrow Airport and London City Airport. The company also operates coaches to Southampton from all major UK cities, such as Edinburgh and Manchester, though longer journeys are often indirect and require a change in London.

Most National Express coaches are accessible; wheelchair users can board via the wheelchair lift which deploys from the coach steps, though coaches only have one wheelchair space so pre-booking is advised. On some vehicles it is possible for customers to remain seated in their wheelchairs and be secured via a tie-down strap system. You will need to notify the assistance team of the size, make and model of your chair to check it can be safely secured. If the wheelchair is not compatible, customers will need to transfer from the wheelchair to a standard coach seat and have the mobility device stored in the hold, though only lightweight manual wheelchairs (under 20

# The Autonomous Cruiser

kg) are allowed in the luggage hold. For safety reasons, only powered wheelchairs operated by dry cell or gel-type batteries can be accepted. Toilets are available on each coach but they are not accessible to wheelchairs. You may store up to two medium cases, each with a maximum weight of 20 kg, though additional luggage can be purchased online.

While National Express do not permit customers to travel in their mobility scooters, they do accept small lightweight models for storage and carriage in the coach luggage hold, provided the Assisted Travel Team are notified at least 36 hours before your journey. The mobility scooter must break down into separate parts, each weighing no more than 20 kg.

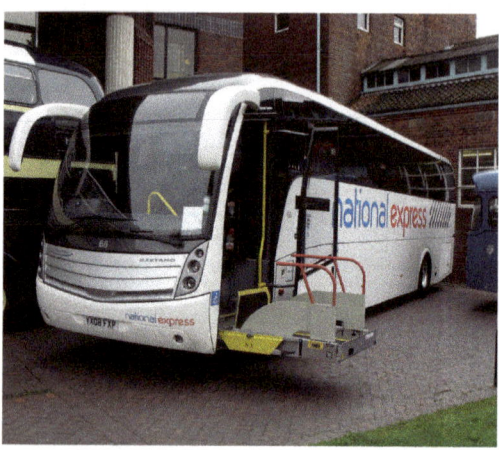

*Credit: Howard Pulling*

For customers with other physical limitations, National Express offers front seat reservations, connection assistance at select stations and staff to help with luggage. Passengers who require oxygen carried in hand-held/personal oxygen bottles are also welcome, but the company cannot carry any large canisters for safety reasons. National Express welcomes trained service dogs on all their coaches, as well as 'Buddy Dogs' (a secondary scheme for Guide Dogs for the Blind Association).

If customers require the use of any of the accessibility features, notify National Express as far in advance as possible by contacting them on 03717 818181 or via email at *addl@nationalexpress.com*.

There are no shuttle buses provided between the coach station and any of the four cruise ship terminals, but there is a taxi rank outside for the short journey. The City Cruise Terminal is the closest at about a 15 minute walk away for those that can manage it, however, it is too far to walk with luggage to any of the other three terminals.

Victoria Coach Station (VCS) is owned and operated by Transport for London and provides its own Mobility Assistance service for National Express customers with reduced mobility. Their Mobility Lounge is available for passengers from 8 am to 10.30 pm. To pre-book Mobility Assistance at VCS, call their help point on 0207 027 2520 at any time of the day or night.

# Directory

## Disabled Coachcard

An annual fee of £10 gives the owner 1/3 off National Express coach travel. The card offers discounts all year round at any time, every day, with no peak or off-peak restrictions.

## Ferry Services

Passenger ferries form vital links through the UK's public transport system, often saving people the need for a much longer journey. For passengers joining the ship from the Isle of Wight (East Cowes), Wightlink Ferries offer several routes. The ferry port has a hearing loop, disabled toilets and ramped access to the ticket office. All car ferries have ramps for easy boarding, lifts to access the lounges, four accessible parking spaces and a disabled or ambulatory toilet (the disabled toilet on Wight Sky, Wight Light and Wight Sun is on the car deck and cannot be accessed during the crossing). Wightlink welcomes service dogs and offers your animal complimentary travel. Red Funnel Ferry has three Red Jet Hi-Speed catamarans on its cross-Solent ferry route between Southampton & West Cowes. The ferry is suitable for wheelchair users, with handrails provided on ramped entrances and walkways, disabled toilet facilities and assistance available. Service dogs are also welcome aboard and are free of charge.

## Transfer Services

The cruise lines do not provide shuttle buses between the coach or train stations and the cruise terminals. However, taxis are available outside both stations and the fare is reasonable for the short sprint across to your terminal.

### Paragon Taxis (*paragontaxis.co.uk*)

Paragon Taxis offers accessible vehicles for long distance transfers to and from Southampton, with each of their vehicles able to take one wheelchair and up to six passengers. They also offer bespoke tours to the local tourist hotspots, such as Stonehenge, Windsor Castle, Winchester and the New Forest. Bookings can be secured by emailing *info@paragontaxis.co.uk* or by phoning 0771 409 0273 or 0787 019 8968.

# The Autonomous Cruiser

**Transmobility Southampton** (*transmobility.co.uk*)
Established in 2008, Transmobility has continued to grow and now boasts the largest fleet of specially adapted vehicles in the South of England, with more than 25 wheelchair-accessible taxis. Offering airport transport, cruise ship transfers and sightseeing tours, they can meet all your needs. Southampton has a footfall of thousands of travellers each day, so put in your request early to avoid disappointment by emailing *info@transmobility.co.uk* or calling 08000 77 87 97.

**Traintaxi** (*traintaxi.co.uk*)
Traintaxi is an invaluable website for accessing local taxi firms that service the railway stations around Britain. The website includes: all train, metro, tram and underground stations in Britain, up to three local taxi or cab firms for each station and all firms that are believed to offer wheelchair-accessible vehicles.

**Uber** (*uber.com*)
Available in more than 700 cities worldwide, Uber is a ridesharing app for fast, reliable rides that are with you in minutes. Simply download the app (available on Android and iOS), tap to request a ride, and it's easy to pay with credit card or cash. Once a booking is confirmed, the passenger can see the driver's photo, name and car registration and can watch their car arrive in real time. You can request an Uber Access car for a forward-facing, wheelchair-accessible vehicle, an UberX car for people with disabilities, service dog owners and riders with foldable wheelchairs, or an Uber Assist car for those who need additional assistance but only need a standard vehicle, such as older people, riders travelling with service dogs, those who have visual or hearing impairments, or riders with foldable wheelchairs.

# Disabled Facilities on Your Favourite Cruise Lines

| Cruise Company | AIDA Cruises [1] |
|---|---|
| Disabled Cabins | - Minimum 32" (81cm) doorways<br>- Balcony cabins have automatic door openers<br>- All barrier-free cabins on *AIDAprima* and *AIDAperla* have automatic cabin and bathroom door openers<br>- Ramped bathroom threshold<br>- Roll-in shower<br>- Folding shower bench<br>- Grab bars<br>- Handheld showerhead<br>- Raised toilets<br>- Lowered sink and vanity unit<br>- Open bed frames |
| Wheelchair or Scooter Access | - Special fast lane check-in for all guests with special needs<br>- Boarding and departure assistance<br>- All post-2010 ships have wheelchair caterpillar tracks for easy transport on gangways<br>- Almost all public areas are accessible<br>- The Theatrium and buffet restaurants have reserved seating for wheelchair users<br>- Accessibility meeting with individual consultation on suitable excursions<br>- Batterie: dry cell, gel, lithium-ion only |
| Pool Hoist | - Pool lifts on *AIDAprima* and *AIDAperla*. |
| Blind & Visual Impairment | - Service dogs welcome<br>- Braille signage throughout the ship<br>- Safety information and a deck plan is available in large print or braille<br>- Qualified readers on request |
| Deaf & Hard of Hearing | - Portable room kit includes tactile alert system and hearing pack on request<br>- Amplified telephone<br>- In-cabin close-captioned television<br>- Audio induction loop systems at guest services and the theatre<br>- Devices have a neck induction loop that transmits to regular hearing aids and implants. The guest's hearing aid will need to be switched to the hearing loop position. |
| Tender | - Guests with assistive devices must be able to board the tender unassisted<br>- Fully collapsible wheelchairs can be placed on tender |

# The Autonomous Cruiser

| Cruise Company | Azamara Cruises |
|---|---|
| **Disabled Cabins** | - Minimum 32" (81cm) doorways<br>- Accessible balcony<br>- Ramped bathroom threshold<br>- Roll-in shower (not *Azamara Quest*)<br>- Folding shower bench<br>- Grab bars<br>- Handheld showerhead<br>- Lowered sink and vanity unit<br>- Lowered closet rods<br>- Lowered safe<br>- Raised toilet seat<br>- Open bed frames |
| **Wheelchair or Scooter Access** | - Accessible transport from the airport to the ship in select ports<br>- Boarding and departure assistance<br>- Gangways are wide enough for most wheelchairs and scooters<br>- No lift access to Deck 11<br>- Wide corridors for 180° turns and accessible routes<br>- Accessible public toilets<br>- Accessible seating at all dining and bar venues<br>- Most decks are accessible via automatic doors<br>- Lowered casino tables<br>- Batteries: dry cell only<br><br>**Private Island:**<br>Labadee is not a tender port and is accessible, with sand wheelchairs and cabanas available. Trams circuit the island. Café Labadee, the Artisan Market, the Native Market and most toilets are accessible. |
| **Pool Hoist** | - No pool lifts |
| **Blind & Visual Impairment** | - Service dogs welcome<br>- Visual tactile alert system<br>- Braille signage throughout the ship<br>- Large print materials<br>- Orientation tours<br>- Qualified readers on request |
| **Deaf & Hard of Hearing** | - Portable room kit with TTY on request, which includes tactile alert system and hearing packs<br>- Amplified telephone<br>- In-cabin closed-captioned television<br>- Sign language (ASL) interpreters (select sailings) |
| **Tender** | - No accessible route to tendering platform<br>- Guests with assistive devices must be able to board tender unassisted<br>- Full time wheelchair users will be unable to go ashore unless roll-on capability is available |

# Directory

| | |
|---|---|
| **Cruise Company** | **Carnival Cruise Line** |
| **Disabled Cabins** | - Minimum 32" (81cm) doorways<br>- Accessible balcony<br>- Ramped bathroom threshold<br>- Roll-in shower<br>- Folding shower bench<br>- Shower seat<br>- Grab bars<br>- Handheld showerhead<br>- Lowered sink and vanity unit<br>- Lowered closet rods |
| **Wheelchair or Scooter Access** | - Accessible transport from the airport to the ship in select ports<br>- Boarding and departure assistance<br>- Gangways are wide enough for most wheelchairs and scooters<br>- No lift access to top decks<br>- Wide corridors and accessible routes<br>- Accessible public toilets<br>- Accessible seating at all dining and bar venues<br>- Batteries: dry cell, gel, absorbed glass mat or lithium-ion only<br><br>**Private Island:**<br>Half Moon Cay requires tendering. The Rum Runners Bar and all the restrooms are wheelchair-accessible. The Taupe cabana is accessible. Sand wheelchairs are available. |
| **Pool Hoist** | - Pool lifts available on select ships - maximum weight: 300 lbs |
| **Blind & Visual Impairment** | - Service dogs welcome<br>- Braille/tactile lift buttons<br>- Audible lift signals<br>- Braille signage<br>- Large print format on select communications<br>- Screen reader software in Internet Cafe |
| **Deaf & Hard of Hearing** | - Portable room kit with TTY on request, which includes tactile alert system and hearing packs<br>- Amplified telephone<br>- In-cabin closed-captioned television<br>- Assistive Listening System (ALS) in the main showroom (select ships)<br>- Sign language (ASL) interpreters (select sailings) |
| **Tender** | - Guests with assistive devices must be able to board tender unassisted<br>- Full time wheelchair users will be unable to go ashore |

# The Autonomous Cruiser

| Cruise Company | Celebrity Cruises [2] |
|---|---|
| Disabled Cabins | - Minimum 32" (81cm) doorways<br>- Accessible balcony<br>- Automatic doors (select ships)<br>- Ramped bathroom threshold<br>- Roll-in shower<br>- Folding shower bench<br>- Grab bars<br>- Handheld showerhead<br>- Lowered sink and vanity unit<br>- Lowered closet rods<br>- Lowered safe |
| Wheelchair or Scooter Access | - Accessible transport to the ship from the airport in select ports<br>- Boarding and departure assistance<br>- Gangways are wide enough for most wheelchairs and scooters<br>- Wide corridors and accessible routes<br>- Accessible public toilets<br>- Accessible seating at all dining and bar venues<br>- Most decks are accessible via automatic doors<br>- Accessible guest relations desk<br>- Dedicated theatre seating<br>- Lowered casino tables<br>- Grab bars in high traffic areas<br>- Batteries: dry cell only |
| Pool Hoist | - Lift to one pool and one hot tub (select ships) |
| Blind & Visual Impairment | - Service dogs welcome<br>- Braille lift buttons and tactile signage throughout the ship<br>- Large print menu and daily schedule on request<br>- Qualified readers on request<br>- Orientation tours (must be requested 45 days in advance) |
| Deaf & Hard of Hearing | - Portable room kit with TTY on request which includes tactile alert system and hearing packs<br>- Amplified telephone<br>- In-cabin closed-captioned television<br>- Assistive Listening System (ALS) in the main theatre<br>- Sign language (ASL) interpreters (select sailings) |
| Tender | - Magic Carpet available on *Edge* and *Apex*, making tendering fully accessible<br>- Accessible routes to tender platform on Solstice class<br>- On other ships, guests with assistive devices must be able to board tender unassisted. Full time wheelchair users will be unable to go ashore |

# Directory

| | |
|---|---|
| **Cruise Company** | **Costa Cruises**[3] |
| **Disabled Cabins** | - Minimum 32" (81cm) doorways<br>- Accessible balcony<br>- Ramped bathroom threshold<br>- Roll-in shower<br>- Folding shower bench<br>- Grab bars<br>- Handheld showerhead<br>- Lowered sink and vanity unit<br>- Lowered closet rods<br>- Emergency call button |
| **Wheelchair or Scooter Access** | - Boarding and departure assistance<br>- Gangways are wide enough for most wheelchairs and scooters<br>- Wide corridors and accessible routes to all public areas<br>- Accessible public toilets<br>- Accessible seating at all dining and bar venues<br>- Dedicated theatre seating<br>- No lift access to top decks (select ships)<br>- Dedicated lift for emergencies<br>- Reserved seating in buffet and on pool decks<br><br>**Private Island:**<br>Catalina Island is a tender port. A wooden walkway connects the entire beach from end to end. Reserved and dedicated beach area next to the pier and lunch area. Accessible toilets. |
| **Pool Hoist** | - Hoist to one pool on *Deliziosa*, *Luminosa*, and *Smeralda* |
| **Blind & Visual Impairment** | - Service dogs welcome<br>- Braille/tactile lift buttons and cabin doors |
| **Deaf & Hard of Hearing** | - Portable room kit with tactile alert system<br>- Guests with hearing disabilities must travel with hearing companion<br>- Infra-red systems available in main show lounge (select ships) |
| **Tender** | - Ship staff will help wheelchair users board the tender |

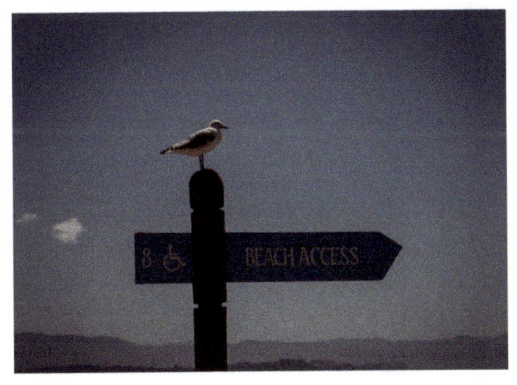

*Credit: Claudio Bianchi, Pixabay*

# The Autonomous Cruiser

| Cruise Company | **Cunard Line** |
|---|---|
| **Disabled Cabins** | - Adapted cabins only<br>- Minimum 32" (81cm) doorways<br>- Flush bathroom threshold<br>- Accessible balcony<br>- Roll-in shower<br>- Folding shower seat<br>- Grab bars<br>- Lowered sink and vanity unit<br>- Raised beds |
| **Wheelchair or Scooter Access** | - Boarding and departure assistance (Southampton only)<br>- Barrier free access<br>- Accessible public toilets<br>- All public rooms are accessible<br>- Dedicated theatre seating<br>- Lowered casino tables<br>- Batteries: gel or dry cell only |
| **Pool Hoist** | - Hoists to at least one of the onboard pools (select ships)<br>- Maximum weight: 308 lbs |
| **Blind & Visual Impairment** | - Service dogs welcome, but only on Southampton to Southampton cruises<br>- Dogs not allowed off at any port of call<br>- Braille lift buttons and audio call signs<br>- Braille signage throughout the ship<br>- Braille and large print format on select communications on request<br>- Audio books<br>- Orientation tour on request |
| **Deaf & Hard of Hearing** | - Portable room kit with TTY on request which includes tactile alert system and hearing packs<br>- In-cabin closed-captioned television<br>- Assistive Listening Systems (ALS) in theatre and planetarium<br>- Audio descriptive emergency warnings<br>- Safety drill in printed format on request<br>- Orientation tour on request |
| **Tender** | - Guests with assistive devices must be able to board tender unassisted<br>- Full time wheelchair users will be unable to go ashore |

> **Don't Ask:**
> *What elevation is this beach?*

# DIRECTORY

| Cruise Company | Disney Cruise Line | |
|---|---|---|
| **Disabled Cabins** | - Minimum 32" (81cm) doorways<br>- Open bed frames<br>- Ramped bathroom thresholds<br>- Roll-in shower<br>- Folding shower seat<br>- Grab bars<br>- Handheld showerhead | - Lowered sink and vanity unit<br>- Lowered towel & closet rods<br>- Second telephone<br>- Emergency call buttons<br>- Raised toilet seat on request<br>- Transfer bench on request |
| **Wheelchair or Scooter Access** | - Accessible transport to the ship from the airport in select ports<br>- Gangways are wide enough for most wheelchairs and scooters<br>- Boarding and departure assistance<br>- Midship lifts on *Disney Magic & Disney Wonder* are small and narrow<br>- Accessible public toilets<br>- Dedicated theatre seating<br>- Wheelchair access to outer deck is via forward or aft doors<br>- Experienced youth counsellors for children with special needs<br>- Batteries: gel or dry cell only<br>- Only two 110-volt electrical outlets in a cabin that has a total power capacity of 12 amps. Power back-up is suggested in case of power outage<br><br>**Private Island:**<br>Castaway Cay is fully accessible, with paved pathways, accessible shops and restaurants, wheelchairs for beach access and disabled toilets. An accessible tram runs to Serenity Bay. Cabana 1 has a ramped entrance and access to the beach. | |
| **Pool Hoist** | - Certain pools on each ship have a hoist available, but need to be pre-booked<br>- Maximum weight: 300 lbs | |
| **Blind & Visual Impairment** | - Service dogs welcome<br>- Braille signage<br>- Large print format on select communications<br>- Select information in audio format<br>- Audio description films<br>- Stateroom communication kits on request | |
| **Deaf & Hard of Hearing** | - Portable room kit with TTY on request which includes tactile alert system and hearing packs<br>- Amplified telephone<br>- In-cabin open-captioned television<br>- Assistive Listening Systems (ALS) in all performance venues and guests can request a show script<br>- Walt Disney Theatre has sign language interpreter near the stage on select sailings | |
| **Tender** | - Guests with assistive devices must be able to board tender unassisted<br>- Full time wheelchair users will be unable to go ashore | |

# The Autonomous Cruiser

| Cruise Company | Fred. Olsen Cruise Lines [4] |
|---|---|
| **Disabled Cabins** | - Adapted cabins only<br>- Minimum 32" (81cm) doorways<br>- Ramped bathroom threshold<br>- Roll-in shower<br>- Fixed shower seat<br>- Grab bars<br>- Raised toilet seat or additional mattress available on request |
| **Wheelchair or Scooter Access** | - Boarding and departure assistance<br>- Public areas accessed by shallow ramp or gradual slope<br>- Only one accessible public restroom<br>- Most outside deck doors are non-automated and are very heavy<br>- Lifts have restricted space<br>- Batteries: gel or dry cell only<br>- All ships are dual voltage: 110 volts requiring a US-style flat two-pin plug, and 220 volts requiring a continental round two-pin plug (both have a 60-volt cycle) - an adaptor and/or a transformer may be needed<br>- Mobility aids in excess of 55 lbs cannot be taken ashore in any port unless there is access via an air-bridge or the device can be dismantled by the guest<br>- There are no specially adapted shuttle buses |
| **Pool Hoist** | - No pool lifts<br>- *Balmoral's* pool has a shallow end |
| **Blind & Visual Impairment** | - Service dogs welcome<br>- Cabins are not fitted with emergency equipment (e.g. flashing lights or bed shakers)<br>- Anyone registered blind or visually impaired must travel with a fully sighted companion |
| **Deaf & Hard of Hearing** | - Cabins are not fitted with emergency equipment (e.g. flashing lights or bed shakers)<br>- Infrared hearing loops are fitted on all ships and headsets are available for use in main lounges - devices are Sennheiser RI-150LL Mono Receiver with neck induction loop (a necklace, which hangs around the neck and receives the audio by infrared then re-transmits to a regular heading aid via an induction loop) - the guest's hearing aid will need to be switched to the hearing loop position |
| **Tender** | - Guests with assistive devices must be able to board tender unassisted<br>- Fully collapsible wheelchairs can be placed on tender<br>- Full time wheelchair users will be unable to go ashore |

# Directory

| | |
|---|---|
| **Cruise Company** | **Holland America Line** [5] |
| **Disabled Cabins** | - Minimum 32" (81cm) doorways<br>- Accessible balcony<br>- No bathroom threshold<br>- Roll-in shower<br>- Shower bench<br>- Grab bars<br>- Handheld showerhead<br>- Lowered sink and vanity unit<br>- Lowered closet rods<br>- Raised toilet seat |
| **Wheelchair or Scooter Access** | - Gangways are wide enough for most wheelchairs and scooters<br>- Boarding and departure assistance<br>- Barrier free access<br>- Accessible public toilets<br>- Accessible seating at all dining and bar venues<br>- Automated doors on Lido level to the main pool and the aft pool deck<br>- Dedicated theatre seating<br>- Lowered casino tables<br>- Batteries: gel or dry cell only<br>- Chargers must be adaptable to 110 volts<br><br>**Private Island:**<br>Half Moon Cay requires tendering. One Taupe cabana, the Rum Runners Bar and all the restrooms are wheelchair-accessible and there are sand wheelchairs. |
| **Pool Hoist** | Pool lifts on *Amsterdam*, *Koningsdam*, *Volendam*, *Nieuw Statendam* & *Ryndam* |
| **Blind & Visual Impairment** | - Service dogs welcome<br>- Dogs are not allowed off at ports of call<br>- Large print or braille menus (45 days' notice required)<br>- Windows-Eyes software available throughout the ship<br>- Orientation tour on arrival |
| **Deaf & Hard of Hearing** | - Portable room kit with TTY on request which includes tactile alert system and hearing packs<br>- Amplified telephone<br>- In-cabin closed-captioned television<br>- Assistive Listening System (ALS) in showroom<br>- Written safety information and lifeboat drill instructions<br>- Orientation tour on arrival |
| **Tender** | - Wheelchair-accessible tender transfer service on all ships (except *Amsterdam*, *Veendam* and *Volendam*)<br>- Transfers will be dependent on weather and sea conditions<br>- The final decision lies with the Staff Captain<br>- Maximum weight of equipment must not exceed 100 lbs without battery |

# The Autonomous Cruiser

| Cruise Company | MSC Cruises [6] |
|---|---|
| Disabled Cabins | - Minimum 35" (89cm) doorways<br>- No bathroom threshold<br>- Roll-in shower<br>- Folding shower bench<br>- Grab bars<br>- Handheld showerheads<br>- Lowered sink and vanity unit<br>- Lowered closet rods<br>- Raised toilet seat |
| Wheelchair or Scooter Access | - Gangways are wide enough for most wheelchairs and scooters<br>- Boarding and departure assistance<br>- Barrier free access<br>- Accessible public toilets<br>- Accessible seating at all dining and bar venues<br>- Automated doors<br>- Dedicated theatre seating<br>- Batteries: gel or dry cell only<br>- Step free excursions on select itineraries<br><br>**Private Island:**<br>Ocean Cay Marine Reserve has its own berth and is completely ADA compliant, with accessible dining, bars and toilets. Tram service and hard paths throughout. Cabanas are on the beach and have a small lip access. Beach wheelchairs available. Late night stays on select cruises. |
| Pool Hoist | - Pool lift on MSC *Seaside* and MSC *Seaview* |
| Blind & Visual Impairment | - Service dogs welcome<br>- Braille lift buttons<br>- Braille signage in public areas and entrance to cabins (select ships)<br>- All lifts have visual, audio and braille deck indicators<br>- Large print menus and daily schedules on request |
| Deaf & Hard of Hearing | - Portable room kit with TTY on request which includes tactile alert system and hearing packs<br>- In-cabin closed-captioned television<br>- Wireless amplifiers and indicator lights in theatres<br>- All lifts have visual, audio and braille deck indicators<br>- Guests with hearing disabilities must travel with hearing companion |
| Tender | - The crew offers assistance for all wheelchair users on tenders, but it is not a guarantee that a full-time wheelchair user can go ashore<br>- Transfers will be dependent on weather and sea conditions<br>- The final decision lies with the Staff Captain |

# Directory

| Cruise Company | Norwegian Cruise Line |
|---|---|
| **Disabled Cabins** | - Minimum 36" (91cm) doorways    - Lowered closet rods<br>- Accessible balcony    - Raised toilet seat<br>- Roll-in shower    - Raised beds<br>- Shower bench    - Emergency pull cord (select ships)<br>- Grab bars |
| **Wheelchair or Scooter Access** | - Accessible transport to the ship from the airport in select ports<br>- Boarding and departure assistance<br>- Accessible public toilets<br>- Dedicated theatre seating<br>- Batteries: gel or dry cell only<br>- Chargers must be adaptable to 110 volts<br>- Embarkation meeting with Access Officer who will oversee all your disability needs during your cruise<br><br>**Private Island:**<br>Great Stirrup Cay has sand wheelchairs. The bar and dining facilities are wheelchair-accessible, as are the toilets. Harvest Caye is fully ADA compliant. |
| **Pool Hoist** | - Pool lifts on every ship<br>- Certified lifeguards at all family pools |
| **Blind & Visual Impairment** | - Service dogs welcome<br>- Braille/tactile signage throughout ship<br>- Alarm buttons next to bed (select ships)<br>- Embarkation meeting with Access Officer who will oversee all your disability needs during your cruise<br>- Orientation tour on request |
| **Deaf & Hard of Hearing** | - The Sky, Sun, and Pride of America have hard wired visual & tactile alert systems<br>- On other ships, a portable room kit and TTY is available on request which includes a tactile alert system & hearing packs<br>- Amplified telephones<br>- In-cabin closed-captioned television<br>- Assistive Listening System (ALS) and pagers for ship announcements on request<br>- Emergency drills on request<br>- Sign language (ASL) interpreters (select sailings)<br>- Embarkation meeting with Access Officer who will oversee all your disability needs during the cruise.<br>- Orientation tour on request |
| **Tender** | - Full time wheelchair users may be able to go ashore if their equipment weighs less than 100 lbs<br>- Transfers will be dependent on weather and sea conditions<br>- The final decision lies with the Staff Captain<br>- If tendering at Harvest Caye, two of the tenders assigned are wheelchair-accessible, with roll-off capabilities |

# The Autonomous Cruiser

| Cruise Company | P&O Cruises |
|---|---|
| Disabled Cabins | - Minimum 32" (81cm) doorways<br>- Automatic doors (select ships)<br>- Accessible balcony<br>- Roll-in shower<br>- Shower seat<br>- Grab bars<br>- Raised toilet seat (on request)<br>- Emergency pull cord<br>- Lowered closet rods (Iona)<br>- Accessible cabin safe |
| Wheelchair or Scooter Access | - Boarding and departure assistance<br>- Most public areas and venues have level or ramped access<br>- Raised door thresholds throughout the ship<br>- Certain areas of the ship are narrow<br>- Accessible public toilets<br>- Easy reach lift buttons<br>- Dedicated theatre seating<br>- Batteries: gel, dry cell, sealed lead acid or lithium-ion only |
| Pool Hoist | - All ships have hoists to at least one onboard pool and hot tub |
| Blind & Visual Impairment | - Service dogs welcome<br>- Large print and braille throughout<br>- Orientation tour<br>- Audio books |
| Deaf & Hard of Hearing | - Limited wireless visual alert systems and special text phones<br>- Hearing packs available<br>- In-cabin closed-captioned television<br>- Assistive Listening System (ALS) in some of the show lounges<br>- Hearing loop facility at guest services' |
| Tender | - Guests with assistive devices must be able to board tender unassisted<br>- Full time wheelchair users will be unable to go ashore |

# Directory

| Cruise Company | Princess Cruises |
|---|---|
| Disabled Cabins | - Minimum 32" (81cm) doorways<br>- Ramped bathroom thresholds<br>- Roll-in shower<br>- Folding shower bench<br>- Grab bars<br>- Handheld showerheads<br>- Lowered sink and vanity unit<br>- Bath distress alarms<br>- Lowered closet rods<br>- Easy access desk |
| Wheelchair or Scooter Access | - Gangways are wide enough for most wheelchairs and scooters<br>- Boarding and departure assistance<br>- Mechanical gangway for easy embarkation and disembarkation<br>- Most areas have barrier free access<br>- Accessible public toilets<br>- Accessible seating at all dining and bar venues<br>- Dedicated theatre seating<br>- Lowered casino table<br>- Accessible guest service desk<br>- Batteries: dry cell only<br><br>**Private Island:**<br>Princess Cays is a tender port. The island has hard paths and ramps for easy access. Disabled toilets on both sides of the island. |
| Pool Hoist | - Lifts for pool and one hot tub |
| Blind & Visual Impairment | - Service dogs welcome<br>- Braille lift buttons and audible arrival sounds<br>- Braille emergency information<br>- Infrared listening assistance systems in all theatres<br>- Audio books |
| Deaf & Hard of Hearing | - Portable room kit with TTY on request which includes tactile alert system and hearing packs<br>- Amplified telephone<br>- In-cabin closed-captioned television<br>- Assistive Listening System (ALS) in the main theatre.<br>- JAWS software with a KOSS_TD/80 headset on terminal in each Internet Cafe<br>- Sign language (ASL) interpreter (select sailings) |
| Tender | - Guests with assistive devices must be able to board tender unassisted<br>- Full time wheelchair users will be unable to go ashore |

# The Autonomous Cruiser

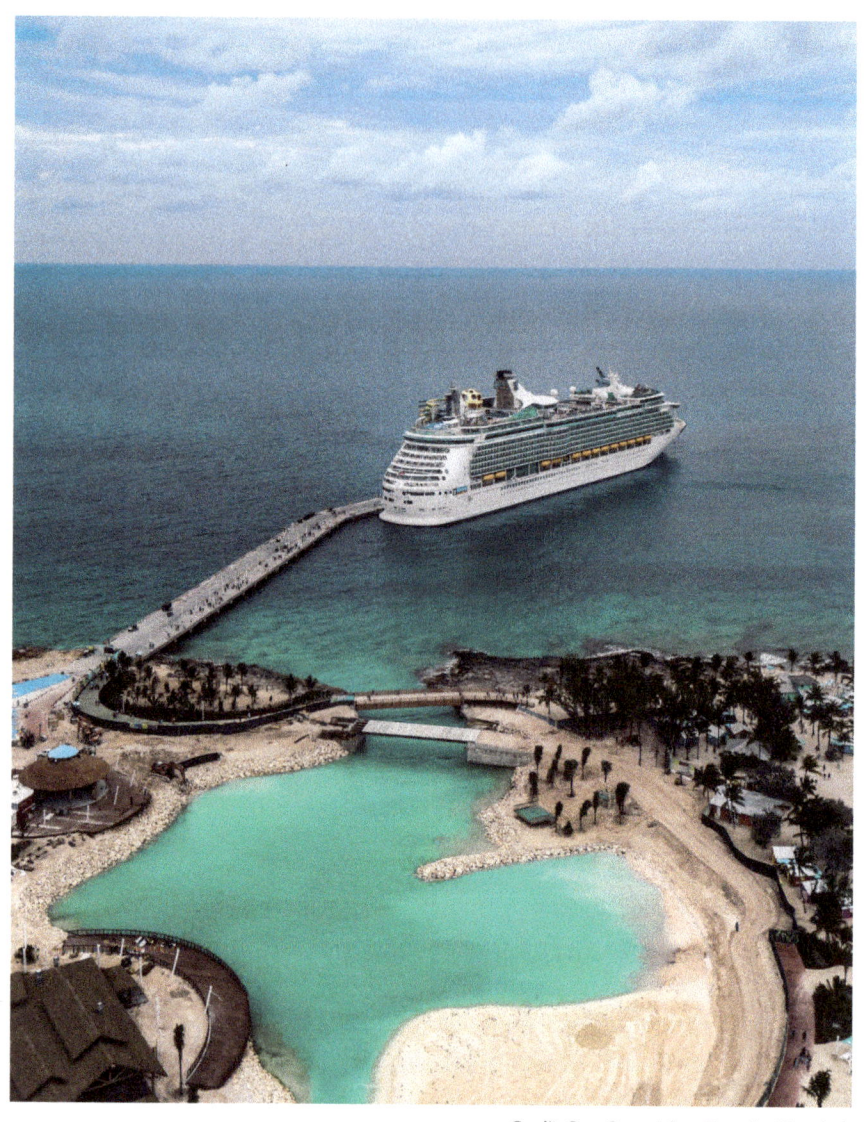

Credit: CocoCay - Adam Gonzales, Unsplash

# Directory

| Cruise Company | Royal Caribbean International [7] |
|---|---|
| Disabled Cabins | - Minimum 32" (81cm) doorways    - Grab bars<br>- Accessible balcony    - Handheld showerhead<br>- Automatic doors (select ships)    - Lowered sink and vanity unit<br>- Ramped bathroom thresholds    - Lowered closet bars<br>- Roll-in shower    - Lowered safe<br>- Folding shower bench    - Raised toilet seat (on request) |
| Wheelchair or Scooter Access | - Accessible transport to the ship from the airport in select ports<br>- Gangways are wide enough for most wheelchairs and scooters<br>- Boarding and departure assistance<br>- Wide corridors for 180° turns<br>- Barrier free access<br>- Accessible public toilets<br>- Most decks have automatic doors<br>- All public rooms feature entrances with gradual inclines<br>- Dedicated theatre seating<br>- Accessible seating at all dining and bar venues<br>- Lowered casino tables and slot machines<br>- Accessible guest service desk<br>- Batteries: gel or dry cell only<br><br>**Private Islands:**<br>CocoCay has docking facilities for two ships and is partly accessible. Trams, pool lifts, beach wheelchairs, dining venues and shops are accessible, as are the toilets. It will offer a limited number of late-night stays.<br>Labadee has good pathways, a tram and toilets that are accessible. Dining, bar, and shopping facilities are all barrier-free. |
| Pool Hoist | - Lift for one pool and one hot tub on every ship<br>- Lifeguard on duty |
| Blind & Visual Impairment | - Service dogs welcome    - Braille/tactile lift buttons and audio call signals<br>- Dogs not allowed off at ports of call    - Large print menus and daily schedule (30 days' notice required)<br>- Portable room kit including tactile alert system and hearing packs    - Qualified readers<br>- Braille/tactile signage    - Orientation tour |
| Deaf & Hard of Hearing | - Portable room kit with TTY on request which includes tactile alert system and hearing packs<br>- Amplified telephones in cabin and public areas<br>- In-cabin closed-captioned television<br>- Assistive Listening System (ALS) in the main theatre on every ship and Studio B on select ships<br>- Sign language (ASL) interpreters (60 day notice required) |
| Tender | - Guests with assistive devices must be able to board tender unassisted<br>- Full time wheelchair users will be unable to go ashore (with the exception of Ovation of the Seas, which offers wheelchair access to tenders) |

# The Autonomous Cruiser

| Cruise Company | Saga Cruises |
|---|---|
| Disabled Cabins | - Minimum 32" (81cm) doorways<br>- Roll-in shower<br>- Shower stool (on request)<br>- Grab bars<br>- Handheld showerhead<br>- Lowered sink and vanity unit<br>- Lowered closet bars<br>- Raised toilet seat (on request) |
| Wheelchair or Scooter Access | - No boarding or departure assistance unless you have registered for the services<br>- Spacious corridors for 180° turns<br>- Accessible public toilets<br>- Dedicated theatre seating<br>- Batteries: gel or dry cell only |
| Pool Hoist | - No pool lifts<br>- Pools have shallow end |
| Blind & Visual Impairment | - Service dogs welcome<br>- Boarding and departure assistance<br>- Large print format for all daily publications<br>- Braille playing cards<br>- Orientation tour on request |
| Deaf & Hard of Hearing | - Portable room kit with TTY on request which includes tactile alert system and hearing packs<br>- Boarding and departure assistance<br>- Safety drill is subtitled on cabin television<br>- Hearing loop system in main entertainment areas<br>- Orientation tour on request |
| Tender | - Guests with assistive devices must be able to board tender unassisted<br>- Full time wheelchair users will be unable to go ashore (except on *Spirit of Discovery* and *Spirit of Adventure*, where tenders are wheelchair-accessible) |

# Directory

| Cruise Company | Seabourn |
|---|---|
| **Disabled Cabins** | - Minimum 32" (81cm) doorways<br>- Roll-in shower<br>- Shower seat<br>- Grab bars<br>- Handheld showerhead<br>- Lowered towel rails<br>- Lowered closet bars |
| **Wheelchair or Scooter Access** | - No ramped gangways<br>- Boarding and departure assistance<br>- Maximum wheelchair weight: 100lbs without battery<br>- Door assistance might be needed to access outside decks<br>- Deck 3 is inaccessible to wheelchairs (*Encore* & *Ovation*)<br>- Batteries: gel, dry cell or AGM (absorbed glass mat) only<br><br>**Private Island:**<br>Half Moon Cay requires a tender service. The Rum Runners Bar and all the restrooms are wheelchair-accessible, as is The Taupe cabana. There are sand wheelchairs available. |
| **Pool Hoist** | - No pool lifts |
| **Blind & Visual Impairment** | - Service dogs welcome<br>- Large print or braille menus (45 days' notice required)<br>- Downloadable daily news, menus and activities for guests with laptops and Screen Reader software<br>- Orientation tour |
| **Deaf & Hard of Hearing** | - Portable room kit with TTY on request which includes tactile alert system and hearing packs<br>- Visual alarm system throughout the ship<br>- Amplified telephones in cabin<br>- In-cabin close-captioned television with amplified sound<br>- Assistive Listening System (ALS) with portable receivers in showrooms<br>- Written safety instructions and lifeboat drill instructions<br>- Orientation tour on request |
| **Tender** | - Guests with assistive devices must be able to board tender unassisted<br>- Full time wheelchair users will be unable to go ashore |

# The Autonomous Cruiser

| Cruise Company | Virgin Voyages |
|---|---|
| Disabled Cabins | - Minimum 32" (81cm) doorways<br>- Roll-in shower<br>- Shower seat<br>- Grab bars<br>- Handheld showerhead<br>- Emergency pull cord |
| Wheelchair or Scooter Access | - Boarding and departure assistance<br>- Spacious corridors<br>- Accessible public toilets<br>- Dedicated theatre seating<br><br>**Private Island:**<br>Bimini Island is accessible and there are sand wheelchairs at the Beach Club. Late night stays on its four and five-day cruises. |
| Pool Hoist | - Lifted seats for the pool<br>- Wheelchairs cannot access the pool area |
| Blind & Visual Impairment | - Service dogs welcome<br>- Boarding and departure assistance<br>- Braille signage throughout<br>- Large print menus<br>- Limited number of portable kits with TTY on request |
| Deaf & Hard of Hearing | - Limited number of portable TTY room kit on request which includes tactile alert system and hearing packs<br>- Amplified telephones in cabin<br>- In-cabin close-captioned television<br>- Assistive Listening Systems (ALS) in the main theatre<br>- Interpreters for the hearing impaired (60 days notice required) |
| Tender | - Virgin currently do not have any tender ports but they insist guests with assistive devices will be helped on the tender should the need arise |

# Directory

1 – AIDA Cruises stipulates that only manual wheelchairs can be accommodated and that disabled guests travel with a companion. You will need the express permission of the company to take an electric wheelchair. The wheelchair may not exceed a certain maximum weight: AIDAaura / -bella / -cara / -diva / -luna / -nova / -vita: up to 160 kg (incl. the wheelchair user) AIDAblu / -mar / -perla / -prima / -sol / -stella: up to 200 kg (incl. the wheelchair user). Toilet attachments, shower stools and portable cabin kits for the deaf can only be reserved via the customer service centre a minimum of 2 weeks before travel.

2 – Celebrity Flora, Celebrity Xploration, Celebrity Xperience and Celebrity Xpedition do not have any accessible cabins and mobility equipment is not allowed on the ships.

3 – Costa Cruises offer the 'cruise only' section of trips free of charge to companions, provided that they travel in the same cabin as a special needs guest. To obtain a free cruise ticket for companions, inform Costa Cruises at the time of the booking confirmation.

4 – Fred. Olsen's fleet of four ships does not have purpose-built accessible cabins, only adapted ones, so you will need to check whether the ship will meet your specific needs before booking. There are complicated rules governing wheelchairs and scooters. There is no overhead air-bridge or sloped gangway at either Liverpool or Rosyth port, so wheelchair users are unable to board. You must be able to manage a stepped gangway with minimum assistance from a crew member or caregiver. The angle of the gangway is subject to tidal conditions. Unless the overseas ports have an overhead air-bridge, full-time wheelchair users may not be able to disembark. Electric wheelchairs and scooters will only be accepted on Braemar if a guest is occupying a designated wheelchair-accessible cabin. Any mobility aid weighing in excess of 55 lb/25 kgs cannot be carried ashore at any port of call unless it can be easily dismantled. You will need to be able to climb the steps of a bus to participate in some shore excursions.

5 – Holland America doesn't allow heavy wheelchairs or scooters on tenders.

6 – MSC's second island, Sir Bani Yas Island Beach Resort, has now been added to the cruise line's portfolio. A purpose-built accessible cruise jetty with berthing for two ships will be available for the start of the 2021 cruise season. A series of hard paths connect all areas of the island. Accessible facilities are available in the Anantara Villa Resort. Beach facilities such as toilets and access to some sun loungers have been made wheelchair-friendly.

7 – Royal Caribbean's private island CocoCay is no longer a tender port since its multi-million dollar facelift. Accessible trams are available all day on regular rotation between the ship and Coco Beach Club, which is also accessible. To access the beach, guests may use a complimentary beach wheelchair. There is a lift in the pool, a lower counter at the bar and ramps to the dining area. Amber Cove in the Dominican Republic, Grand Turk Cruise Centre in Turks, and Caicos and Mahogany Bay in Roatan, are all operated by Carnival - rather than bronzed tropical islands, they are more like high-end shopping malls. All of them feature a two-berth cruise terminal and are totally accessible.

**Autism Friendly:** Celebrity Cruises, Royal Caribbean and Disney offer autism friendly ships for families living with Down's Syndrome, autism and other developmental disabilities. Autism on the Seas 'Staffed Cruises' are offered on select sailings.

**Sensory Inclusive:** Carnival has been certified to assist adults, youth and children with a sensory or cognitive need by KultureCity who offer complimentary Sensory Bags which include comfortable noise-cancelling headphones, fidget tools, and a visual feeling thermometer. Issued on a first-come-first-served basis at Guest Relations or Carnival's Children's Club, the additional VIP lanyard helps staff to easily identify a special guest.

*******

# The Autonomous Cruiser

This chart's aim is to give an overall picture of what provisions are in place for disabled guests, but cabin sizes, layouts and amenities vary, so the information might not pertain to all the cruise ships in a given fleet or even in every room category. The equipment on each ship is not necessarily uniform, so check with the cruise line before making a booking to ensure they can meet your special needs. If a cruise line isn't mentioned it doesn't mean they don't cater to disabled people, but that there are very few provisions for all categories of special needs. Companies such as Hurtigruten, CMV and Regent Seven Seas only have a handful of adapted cabins, with no portable room kits or tactile alert systems in the cabin. Viking's ocean ships only have two ADA compliant cabins, an adapted version of their Penthouse Junior Suite, which allows guests to manoeuvre a wheelchair in the room, out to the balcony and in the bathroom to use facilities such as a roll-in shower, accessible sink and handrails. If you wish to explore further, ring customer service and they will be happy to discuss how they can service your requests.

If you need further information, then the following special needs contacts will be happy to help.

***AIDA Cruises Website:*** *www.aida.de*
***Email:*** *specialneeds@aida.de or barrierefreiheit@aida.de*
***Phone:*** *+49 (0) 381 444 8021*

***Azamara Cruises Website:*** *www.azamara.co.uk*
***Email****: special_needs@azamara.com*
***Tour Assistance:*** *shorexaccess@azamara.com*
*or shorexaccess@azamaraclubcruises.com*
***Phone:*** *UK: 0344 493 4016 - US:1 866 592 7225*

***Carnival Cruise Line Website:*** *www.carnival.co.uk*
***Email****: specialneeds@carnival.com or access@carnival.com*
***Tour Assistance:*** *shoremobilityinfo@carnivalukgroup.com*
***Phone:*** *UK: 0808 234 0680 (toll-free) - US: 001 800 764 7419 or 001 800 438 6744 ext. 70025*

# Directory

**Celebrity Cruises Website:** www.celebritycruises.co.uk
**Email:** specialistservicesuk@celebritycruises.com *or* special_needs@celebrity.com
**Tour Assistance:** shorexaccess@celebrity.com
**Phone:** UK: 01932 834 194 - US: 1 407 566 3602

**Costa Cruises Website:** www.costacruises.co.uk
**Email:** esigenzespeciali@costa.it *or* customerrelations@uk.costa.it
**Phone:** UK: 0800 389 0622 - US: 1 800 462 6782

**Cunard Line Website:** www.cunard.com
**Email:** disability@carnivalukgroup.com
**Tour Assistance:** accessoffice@cunard.com
*or* shoremobilityinfo@carnivalukgroup.com
**Phone:** UK: 0344 338 8641 - US:1 800 728 6273

**Disney Cruise Line Website:** www.disneyholidays.co.uk/disney-cruise-line
**Email:** specialservices@disneycruiseline.com
**Phone:** UK: 0800 169 0742 - US: 001 407 566 3500/3602

**Fred Olsen Cruise Lines Website:** www.fredolsencruises.com
**Email:** specialistsupport@fredolsen.co.uk
**Tour Assistance:** shore.tours@fredolsen.co.uk *or* 0147 3746163
**Phone:** UK: 01473 746 165 or 01473 742 424

**Holland America Line Website:** www.hollandamerica.com
**Email:** halw_access@hollandamerica.com
*or* guestaccessibility@hollandamerica.com
**Tour Assistance:** 001 888 425 9376 or 001 206 626 7320
**Phone:** UK: 0344 338 8605 - US:1 800 547 8493 - 1 206 626 7044

**MSC Cruises Website:** www.msc.com
**Email:** bookingmanagement@msccruises.co.uk
**Phone:** UK: 0203 426 3010 - US: 1 877 665 4655

# The Autonomous Cruiser

**Norwegian Cruise Line Website:** www.ncl.com
**Email:** accessdesk@ncl.com
**Phone:** UK: 0333 241 2319 or 0330 828 0854 - US:1 866 584 9756

**P&O Cruises Website:** www.pocruises.com
**Email:** disability@carnivalukgroup.com
**Tour Assistance:** shoremobilityinfo@carnivalukgroup.com
**Phone:** UK: 0345 355 5111

**Princess Cruises Website:** www.princess.com
**Email:** accessofficeprincess@princesscruises.com
**Phone:** UK: 0344 338 8663 or 0344 338 8660 - US: 1 800 774 6237

**Royal Caribbean International Website:** www.rccl.com
**Email:** special_needs@rccl.com or royalspecialservicesuk@rccl.com
**Tour Assistance:** shorexaccess@rccl.com
**Phone:** UK: 0344 493 4005 - US: 001 866 592 7225

**Saga Cruises Website:** www.saga.co.uk
**Email:** cruise@saga.co.uk
**Phone:** UK: 0800 373 034

**Seabourn Website:** www.seabourn.com
**Email:** access@seabourn.com or guestrelations@seabourn.com
**Phone:** UK: 0845 070 0500 - US: 001 866 530 2193

**Virgin Voyages Website:** www.virginvoyages.com
**Email:** sailorservices@virginvoyages.com
**Phone:** UK: 0203 003 4919 - US: 001 954 488 2955

> **Don't Ask:**
> Will the snow be cold?

# Directory

# Smoking Facilities

| Cruise Line | American Cruise Lines |
|---|---|
| Cigarette smoking areas | - Designated areas at discretion of the captain |
| E-Cigarettes/Vaping smoking areas | - Designated areas at discretion of the captain |
| Cigar and pipe smoking areas | - Designated areas at discretion of the captain |

| Cruise Line | Azamara Club[1] |
|---|---|
| Cigarette smoking areas | - Starboard forward section of pool deck |
| E-Cigarettes/Vaping smoking areas | - Starboard forward section of pool deck |
| Cigar and pipe smoking areas | - Starboard forward section of pool deck |

| Cruise Line | Carnival[2] |
|---|---|
| Cigarette smoking areas | - Carnival's Dance Club<br>- Carnival's Jazz Club<br>- Designated areas casino & attached bar<br>- (Indoor smoking spaces do not extend to *Horizon*, *Panorama*, *Sunshine* or *Vista*)<br>- Designated open deck areas on all ships (starboard side) |
| E-Cigarettes/Vaping smoking areas | - Carnival's Dance Club<br>- Carnival's Jazz Club<br>- Designated areas casino & attached bar<br>- (Indoor smoking spaces do not extend to *Horizon*, *Panorama*, *Sunshine* or *Vista*)<br>- Designated open deck areas on all ships (starboard side) |
| Cigar and pipe smoking areas | - Designated areas of open decks |

| Cruise Line | Celebrity |
|---|---|
| Cigarette smoking areas | - Port side of pool deck and sun decks<br>- Port side of Sunset Bar on Celebrity Century & Celebrity Millennium class ships<br>- Port side, aft and outside of Winter Garden on *Celebrity Mercury & Galaxy* |
| E-Cigarettes/Vaping smoking areas | - Port side of pool deck and sun decks<br>- Port side of Sunset Bar on Celebrity Century & Celebrity Millennium class ships<br>- Port side, aft and outside of Winter Garden on *Celebrity Mercury & Galaxy* |
| Cigar and pipe smoking areas | - Designated areas of the open decks |

# The Autonomous Cruiser

| Cruise Line | Celestyal Cruises |
|---|---|
| Cigarette smoking areas | - Designated areas of the open decks |
| E-Cigarettes/Vaping smoking areas | - Designated areas of the open decks |
| Cigar and pipe smoking areas | - Designated areas of the open decks |

| Cruise Line | Costa Cruises |
|---|---|
| Cigarette smoking areas | - Designated area of open decks<br>- Cabin balconies<br>- Cigar Bar |
| E-Cigarettes/Vaping smoking areas | - Cabin balconies<br>- Cigar Bar |
| Cigar and pipe smoking areas | - Designated areas of the ship<br>- Cigar Bar |

| Cruise Line | Crystal Cruises[3] |
|---|---|
| Cigarette smoking areas | - Connoisseur Club<br>- VIP Casino during play<br>- Decks 8, 9 & 10 aft (*Serenity and Symphony*, Deck 11 aft is also a smoking area (*Serenity* only)<br>- Port side of Seahorse Pool<br>- Port side of Promenade Deck |
| E-Cigarettes/Vaping smoking areas | - Connoisseur Club<br>- VIP Casino during play<br>- Decks 8, 9 & 10 aft (*Serenity* and *Symphony*, Deck 11 aft is also a smoking area (*Serenity* only)<br>- Port side of Seahorse Pool<br>- Port side of Promenade Deck |
| Cigar and pipe smoking areas | - Connoisseur Club<br>- Decks 8, 9 & 10 aft (*Crystal Serenity* and *Symphony*)<br>- Deck 11 aft (*Crystal Serenity*) |

| Cruise Line | Cunard |
|---|---|
| Cigarette smoking areas | - Designated areas on starboard side of open decks<br>- Upper level of G32 nightclub (*Queen Mary 2*) |
| E-Cigarettes/Vaping smoking areas | - Designated areas on starboard side of open decks<br>- Upper level of G32 nightclub (*Queen Mary 2*)<br>- Cabins & balconies |
| Cigar and pipe smoking areas | - Churchill's Cigar Lounge |

# Directory

| Cruise Line | Disney Cruise Line |
|---|---|
| Cigarette smoking areas | - Starboard side of open Deck 4 between 6 pm–6 am (*Magic* & *Wonder*)<br>- Open Decks 9 & 10 (excluding Mickey's Pool)<br>- Port side of Deck 4 between 6 pm–6 am (*Dream* & *Fantasy*)<br>- Port side of open Deck 12 aft by Meridian Lounge<br>- Port side of open Deck 13 forward by Currents Bar |
| E-Cigarettes/ Vaping smoking areas | - Starboard side of open Deck 4 between 6 pm–6 am (*Magic* & *Wonder*)<br>- Open Decks 9 & 10 (excluding Mickey's Pool)<br>- Port side of Deck 4 between 6 pm–6 am (*Dream* & *Fantasy*)<br>- Port side of open Deck 12 aft by Meridian Lounge<br>- Port side of open Deck 13 forward by Currents Bar |
| Cigar and pipe smoking areas | - Designated areas of open deck |

| Cruise Line | Fred. Olsen |
|---|---|
| Cigarette smoking areas | - Cabin balconies<br>- Designated areas on open decks |
| E-Cigarettes/ Vaping smoking areas | - E-cigarettes in cabin (must not emit vapour)<br>- Cabin balconies<br>- Designated areas on open decks |
| Cigar and pipe smoking areas | - Designated areas of open decks |

| Cruise Line | Hapag-Lloyd Cruises[4] |
|---|---|
| Cigarette smoking areas | - Outer terrace port side Yacht Club (*Europa 2*)<br>- Outer deck of the Sansibar (*Europa, Europa 2*)<br>- Designated areas of the open deck (*Europa, Europa 2, Bremen, Hanseatic*)<br>- Herrenzimmer (*Europa 2*)<br>- Havana Bar (*Europa*)<br>- Cabin balcony (*Europa* & *Europa 2*)<br>- Cabin veranda (*Bremen*)<br>- Smoker's Lounge Deck 4 (*Hanseatic Nature* & *Inspiration*) |
| E-Cigarettes/ Vaping smoking areas | - Outer terrace port side Yacht Club (*Europa 2*)<br>- Outer deck of the Sansibar (*Europa, Europa 2*)<br>- Designated areas of the open deck (*Europa, Europa 2, Bremen, Hanseatic*)<br>- Herrenzimmer (*Europa 2*)<br>- Cabin veranda (*Europa* & *Europa 2*)<br>- Cabin veranda (*Bremen*) |
| Cigar and pipe smoking areas | - Outer deck of the Sansibar<br>- Havana Bar (*Europa*)<br>- The Collins (*Europa 2*)<br>- Smoker's Lounge (*Hanseatic Nature* & *Inspiration*) |

# The Autonomous Cruiser

| | | |
|---|---|---|
| | **Cruise Line** | **Holland America** |
| **Cigarette smoking areas** | | - Designated areas of open decks<br>- Designated area in the casino (players only on specific nights (*Koningsdam, Nieuw Statendam, Amsterdam, Maasdam, Volendam, Zaandam, Rotterdam, Veendam*) |
| **E-Cigarettes/Vaping smoking areas** | | - Designated areas of open decks<br>- Cabins (not balconies) |
| **Cigar and pipe smoking areas** | | - Designated areas of open decks Oak Room (*Noordam*) |
| | **Cruise Line** | **Hurtigruten**[4] |
| **Cigarette smoking areas** | | - Designated areas of outside decks except when in port |
| **E-Cigarettes/Vaping smoking areas** | | - Designated areas of outside decks except when in port |
| **Cigar and pipe smoking areas** | | - Designated areas of outside decks except when in port |
| | **Cruise Line** | **Louis Cruise Lines** |
| **Cigarette smoking areas** | | - Open decks<br>- Designated areas of public rooms |
| **E-Cigarettes/Vaping smoking areas** | | - Open decks<br>- Designated areas of public rooms |
| **Cigar and pipe smoking areas** | | - Open decks |
| | **Cruise Line** | **Marella Cruises** |
| **Cigarette smoking areas** | | - Designated areas of open decks |
| **E-Cigarettes/Vaping smoking areas** | | - Designated areas of open decks<br>- Casino and adjoining bars |
| **Cigar and pipe smoking areas** | | - Designated areas of open decks |
| | **Cruise Line** | **MSC Cruises** |
| **Cigarette smoking areas** | | - Casinos and dedicated lounges<br>- Designated side of Sun Deck<br>- Smoking only allowed on port side of designated outside decks (*Devina*) |
| **E-Cigarettes/Vaping smoking areas** | | - Casinos and dedicated lounges<br>- Designated side of Sun Deck<br>- Smoking only allowed on port side of designated outside decks (*Devina*) |
| **Cigar and pipe smoking areas** | | - The Cigar Lounge |

# Directory

| Cruise Line | Norwegian Cruise Line (NCL) |
|---|---|
| Cigarette smoking areas | - Limited areas of open decks excluding food service areas<br>- Designated area of casino (players only)<br>- Smoking Lounge within casino (*Bliss, Joy, Encore*)<br>- Guests in Garden Villas may smoke in private garden or on private sun deck |
| E-Cigarettes/Vaping smoking areas | - Limited areas of open decks excluding food service areas<br>- Designated area of casino (players only)<br>- Smoking Lounge within casino (*Bliss, Joy, Encore*) |
| Cigar and pipe smoking areas | - Limited areas of the open deck<br>- Humidor Cigar Lounge (*Bliss, Joy, Epic, Escape, Getaway*).<br>- Cigarettes, pipes, vapes and e-cigarettes are not allowed in the cigar lounge |

| Cruise Line | Oceania Cruises |
|---|---|
| Cigarette smoking areas | - Designated areas on Deck 9<br>- Port, aft corner of Horizons on Deck 10<br>- Starboard forward corner of Pool Deck |
| E-Cigarettes/Vaping smoking areas | - Designated areas on Deck 9<br>- Port, aft corner of Horizons on Deck 10<br>- Starboard forward corner of Pool Deck |
| Cigar and pipe smoking areas | - Starboard, forward corner of the Pool Deck |

| Cruise Line | P&O Cruises |
|---|---|
| Cigarette smoking areas | - Designated areas of open decks |
| E-Cigarettes/Vaping smoking areas | - Designated areas of open decks |
| Cigar and pipe smoking areas | - Designated areas of open decks |

| Cruise Line | Ponant |
|---|---|
| Cigarette smoking areas | - Designated areas of open decks |
| E-Cigarettes/Vaping smoking areas | - Designated areas of open decks |
| Cigar and pipe smoking areas | - Designated areas of open decks |

| | |
|---|---|
| **Cruise Line** | **Princess Cruises** |
| **Cigarette smoking areas** | - Churchill's Cigar Lounge<br>- Designated areas of open decks<br>- Section of nightclub<br>- Designated slot machine area (excluding non-smoking casino nights) |
| **E-Cigarettes/Vaping smoking areas** | - Cabins (not balcony)<br>- Designated areas of open decks<br>- Section in nightclub<br>- Designated slot machine area (excluding non-smoking casino nights) |
| **Cigar and pipe smoking areas** | - Designated areas of open decks unless there is a cigar lounge<br>- Churchill's Cigar Lounge |
| **Cruise Line** | **Regent Seven Seas (RSSC)** [5] |
| **Cigarette smoking areas** | - Designated areas of open decks Connoisseur Club |
| **E-Cigarettes/Vaping smoking areas** | - Electronic cigarettes are permitted throughout the ship, with the exception of the enclosed dining areas |
| **Cigar and pipe smoking areas** | - Connoisseur Club (pipes & cigars)<br>- Designated area of open decks for cigars only (opposite pool bar)<br>- Pipe smoking is not allowed on open decks |
| **Cruise Line** | **Royal Caribbean** |
| **Cigarette smoking areas** | - Designated areas of open decks<br>- Designated area of casino (excluding departures from Australia and the UK) (Cruises from China & Hong Kong will have a non-smoking area) |
| **E-Cigarettes/Vaping smoking areas** | - Designated areas of open decks<br>- Designated area of casino (excluding departures from Australia and the UK) (Cruises from China & Hong Kong will have a non-smoking area) |
| **Cigar and pipe smoking areas** | - Designated area of open decks<br>- Connoisseur Club (Freedom & Voyager Class ships) |
| **Cruise Line** | **Saga Cruises** |
| **Cigarette smoking areas** | - Designated areas of open decks |
| **E-Cigarettes/Vaping smoking areas** | - Designated areas of open decks |
| **Cigar and pipe smoking areas** | - Designated areas of open decks |

# Directory

| | |
|---|---|
| **Cruise Line** | **Seabourn**[4] |
| Cigarette smoking areas | - Starboard side of Sky Bar on Deck 9 (Deck 10 on *Encore* & *Ovation*)<br>- Starboard side of the open terrace aft of The Club (Deck 5)<br>- Starboard side of the open terrace aft of *Seabourn Square* (Deck 7) |
| E-Cigarettes/ Vaping smoking areas | - All suites<br>- Starboard side of Sky Bar on Deck 9 (Deck 10 on *Seabourn Encore*)<br>- Starboard side on the open terrace aft of The Club (Deck 5)<br>- Starboard side of the open terrace aft of Seabourn Square (Deck 7) |
| Cigar and pipe smoking areas | - Open terrace aft of Seabourn Square (Deck 7) |

| | |
|---|---|
| **Cruise Line** | **SeaDream Yacht Club** |
| Cigarette smoking areas | - Designated areas of open decks on Decks 3, 4 & 6 except during meal times |
| E-Cigarettes/ Vaping smoking areas | - Designated areas of open decks on Decks 3, 4 & 6 except during meal times |
| Cigar and pipe smoking areas | - Designated areas of open decks |

| | |
|---|---|
| **Cruise Line** | **Silversea** |
| Cigarette smoking areas | - Designated areas of open decks outside La Terrazza, outside the Panorama Lounge and the Pool Bar as well as on open Decks 9 & 10 (*Silver Spirit*, *Shadow* and *Whisper*)<br>- Designated area of open decks on Deck 9 (*Silver Cloud* and *Wind*)<br>- Designated area of open decks 5 & 6 (*Silver Explorer*)<br>- Connoisseur's Corner |
| E-Cigarettes/ Vaping smoking areas | - Designated areas of open decks outside La Terrazza, outside the Panorama Lounge and the Pool Bar as well as on open Decks 9 & 10 (*Silver Spirit*, *Shadow* and *Whisper*)<br>- Designated area of open decks on Deck 9 (*Silver Cloud* and *Wind*)<br>- Designated area of open decks 5 & 6 (*Silver Explorer*)<br>- Connoisseur's Corner |
| Cigar and pipe smoking areas | - Connoisseur's Corner<br>- Designated areas of open Decks 9 & 10 (*Silver Spirit*, *Shadow* and *Whisper*)<br>- Designated area of open Deck 9 (*Silver Cloud* and *Wind*)<br>- Designated areas open decks 5 & 6 (*Silver Explorer*) |

| Cruise Line | Star Clippers |
|---|---|
| Cigarette smoking areas | - Designated area of open deck<br>- Designated section in Piano Bar |
| E-Cigarettes/Vaping smoking areas | - Designated area of open deck<br>- Designated section in Piano Bar |
| Cigar and pipe smoking areas | - Designated area of open deck |

| Cruise Line | Viking Cruises |
|---|---|
| Cigarette smoking areas | - Designated area on starboard side of open Deck 8 |
| E-Cigarettes/Vaping smoking areas | - Designated area on starboard side of open Deck 8 |
| Cigar and pipe smoking areas | - Designated area on starboard side of open Deck 8 |

| Cruise Line | Windstar |
|---|---|
| Cigarette smoking areas | - Designated areas of open decks |
| E-Cigarettes/Vaping smoking areas | - Designated areas of open decks |
| Cigar and pipe smoking areas | - Designated areas of open decks |

1 – Azamara: Smoking, including electronic cigarettes, is not allowed at any point during an Azamara cruise unless specifically stated by the tour operator.
2 – Carnival: On some Australian itineraries aboard Carnival Legend, smoking is prohibited in all indoor public and private spaces.
3 – Crystal: Crystal Esprit is a non-smoking vessel.
4 – Some cruise lines with small vessels like Hapag-Lloyd, Hurtigruten and Seabourn strictly forbid smoking on all external decks while bunkering (refuelling), which can take up to seven hours.
5 – Regent Seven Seas: Guests choosing to disregard the smoking policy on Oceania and Regent will be disembarked at the next port of call at their expense, without refund or credit for any unused portion of their cruise. There may also be fines imposed to cover the cost associated with cleaning of the passenger's cabin or balcony.

# Travel Planning Disability Resources

There are a wealth of companies willing to help you plan your holiday - they have the resources, experience and knowledge that can help answer any questions you have. Research is one of the most important elements of any trip and these companies are committed to supporting travellers with disabilities and have in-depth specialised knowledge that will help you in booking the perfect getaway. Here are just a few of the best resources available.

# Directory

## Accessible Shore Excursions

**Best Bets Travel** (*bestbetstravel.com*)
The Travel Institute has recognised Best Bets Travel as an Accredited Disability Agent, an Autism Friendly Agent and an Accessible Travel Specialist. Whether you want a wheelchair-accessible cruise, an ASL interpreter for deaf travellers, use dialysis or oxygen or want to book a tour for slow walkers or the visually impaired, Bets Bets have it covered.

**Disabled Accessible Travel** (*disabledaccessibletravel.com*)
Europe's leading accessible travel agent, offering a wide range of bespoke services to any type of traveller in need of adapted solutions, including accessible cruise port transfers and accessible shore excursions. Taking on the challenges others wouldn't, the team offers amazing experiences on Easter Island, Machu Picchu, Saigon to name a few. If you can dream it, they will make it a reality.

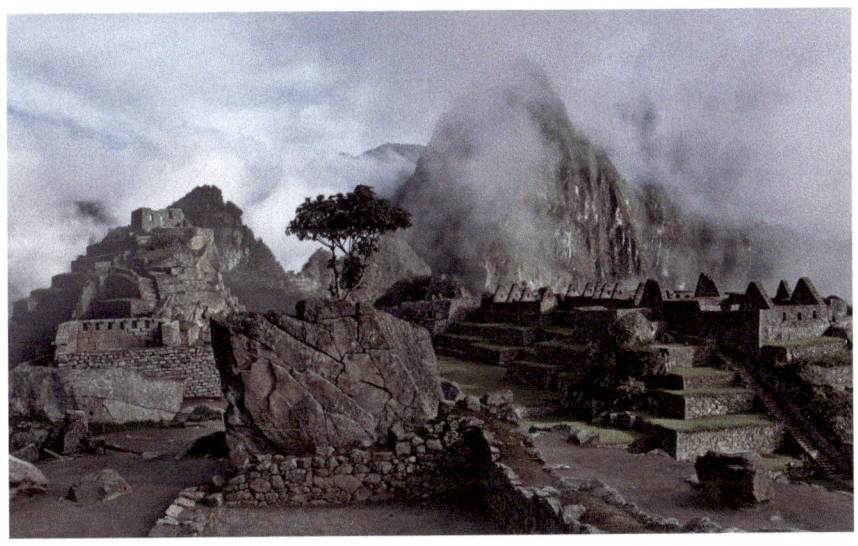

*Credit: Machu Picchu - Tomas Sobek, Unsplash*

**Sage Traveling** (*sagetraveling.com*)
John Sage, the founder and owner of Sage Traveling, sustained a spinal cord injury when he was only 22 years old and is now a full-time wheelchair user, giving him a unique perspective of all the challenges that disabled travellers

can encounter during their trip. Sage Travelling offers custom accessible cruise itineraries and shore excursions for people with special mobility needs, including wheelchair, scooter, cane and walker users and senior travellers.

**Wheel the World** (*gowheeltheworld.com*)
An incredible team of people, some with disabilities, but all dedicated in developing the best tailored accessible travel experiences all over the world

## Accessible Travel News, Reviews & Practical Advice

**Amputee Coalition** (*amputee-coalition.org*)
The Amputee Coalition's objective is to enable amputees to fulfil their aspirations through education, support and advocacy and to enhance awareness of preventative limb loss. Check out their page on 'Travel Questions/Concerns'.

**Coloplast** (*coloplast.co.uk/wheelmate*)
Coloplast develops ostomy, continence, urology and wound care products and services that make life easier for people with intimate healthcare needs. Their WheelMate app is free and provides a dynamic overview of the nearest public conveniences to help you plan your day.

**Emerging Horizons** (*emerginghorizons.com*)
An accessible travel news source offering articles, tips, advice and practical solutions for barrier-free holidays.

**Mobility International** (*miusa.org*)
A cross-disability organisation whose focus is to serve people with a broad range of disabilities. With innovative programs, they are intent on creating a new age where people with disabilities have equal rights to travel experiences as anyone else.

**Norwegian Association of Disabled** (*nhf.no*)
The advocacy organisation of people with disabilities whose vision is a society for all, where people with disabilities have equal opportunities as other people have to live according to their own wishes, abilities and interests.

**Silver Travel Advisor** (*silvertraveladvisor.com*)
Winner of the Gold Award for Best Travel Reviews Website for the second year running, the company is committed to continuing to bring the best news, reviews and advice for the mature traveller.

**Society for Accessible Travel & Hospitality** (*sath.org*)
An educational non-profit membership organisation whose main objective is to raise awareness of the needs of all special needs travellers, remove disability discrimination and expand accessible travel opportunities worldwide.

**Tom's Port Guides** (*tomsportguides.com*)
Tom's Port Guides offers free maps and comprehensive planning details for exploring tourist sites with knowledge and confidence.

# The Autonomous Cruiser

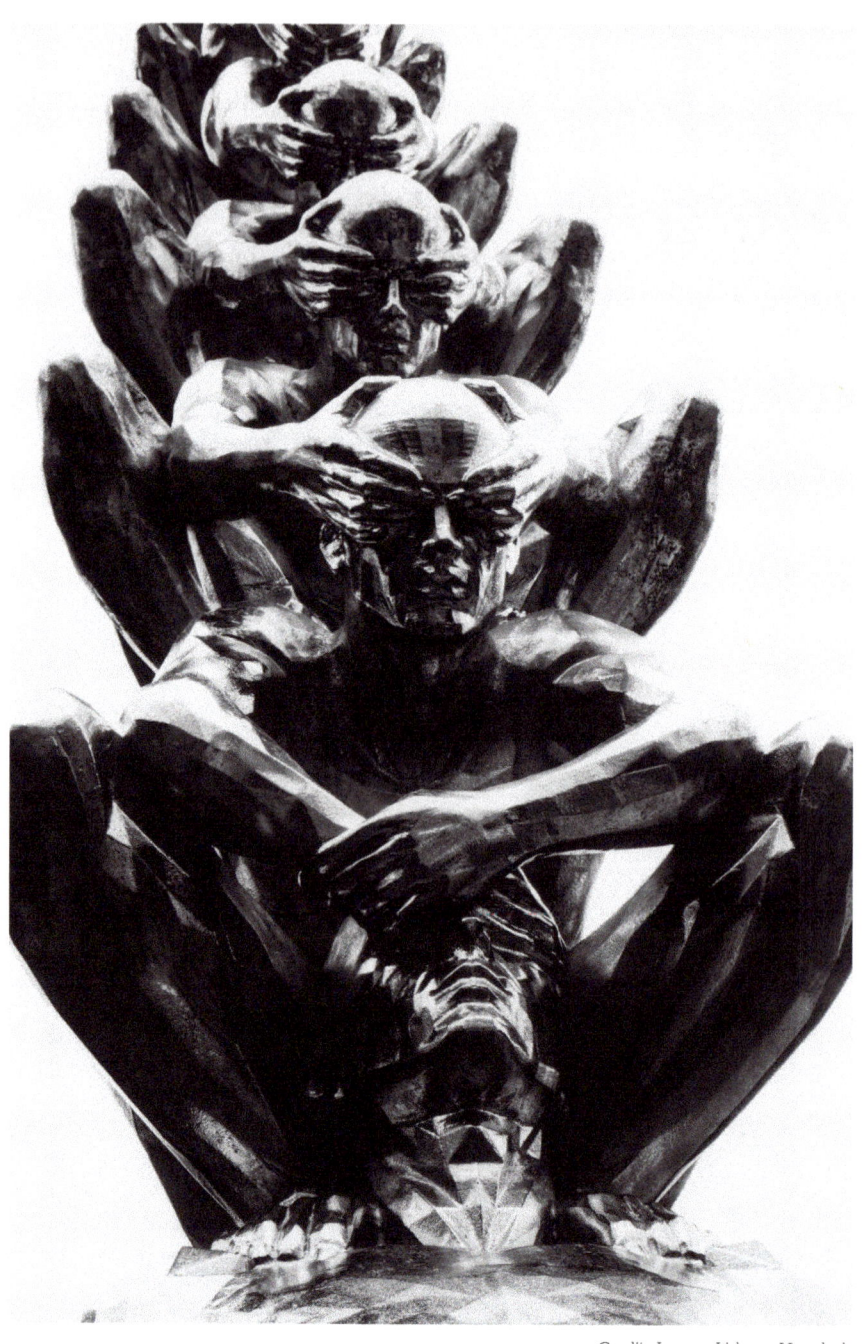

*Credit: Jeremy Lishner, Unsplash*

# Directory

## Blind/Impaired Sight

**Mind's Eye Travel** (*mindseyetravel.com*)
A specialised company creating tours for people who are blind or visually impaired. Services include sighted guide assistance, help with boarding passes, cruise line bag tags, embarkation, disembarkation, ship orientation and shore excursions.

**Royal National Institute of Blind People** (*RNIB*) (*rnib.org.uk*)
Planning to travel or take a holiday when you're blind or partially sighted can seem daunting. Guest travel blogger for RNIB, Kate Bosley talks about some of her best travel experiences and the biggest challenges she faced. She also writes for 'Limitless Travel', an organisation that looks after and supports people who want to travel but who have disabilities of various sorts.

**Travel Eyes** (*traveleyes-international.com*)
Travel Eyes is the world's first commercial tour operator set up by blind impresario Amar Latif, whose goal is to provide independent group travel for people who are blind or partially sighted.

## Breathing Disorders & Oxygen

**Advanced Aeromedical** (*aeromedic.com*)
Advanced Aeromedical provides portable oxygen concentrator rentals for people travelling within the US and internationally.

**Omega Advanced Aeromedical** (*omegaoxygen.com*)
Omega Advanced Aeromedical specialises in travel oxygen equipment, working closely with the world's cruise and travel companies. Their cruise oxygen teams will deliver all your equipment direct to your cabin as well as liaising with the onboard crew to ensure all is ready for your arrival, ensuring a smooth start to your holiday.

**OxygenWorldwide** (*oxygenworldwide.com*)
Operational since 1993, the company delivers oxygen worldwide to meet your individual needs. The website is available in multiple languages, and their customer service staff are often multilingual, something that is particularly important if you have problems while away.

### Sea Puffers Pulmonary Cruises & Vacations (*seapuffers.com*)
Respiratory therapists will call, discuss and arrange all your cruise, oxygen and equipment needs so you can relax knowing your special needs will be met.

### Travel O2 (*travelo2.com*)
Travel O2 provides all of your travel oxygen needs in more than 215 countries. With their new Sequal Eclipse portable oxygen concentrator, you can travel wherever and whenever you want without the need for any other type of oxygen, as this ground-breaking equipment has both Continuous Flow and Pulse Dose options for all your oxygen needs. Approved by the FAA and approved for airlines, as well as cruise ships and foreign travel, the Sequal Eclipse is the only continuous flow portable oxygen concentrator on the market.

### UK CPAP (*ukcpap.co.uk*)
Although a serious disorder, Sleep Apnea can be controlled by using a CPAP (continuous positive airway pressure) machine. Renting can help you decide on the best solution before purchase. UKCPAP has hire periods that range from one to six months and come as a complete package. Before effecting a rental contract, ask whether the machine's electrical system will need a converter or adaptor for your chosen ship.

## Car Services

### Driving Miss Daisy (*drivingmissdaisy.co.uk*)
A safe and reliable companion and driving service, providing wheelchair-accessible vehicles that will take you to your chosen departure airport, cruise terminal or coach pick-up point.

### Holiday Taxis (*holidaytaxis.com*)
A worldwide transport service, offering you quality, safe and licensed vehicles for airport to city and resort transfers in over 21,000 destinations in over 150 countries around the world.

### Medical Travel (*medicaltravel.org*)
Family-owned Florida Van Rentals is the leading handicap van rental company in Florida. They rent wheelchair and scooter accessible vans in almost every

major city in Florida. If you are fly-cruising, Florida Van Rentals will deliver the vehicle to you seven days a week so you can explore the port on your own terms.

**Wheelchair-accessible Holiday Taxis (***wheelchairaccessibleholidaytaxis.com***)**
An online taxi booking service specialising on making transfers and tailor-made tours as easy and accessible as possible.

## Cognitive, Intellectual and Developmental Disabilities

**Alzheimer's Society (***alzheimers.org.uk***)**
Find tailored information and advice that is right for you with their quick and easy to use website, full of information, publications and factsheets. Their 'Staying Independent' section has tips and information on travelling when dementia is involved.

**Autism on the Seas (***autismontheseas.com***)**
Autism on the Seas has teamed up with Royal Caribbean International since 2007. It is resolute in its mission of delivering the most comprehensive accessible cruise holidays with the right accommodation and services to meet their guest's special needs. Professional staff accompany you on your cruise to provide amazing travel experiences onboard Royal Caribbean, Celebrity, Norwegian, Disney and Carnival Cruise Lines.

**Autism Speaks (***autismspeaks.org***)**
Using the planning and information resources on the website, the company aims to open new travel opportunities for children and adults with autism.

**MS Focus At Sea (***msfocus.org***)**
MS Focus At Sea (formerly Cruise for a Cause) is an annual educational event featuring presentations from MS experts, interactive exercise sessions and social gatherings. During your days at sea, the company offers onboard workshops and discussion groups while leading neurologists and other healthcare professionals present the latest information on MS research and treatment, and offer practical advice to help you live comfortably with MS. In addition, onboard support group meetings serve to motivate and inspire both people with MS and caregivers.

**MS Society** (*mssociety.org.uk*)
A community that helps you through the highs and lows of living with MS. They are researching, writing, campaigning, fighting and providing award-winning support and information.

**National Autistic Society** (*autism.org.uk*)
The UK's largest provider of specialist autism services whose aim is to bring passion and expertise to the lives of autistic people every year. Their website's 'Holidays: preparation and practicalities' section highlights practical considerations when planning a trip and you will find the autism card by visiting their shop.

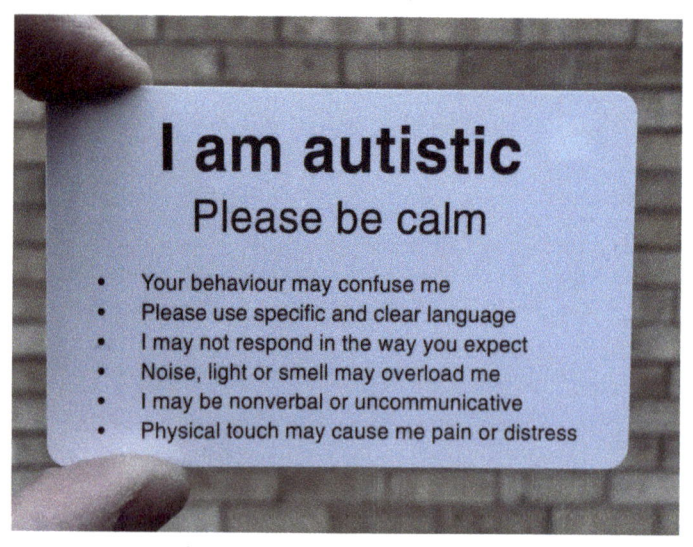

*Credit: Hackney Autism Communications Card - Panda Mery, Flickr*

## Companion/Carer Service

**Able Community Care** (*ablecommunitycare.com*)
Able Community Care can provide holiday carers or companions for older people or those with disabilities to enable them to take any holiday of their choice. Your travel buddy can provide personal and domestic care, assistance and holiday companionship. The company will do their best to find a companion that suits your preference and personality, someone who loves travel, can assist on day trips and can share your adventure.

# DIRECTORY

**Dignity Travel** (*dignitytravel.biz*)
Dignity Travel strives to make sure that you have a stressless travel experience, presented in a dignified, fun and adventurous manner. They understand that not everyone has someone to travel with, or your care partner may want an opportunity to relax as well. Therefore, they arrange for experienced travel companions who are able to assist you while travelling, provide a break to the person that cares for you or simply support your normal care partner. Travel companions can help you with daily care needs, toileting, dressing, transfers and any other assistance which might be needed.

**Helping Hands** (*helpinghandshomecare.co.uk*)
Helping Hands provides a holiday care service that's fully tailored to your requirements. They work with you, your family, your GP and professionals from a variety of other healthcare organisations to ensure your medical needs are met. They provide assistance with all essential elements of care and take responsibility for ensuring your medication is correctly administered. Their carers will provide support on the journey, allowing you to fully relax during your holiday.

**Independent Travel Care** (*independenttravelcare.com*)
Providing experienced personal care assistants and travel companions for ageing or physically disabled travellers, Independent Travel Care allows you to travel with confidence, knowing someone is there to help throughout your cruise.

**Live In Care** (*https://livein.care/holiday-companionship-care-breaks*)
Live In Care provides a personal care service that helps you remain independent and allows you to take a holiday without cause for concern. Their essential care companion will travel with you and can stay in your cabin so that they are there to assist with any difficulties that may arise. Your care companion is also a friend to share your experiences with and provide engaging company so that you will never feel alone while travelling.

**Medical Travel Companions** (*medicaltravelcompanions.com*)
Offering non-emergency travel companions for travellers who need extra help on their trip abroad. Companions are matched to the customer's requirements, offering support to individuals, families or groups.

## Deaf/Impaired Hearing

**Caroline's Rainbow Foundation**
(*carolinesrainbowfoundation.org/deaf-travellers*)
Invaluable deaf travel tips and information for journeys by train, plane and automobiles.

**D-Travel Agency** (*dtravelagency.com*)
D-Travel Agency's objective is to nurture and cultivate partnerships with travel and tour suppliers to ensure sign language is included in their travel itineraries, tours and services they can offer to deaf travellers.

**Deaf Travel** (*deaftravel.co.uk*)
A unique travel website full of information and advice for the deaf community. The website shows that being deaf and using sign language to communicate is no barrier to independent travel.

**Deaf Ventures Travel** (*deafventurestravel.com*)
With over 40 years of travel industry experience, founder Chanin Nickerson, a Child of Deaf Adults (CODA) and partially deaf herself, set up DeafVentures Travel to develop fun, exciting and amazing travel opportunities for the deaf community.

**Rexy Edventures** (*rexyedventures.com*)
Deaf travel inspiration through the adventures, recommendations and advice of a seasoned, profoundly deaf backpacker travelling the unexpected.

## Diabetes

**Diabetes.co.uk** (*diabetes.co.uk*)
Europe's largest diabetes community website with a focus on providing a comprehensive, supportive and independent experience for their visitors across the globe. They have loads of valuable information on their website, with daily news and guides on diabetes management, and even a 'Diabetes Travel Tips' section.

# Directory

**Diabetes UK** (*diabetes.org.uk*)
The organisation campaigns for and supports everyone affected by diabetes and is funding research that will one day lead to a cure. Read the latest stories on diabetes, search through the news archive and visit their 'Travel and Diabetes' section.

## Dialysis

**Cruise Dialysis** (*cruisedialysis.co.uk*)
Cruise Dialysis offers a wide range of cruises with onboard haemodialysis that mirrors your treatment back home. An experienced dialysis team and nephrologist are on the ship throughout your cruise so you can rest assured that you're getting the best attention at all times. They have so many wonderful ships and destinations to choose from, including sailings from Bristol, Tilbury and Southampton, with more itinerary choices than ever before but places are limited to a maximum of 12-16 patients so book early to avoid disappointment.

> Following a meeting between NHS England, the BKPA and Lisa Parnell of Cruise Dialysis, NHS England has chosen to exercise its discretionary rights to partially reimburse the cost of healthcare onboard cruise ships subject to certain conditions: If the majority of ports visited during your cruise are within the European Economic Area (EEA) (or a country with which the NHS has formal healthcare agreements, i.e., those covered under Article 56 or those countries with which England has bilateral agreements) then you will be reimbursed the amount of the National Tariff. For more information, please contact NHS England *england.contactus@nhs.net*.

**Dialysis at Sea** (*dialysisatsea.com*)
Dialysis at Sea Cruises is the largest provider of dialysis services aboard cruise ships in the world, providing a renal care specialist team consisting of a nephrologist, dialysis nurses and certified technicians on select cruise sailings with Royal Caribbean and Celebrity Cruise Lines. They provide the most advanced equipment and supplies, which are housed and maintained with Dialysis at Sea Cruises and undergo strict maintenance protocols for the most optimum performance.

### Dialysis Cruises (*en.diacare.ch*)
German-based Dialysis Cruises provides a complete cruise holiday for haemodialysis patients. Dialysis machines and equipment are a permanent part of their ships' medical centres and treatments are made available for destinations all over the world. The machines meet the highest dialysis standards, have volumetric control, sodium modelling and can handle your individual dialysis prescription. Experienced renal medical staff are on hand to take care of you from the beginning to the end of your cruise.

### Global Dialysis (*globaldialysis.com*)
Global Dialysis is the premier resource for haemo, home and peritoneal dialysis around the world. Established in 2000, with more than 16,800 dialysis centres in 161 countries, Global Dialysis is the world's leading specialist in holiday dialysis and travel, providing an independent resource for information. Global Dialysis maps are easy to use, accessible and there is a free listing for every dialysis centre in the world, which is updated daily by unit managers, volunteers and their users' feedback.

## Epilepsy

### Epilepsy Action (*epilepsy.org.uk*)
Epilepsy Action is a charity that improves the lives of everyone affected by epilepsy. They offer advice, improve healthcare, fund research and campaign for change. Check out their 'Travel Advice' Section for amazing information about travelling with epilepsy.

### Epilepsy Society (*epilepsysociety.org.uk*)
Epilepsy Society is the UK's leading provider of epilepsy services. Through their cutting-edge research, awareness campaigns, information resources and expert care, they work for everyone affected by epilepsy in the UK. Crammed with information, articles, personal stories and blogs, including a 'Travel and Holidays' section, there is something for everyone learning to live with the condition.

# Directory

## Equipment Rental

**British Red Cross** (*redcross.org.uk*)
You can now borrow or hire a wheelchair from the British Red Cross for a single trip for up to six weeks. They can provide self-propelled chairs (push yourself) or transit chairs (companions push) to suit your size and weight. They also offer a leg extension if your leg is in a cast. The fee depends on where you live, but in most places they only ask for a donation.

**Mobility at Sea** (*mobilityatsea.co.uk*)
Mobility at Sea provides a host of mobility aids, from walking frames to wheelchairs, and living aids, from toilet raisers to adjustable beds, that can all be delivered to your cabin prior to embarkation and simply left onboard at the end of the cruise. Passengers can be met inside the cabin or cruise terminal if a demonstration of equipment is needed. The company can even arrange a cruise carer if needed.

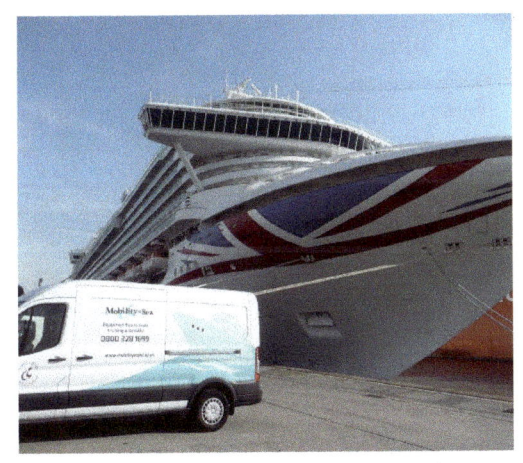

*Credit: Mobility at Sea*

**Mobility Equipment Hire Direct** (*mobilityequipmenthiredirect.com*)
With a network that spans the British Isles and several overseas countries, the company offers a nationwide delivery service of mobility equipment including wheelchairs, hoists, mobility scooters, shower chairs, walkers, standing electric hoists, hospital beds and pressure relief mattresses.

**Scootaround** (*scootaround.com*)
The company's vast network of locations allows them to supply most major cruise ports worldwide with mobility rentals and accessibility solutions, including scooters, wheelchairs, power chairs, and oxygen concentrators. They serve over 20 cruise lines at nearly 50 major ports throughout the United States, Canada and Europe. Customers can arrange rentals 24/7, with your cruise mobility equipment delivered directly to your home, hotel, port or cabin.

**Special Needs at Sea** (*specialneedsatsea.com*)
One of the top mobility equipment delivery sites dedicated to fulfilling the special needs of travellers who may require mobility aids, oxygen units or audio and visual aid rentals. Available in 215 ports across 68 countries, a company ambassador will ensure your rental equipment is delivered directly to your stateroom.

### Travel Equipment Insurance

**Blue Badge Mobility Insurance** (*bluebadgemobilityinsurance.co.uk*)
As well as offering travel health insurance, Blue Badge Mobility Insurance offers up to 90 days of cover for your mobility scooters, power chairs, manual wheelchairs and disability adapted trikes. They also have care worker and personal assistant cover so you can go away with complete peace of mind.

**Chartwell Insurance** (*chartwellinsurance.co.uk*)
Offers insurance covering all powered mobility equipment that is designed around your needs. Although losing your scooter or wheelchair is unimaginable, consider the shock and devastation if you found out you were responsible, or partly responsible, for causing an accident, and that the liability costs could run into thousands of pounds. Chartwell Insurance takes that burden away by offering a selection of reasonably priced plans that will cover your personal safety, other people's safety and the value of the vehicle.

**Fish Insurance** (*fishinsurance.co.uk*)
For over 40 years, Fish Insurance has been providing specialist insurance in the UK and abroad for people with pre-existing medical conditions, disabilities or mobility issues. They provide specialist insurance cover for manual

wheelchairs, powered wheelchairs, mobility scooters, in-home products such as stairlifts and hoists, as well as protection for wheelchair-accessible vehicles (WAV). Their cover also extends to covering orthotics and prosthetic limbs valued up to £80,000.

**Surewise.com** (*surewise.co.uk*)
A dedicated team based in Hadleigh, Essex, all united by a passion for building trust, care and fairness within the insurance sector. They are committed to helping and protecting their customers against the unexpected and unforeseen. Electric mobility equipment cover includes accidental and malicious damage, fire, flood, storm damage, theft, liability insurance and worldwide travel costs up to 21 days (excluding North America and Canada). A manual wheelchair is automatically covered within their policy and they also cover your wheelchair accessories, replacing them if they are damaged or stolen along with your wheelchair.

## Travel Health Protection Comparison Site

There is no singular comparison site that scans every insurance site so visit several and look at the options available before making your choice. As good as these sites are for finding the best insurance provider not every company chooses to be featured. Just remember insurance doesn't have to be complicated, it just has to be good.

**All Clear Travel** (*allcleartravel.co.uk*)

**Find Me Expat Insurance** (*findmeexpatinsurance.com*)

**Insure My Trip** (*insuremytrip.com*)

**Medical Travel Compared** (*medicaltravelcompared.co.uk*)

**Money Supermarket** (*moneysupermarket.com/travel-insurance*)

**Paying Too Much** (*payingtoomuch.com*)

**SquareMouth** (*squaremouth.com*)

## Travel Health Protection

Most people who suffer from pre-existing medical conditions do not qualify for standard travel insurance, but there are a host of specialist insurers who offer specific policies for older travellers or those with disabilities including long stay trips with no upper age limit. You should always check the small print and policy exemptions relating to drugs or pre-existing medical conditions.

> **Don't Ask:**
> Why didn't you tell me it would be hot? (said while cruising in the Amazon)

**All Clear Travel** (*allcleartravel.co.uk*)
With cover for a range of medical conditions including arthritis, epilepsy, stroke, heart condition and cancer and no upper age limit, All Clear Travel has a specialised cruise cover that is right for you.

**Avanti Travel Insurance** (*avantitravelinsurance.co.uk*)
Not only do Avanti Travel Insurance offer cover with no age limit for pre-existing health conditions, they have a 24/7 medical help line and pay out unlimited medical expenses with their Deluxe policy. Their policy safeguards single trips of up to 550 days with no upper age limit and with protection against pre-existing conditions.

**Boots Travel Insurance** (*bootstravelinsurance.com*) considers any medical condition, with no upper age limit, on single-trip policies. They also have specialist cover for people suffering from all types of multiple sclerosis (MS), including benign, relapse remitting, primary progressive and secondary progressive.

**Chartwell Insurance** (*chartwellinsurance.co.uk*)
Chartwell Insurance offers single-trip policies that have no age limit and cover a maximum duration of 154 days, whilst their multi-trip yearly policies have an age limit of 85 years old, but each trip must be less than 92 days. Both companies automatically provide £1500 for accidental loss, theft or damage of luggage, and if you lose your medication while away, the policy will cover the cost of an urgent replacement, up to £300.

# Directory

**Fish Insurance** (*fishinsurance.co.uk*)
Fish Insurance work hand in hand with Ancile Insurance and their experts will make sure you get the cover that is right for you. With no age limit, and cover for 94 days their range of pre-existing conditions includes cover for Parkinson's disease, cerebral palsy, muscular dystrophy and diabetes.

**Free Spirit** (*freespirittravelinsurance.com*)
Free Spirit is arranged by travel insurance specialist P J Hayman, one of the largest specialist travel insurance providers for people with medical conditions and disabilities. With no upper age limit on single or multi-trips their cover also includes medical aids and medications. Their 'Super Duper' cover is rated five star by Defaqto

**Get Going Travel Insurance** (*getgoinginsurance.co.uk*)
Offering single, multi and longstay trip cover for travellers over 80, they offer comprehensive cover for pre-existing conditions including cancer, cystic fibrosis and diabetes.

**Good to Go Insurance.Com** (*goodtogoinsurance.com*)
Winner of several industry awards Good to Go Travel Insurance design policies that offer the right cover for people travelling with all types of medical conditions including those on a course of radiotherapy or chemotherapy, up to a high level of severity or even a terminal prognosis.

**Insure and Go** (*insureandgo.com*)
Insure and Go provide hassle-free specialist cruise travel insurance with no upper age limit and cover for pre-existing conditions. Their cover also provides for a number of cruise specific eventualities such as cabin confinement, holiday interruption and itinerary changes.

**Insurancewith** (*insurancewith.com*)
Award-winning medical travel insurance provider covering over 5000 medical conditions and offering reasonable quotes that have undercut high street brands by up to 98%. There is no upper age limit for single trip policies depending on your age, destination and trip duration.

**Just Travel** (*justtravelcover.com*) provides single-trip cover for up to 365 days, for people up to 70 years old, and will protect all pre-existing medical conditions, including terminal prognosis.

**PJ Hayman** (*pjhayman.com*)
P J Hyman offers single trips of up to 186 days, has no upper age limit and, for an additional premium, will consider a traveller with a pre-existing medical condition.

**Saga** (*saga.co.uk/insurance*)
Saga offers single policies with cover for up to 120 days anywhere in the world. Specialising in travel for the over 50s with no upper age limit they also cover for many pre-existing medical conditions. The company have recently announced that treatment abroad for Covid-19 and repatriation to the UK will be included as standard on their travel policies if a guest contracts the virus.

**Travel Insurance 4Medical** (*travelinsurance4medical.co.uk*)
A specialist insurance company that offers cruise cover for people up to the age of 100 and for those with pre-existing conditions including cancer, multiple sclerosis and Alzheimer's.

## Wheelchair Accessibility Resources

**Disabled Travelers Guide** (*disabledtravelersguide.com*)
Nancy & Nate Berger share their experiences and offer help and advice to disabled travellers.

**Gimp on the Go** (*gimponthego.org*)
Full of travel tips, advice and resources for those with special needs, including access to accessible ground transportation and tour agents at the more popular cruise ports.

**Queen Elizabeth's Foundation for Disabled People**
(*qef.org.uk/accessibleaviation*)
Useful flight video guides, made in partnership with the UK Civil Aviation Authority, that gives wheelchair users practical information about travelling by air and the support available to them.

# Directory

**Spin the Globe** (*spintheglobe.net*)
Sylvia Longmire has visited 51 countries, 43 of those as a wheelchair user, and the majority as a solo traveller. Her goal is to share destination accessibility with fellow wheelchair users around the world.

**Wheelchair Travel** (*wheelchairtravel.org*)
Offering practical information, advice and resources to help you plan a wheelchair-friendly holiday, using accessible city guides and information on air, train and hotel travel.

**Wheelchair Travelling** (*wheelchairtravelling.com*)
Thousands of resources, reviews, guides and tips to empower people with impaired mobility to experience the world of accessible travel.

**Wheelchair World** (*wheelchairworld.org*)
A collection of reviews, articles, blogs and information that help people with limited mobility and wheelchair users to be more aware of their destination's accessibility.

**Wheelmap** (*wheelmap.org*)
An online map for finding and marking accessible places worldwide, including bars, restaurants, toilets, museums, banks, cinemas and supermarkets, with two million places already registered. Also available as an app for iOS, Android and Windows phones.

## Accessible Travel Agents

**accessible Go** (*accessiblego.com*)
A great user-friendly website offering the chance to search, review and book an accessible hotel, cruise or mode of transport in 30 of the most visited U.S cities.

**Accessible Journeys** (*accessiblejourneys.com*)
A holiday planner and tour operator specifically for wheelchair travellers, their families and friends, with an option to design custom accessible trips.

**Accessible Travel & Leisure (***accessibletravel.co.uk***)**
Wheelchair user Andy Wright is a family man who has experienced the challenge of travelling with a disability. He decided to combine his travel experience with his personal knowledge of disability and founded a tour operator to provide trustworthy accessible holidays. Looking after *all* holidaymakers irrespective of their special requirements Andy has provided holidays for thousands of clients with wide-ranging, diverse medical conditions and illnesses. Nobody is excluded.

**Accessible Travel Solutions (***accessibletravelsolutions.com***)**
With years of experience in the accessible travel industry, Accessible Travel Solutions are passionate in providing travellers the best in barrier-free travel services.

**Best Bets Travel (***bestbetstravel.com***)**
The Travel Institute has recognised Best Bets Travel as an Accredited Disability Agent, an Autism Friendly Agent and an Accessible Travel Specialist. Whether you want a wheelchair-accessible cruise, an ASL interpreter for deaf travellers, use dialysis or oxygen or want to book a tour for slow walkers or the visually impaired, Bets Bets have it covered.

**Connie George Travel Associates (***cgta.com***)**
Connie George Travel Associates recognises that every traveller with special needs is unique, and tailors cruises and tours to holidaymakers that are deaf, wheelchair users, and slow walkers.

**Deaf Globetrotters (***deafglobetrotters.com***)**
A full-service travel agent for the deaf and hearing impaired that offers ocean and river cruising opportunities. A complete travel management service, they will dig deep to offer the best fares and create your trip from start to finish.

**Dignity Travel (***dignitytravel.biz***)**
Dignity Travel is committed to opening the world of travel to anyone with a chronic illness, a walking or physical disability or are wheelchair bound. Their cruises are designed to provide unique experiences, travel companions and care assistance if needed, while also delivering accessible accommodation, transportation and sightseeing opportunities.

# Directory

*Two modern day heroes, Timothy Holtz and Edward Gillespie, conceived, started and run Dignity Travel, delivering to all their guests with a disability or chronic illness the chance to travel in a dignified, fun and adventurous manner. They make the impossible happen.*

*Timothy is the company president and his past accessible travel expertise with Flying Wheels Travel was preceded by almost ten years' experience of working with people who had a chronic illness or disability with the National Multiple Sclerosis Society. Timothy developed respected and award-winning syllabi and benefits for people living with MS and offering travel prospects, weekend sabbaticals and advocacy for people with varying impairments.*

*For nearly ten years, Edward, a trained physical therapist, was a volunteer with the National MS Society, assisting people with multiple sclerosis at MS Camp and getaways. In 2008 he was recognized as a Volunteer All-star by the MS Society and is highly respected and admired by his colleagues and clients. Edward was struck by how many limitations there were for the physically disadvantaged to travel and 2012 saw him partner with long-time friend and colleague Timothy in bringing their dream of making the impossible a reality. Edward extends his expertise to coordinating, hosting and providing personal care assistance on group tours.*

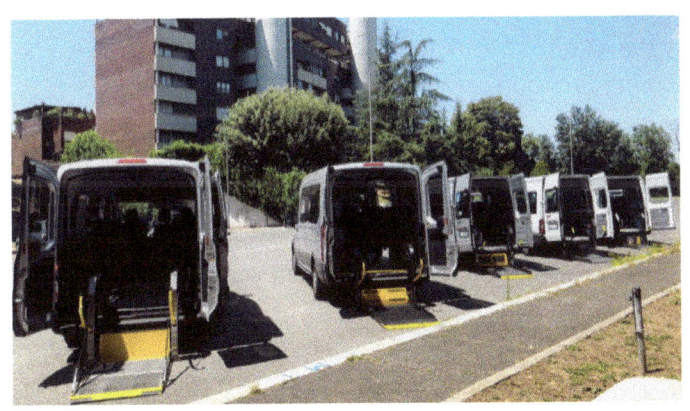

*Credit: Disabled Accessible Travel*

**Disabled Access Holidays** (*disabledaccessholidays.com*)
Offering wheelchair-accessible holidays to disabled travellers, including arranging wheelchair assistance and flights from any UK Airport, wheelchair adapted taxi transfers, mobility equipment hire and guaranteed accessible cabins.

**Disabled Accessible Travel** (*disabledaccessibletravel.com*)
Europe's leading accessible travel agent, offering a wide range of bespoke services to any type of traveller in need of adapted solutions, including accessible cruise port transfers and accessible shore excursions.

**Disabled Cruise Club** (*disabledcruiseclub.com*)
With years of cruise experience and detailed knowledge of the cruise lines, destinations and ports, the Disabled Cruise Club are the UK's only cruise club catering exclusively for those with disabilities and is a specialist in accessible cruises offering the best advice in finding you the perfect cruise ship and itinerary. They can arrange disabled equipment, adapted excursions, adapted transfers & assistance at ports.

**DisabledHolidays.com** (*disabledholidays.com*)
One of the UK's largest accessible holiday specialists, guaranteeing accessible accommodation and organising flights, adapted transfers, luggage delivery, disabled travel insurance and equipment hire. Originally called The Disabled Holiday Directory, the company was launched by Sian Lavis who has suffered since childhood with peroneal muscular atrophy, more commonly known as Charcot-Marie Tooth disease (CMT). She has subsequently helped hundreds of travellers find the right holidays to suit their handicap. In June 2008, Sian retired and sold the website to its current owner who is committed to continuing the ethos of the founder.

**Easy Access Travel** (*easyaccesstravel.com*)
Debra Kerper suffers from Lupus and is a bilateral amputee. Her company, Easy Access Travel, is dedicated to organising group trips and meeting the special needs of disabled and mature travellers. An extensive traveller herself, Debra has been on more than 90 cruises doing hands-on research, ship inspections, visiting tourist spots and gathering information from people she knows and trusts.

**Exceptional Vacations** (*exceptional-vacations.com*)
Dedicated in arranging high quality holiday experiences for individuals with developmental disabilities and special needs.

# DIRECTORY

**Kirstin's Deaf Travel (***kirstinstravel.com***)**
This travel agent specialises in tour packages for the deaf. Guests can choose from ocean or river cruises in Europe, America, the Caribbean and Asia. Although most of the tours are organised as group packages, individual and customised cruises can also be arranged.

**Mind's Eye Travel (***mindseyetravel.com***)**
An organisation that creates tours for people who are blind or visually impaired. Their prices include sighted guide assistance and help with boarding passes, cruise line bag tags, embarkation, disembarkation, orientation while on the ship, shore excursions and airline bookings.

**Sage Traveling (***sagetraveling.com***)**
John Sage, the founder and owner of Sage Traveling, sustained a spinal cord injury when he was only 22 years old and is now a full-time wheelchair user, giving him a unique perspective of all the challenges that disabled travellers can encounter during their trip. Sage Travelling offers custom accessible cruise itineraries and shore excursions for people with special mobility needs, including wheelchair, scooter, cane and walker users and senior travellers.

*At the age of 22, John Sage was injured in a skiing accident and sustained a T-4 incomplete spinal cord injury resulting in his need to use a wheelchair. John quickly adapted to his new lifestyle and retained his passion for travel, visiting Europe 16 times and enjoying 140+ cities.*

*After his sixth trip to Europe, he realised there had to be a better way to plan a wheelchair-accessible trip. He spent dozens of hours researching trips to southern France and Italy and was still met by a few nasty surprises. The existing internet accessibility information was sporadic, vague, non-existent and at times completely incorrect! Some sites described Venice as "totally inaccessible for wheelchairs", yet with the right information it can be visited by wheelchair users!*

*It's taken years, a lot of hard work and numerous personal visits to the top European destinations to make Sage Traveling a leading expert in disabled European travel.*

*"I have had the best experiences of my life travelling the world and living out my dreams. Travelling is my passion and I look forward to making your dream accessible vacation a reality!" - Founder & Owner, John Sage*

**Travel-For-All** (*travel-for-all.com*)
A global leader in wheelchair-accessible travel, their agents custom design each trip to match their guest's special needs. Working with a hand-picked group of suppliers, Travel-For-All will create the most accessible holiday possible.

**Wheelchair Escapes** (*wheelchairescapes.com*)
An experienced Certified Accessible Travel Specialist whose focus is on meeting the specific travelling needs of wheelchair users and their families.

## Independent Cruise Specialists

Cruise Lines International Association (CLIA) is the largest cruise industry trade association across the world, and the leading authority of the cruise community. A major priority of CLIA is the safety of all guests and crew and their members are proactive in accommodating passengers with disabilities. The members listed below work together to provide each guest with an amazing experience.

**Barrhead Travel** (*barrheadtravel.co.uk*)
With 900 employees across 76 UK outlets and with 45 years' experience, Barrhead Travel is now one of the UK's leading independent travel groups and have expert travel specialists focusing on accessible travel. Their specialist department offers impartial advice, innovative holiday options and excellent value and is the reason they've been voted UK Travel Agent of the Year at the Travel Trade Gazette Awards for seven years in a row.

**Bolsover Cruise Club** (*bolsovercruiseclub.com*)
This award-winning company is officially the UK's No.1 Cruise Agent. Unlike other high street travel agents, they are exclusively a cruise only specialist, dealing solely with premium cruise brands. Their sales consultant team has specialist knowledge of cruising having sailed on hundreds of ships for around 16,000 nights in total and they are experienced in understanding which ships, and indeed destinations, are most suited in terms of accessibility.

# Directory

**Cruise 118** (*cruise118.com*)
Voted Favourite Cruise Agent of the Year in World of Cruising's Wave Awards in 2019, Cruise 118 is one of the UK's largest cruise retailers. Their dedicated Cruise Concierge team will give you access to all the best deals and discounts including exclusive offers that are not available elsewhere. Their website offers detailed information on the cruise lines and their ships and lists more than 53,000 passenger reviews.

**Cruise 1st** (*cruise1st.co.uk*)
Another company voted Favourite Cruise Agent of the Year in World of Cruising's Wave Awards in 2019, Cruise 1st makes it their aim to bring you the best cruise deals on the market. Because of their strong relationships with the major cruise lines they can deliver the best cruise holiday options at the lowest price including accessible shore excursions.

**Iglu** (*iglucruise.com*)
Trading for more than 17 years, this company is the UK's largest independent cruise agent after buying out Planet Cruise in 2013. Offering more than 8000 cruises to over 3000 ports from more than 40 cruise lines, their website and in-house specialists are dedicated to finding the best deal for you. For those with special requirements, Iglu suggests you contact the ship first to ensure it suits your needs, after which Iglu's Special Assistance team will help with further details.

**The Luxury Cruise Company** (*theluxurycruisecompany.com*)
Combined, their cruise consultants have almost 200 years' experience of selling cruises, have crossed every ocean and tested every cruise line; giving them the edge over their competitors when it comes to knowledge and experience. A division of Wexas Travel, they offer ocean, river and exploration-style cruises worldwide and specialise in arranging hand-picked cruise itineraries aboard some of the world's finest vessels. They are one of a few companies that organise ship visits throughout the year.

**Mundy Cruising** (*mundycruising.co.uk*)
With over 45 years of experience and meticulous planning, nobody knows more about the luxury cruise market than Mundy Cruising. They were the first cruise specialist in the UK, and have maintained their position through

ingenuity, customer focus, personal service and tailoring your holiday to your own specifications. Their agents have first-hand knowledge of the ships and their accessibility features.

**Ponders Travel** (*ponderstravel.co.uk*)
Managing Director Clare Dudley is Director of the trade body Leading Cruise Agents and offers up a wealth of experience with all luxury cruise lines, river cruising, soft adventure, round the world epics and cargo ships. Her experienced staff will match your needs with the right cruise at a highly competitive price. Ponders Travel have also designed a series of accessible shore excursions that can provide specially adapted ramped vehicles in a majority of ports that they offer.

**Six Star Cruises** (*sixstarcruises.co.uk*)
Six Star Cruises have established itself as a leading brand in the world of luxury travel, offering bespoke cruise experiences from multi-award-winning lines like Azamara Club Cruises, Crystal Cruises, Oceania Cruises, Regent Seven Seas Cruises, Seabourn, Silversea and Hapag-Lloyd Cruises. Their expert Cruise Concierge team are familiar with each of the luxury cruise lines, their ships and their itineraries, as well as access at each port and which accessible excursions are available. They can also arrange for the hire of any medical equipment, coordinate transfers from your home or the airport to the ship as well as reserving accessible hotel rooms pre or post cruise.

**Vision Cruise** (*visioncruise.co.uk*)
With offices in Australia and America, Vision Cruise is looking to get the best price for your cruise adventure. They are the only travel company with a daily television program on the Holiday and Cruise TV channel, which brings cruising directly to your living room. The shows reimagine cruise ships and capture a vision of your future voyage whether you're a first-time cruiser or a veteran of the seas. The company has a dedicated online accessibility section.

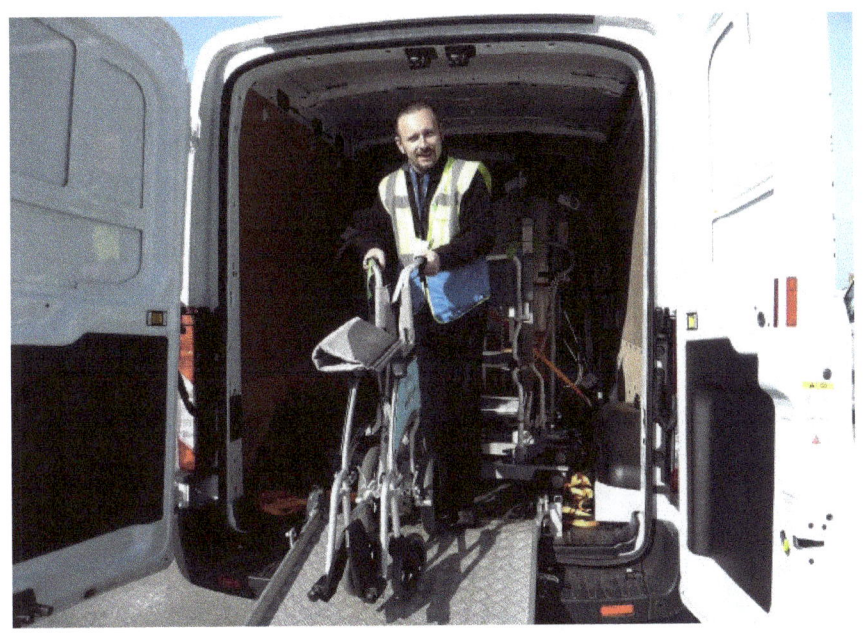

*Credit: Mobility at Sea*

# Travel Planning Website Directory

When planning any trip there are a host of websites that can help you with your research. There are too many to highlight individually but you will find some of the most popular listed.

**Travel Planning:**
*triphobo.com, wendyperrin.com, tripplannera.com, travelleaders.com, adiosadventuretravel.com, travelmuse.com, inspirock.com, tripit.com, minube.net, lifesincrediblejourney.com, greatexpeditions.com, trover.com, nomadicmatt.com, tripadvisor.co.uk, untravel.com, reidsguides.com, fancyhands.com, triposo.com, rome2rio.com, moovitapp.com, mapify.travel, contexttravel.com, timeanddate.com*

# The Autonomous Cruiser

**Travel Guides:** *wikitravel.com, wikivoyage.org, lonelyplanet.com, frommers.com, worldtravelguide.net, timeout.com, afar.com/travel-guides, autoeurope.com/travel-guides, ctwtravels.com, smartertravel.com/destinations, telegraph.co.uk/travel/destinations, fodors.com, https://www.worldnomads.com/explore/guides, roughguides.com, inyourpocket.com, theculturetrip.com, planetware.com*

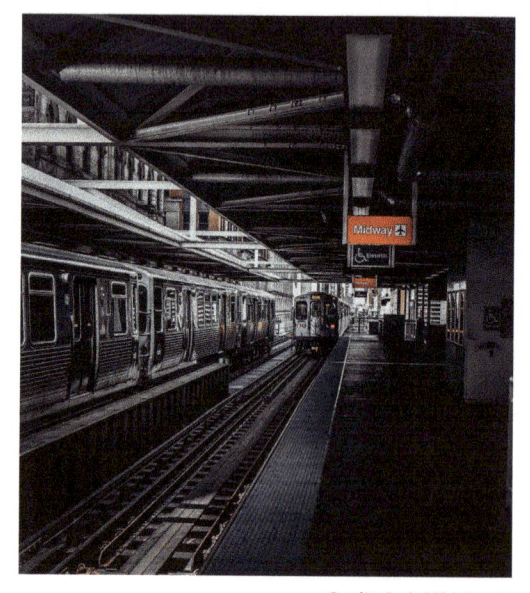

*Credit: Josh Hild, Pexels*

**Hotel Search Engines:** *hotels.com, hotelscombined.com, tripadvisor.com, rome2rio.com, trivago.co.uk, kayak.com, booking.com, expedia.com, agoda.com, priceline.com, hotwire.com, orbitz.com, hoteltonight.com, travelsupermarket.com, opodo.co.uk, liligo.co.uk, travelocity.com, roomkey.com, hipmunk.com, momondo.com, vayama.com, google.com, dohop.com, room77.com, latemaster.com, slh.com, i-escape.com, hotelmix.co.uk, hotely.co.uk*

# Directory

**Flights Travel Search:** momondo.co.uk, kayak.com, priceline.com, tripadvisor.com, expedia.com, travelocity.com, orbitz.com, hotwire.com, flightnetwork.com, google.com/flights, jetabroad.co.uk, skyscanner.net, fareness.com, cheaptickets.com, hipmunk.com, booking.com, agoda.com, skiplagged.com, bookit.com, vayama.com, cheapflights.com, travelzoo.com, dohop.com, cheapoair.co.uk, latemaster.com, seatguro.com, holidaypirates.com, gotogate.com

**Private Jet Charter:** prestigejets.co.uk, ecsjets.com, privatejetcharter.com, vistajet.com, lunajets.com, privatefly.com, flyxo.com, globeair.com, elevatecharter.com, starjets.net, vip-jets.net

**Airport Lounges:** prioritypass.com, loungepass.com, aph.com/airport-lounges.html, loungebuddy.co.uk, holidayextras.co.uk/airport-lounges.html, skyteam.com/lounges

**Train Travel:** eurostar.com, seat61.com, traingenius.com, rome2rio.com, thetrainline.com, omio.co.uk, railpass.com, raileurope.com, eurail.com

**Road Tripping:** roadtrippers.com, theaa.com, autoeurope.com/travel-guides, autoeurope.com/road-trip-planner

**Car Rentals:** autoeurope.co.uk, rentalcars.com, autoslash.com, orbitz.com, expedia.com, travelocity.com, momondo.com, vayama.com, kayak.com, dohop.com

**Tourist Info:** visiteurope.com, rove.me, travel-tourist-information-guide.com, world-guides.com/europe, ctwtravels.com

**Tours, Expeditions & Adventures:** viator.com, triphobo.com, veltra.com, shoretrips.com, contexttravel.com, museumland.com, isango.com, gocollette.com, nordicwildlife.no, tripadvisor.com, tourradar.com, musement.com, disabledaccessibletravel.com, accessibletravelsolutions.com

**Tour Guides:** viator.com, privateguides.com, contexttravel.com, mycreativetours.com, getyourguide.co.uk, toursbylocals.com, takewalks.com, liveprivateguide.com, spottedbylocals.com

# The Autonomous Cruiser

**Intrepid Travel:** *rei.com/adventures, gate1travel.com, iexplore.com, intrepidtravel.com, gadventures.com, djoserusa.com, tripoto.com, tucantravel.com, https://unboundtravel.com, naturetrek.co.uk*

**Eating Out:** *eatwith.com, travelingspoon.com, mamalovesfood.com, restaurantguru.com, timeout.com/restaurants, theculturetrip.com/europe/restaurants, tripadvisor.co.uk/restaurants-g4-europe, eatingeurope.com*

**Accessible Travel Info:** *iglucruise.com/guide-for-disabled-cruisers, travelonthelevel.blogspot.com, disabledtraveladvice.co.uk, parking4less.com/flying-with-a-disability*

**Accessible Travel Blogs:** *wheelchairtraveling.com, curbfreewithcorylee.com, rexyedventures.com, theblimblers.com, simplyemma.co.uk, martynsibley.com, havewheelchairwilltravel.net, accessibletourismresearch.blogspot.com, euansguide.com*

**Cruise Blog:** *cruisefever.net, cruisehive.com, cruiseradio.net, cruzely.com, eatsleepcruise.com, lifewellcruised.com, cruise-addicts.com, cruisebe.com, cruiseportadvisor.com/blog, cruiseline.co.uk/blog, theoceantraveler.com, cruiseindustrynews.com, cruisemaven.com, allthingscruise.com, theblondeabroad.com*

**Solo Travel:** *soloholidays.co.uk/cruise-solos, gutsytraveler.com, singlescruise.com*

**Packing:** *herpackinglist.com, upgradedpoints.com/travel-packing-list, onebag.com/checklist.html, indianajo.com/packing-list-template.html, maketimetoseetheworld.com/cruise-packing-list, travelfashiongirl.com/packing-list, smartertravel.com/cruise-packing-list-what-to-pack-for-a-cruise*

**Weather:** *worldweatheronline.co.uk, weatherspark.com, 1weatherapp.com, yr.no/en, snow-forecast.com, accuweather.com, weather.org, bbc.com/weather, weather2travel.com, edition.cnn.com/weather*

**Festival Finder:** *skiddle.com, festicket.com, jambase.com/festivals, festivalfinder.eu, festivalfinder.com, festivals.com, greenglobaltravel.com/best-festivals-in-the-world*

# Directory

**Creative Photography Apps:** *Instagram, Snapseed, Pixlr, Lapse It, NightCap Pro, Darkroom, Google Photos, Adobe Photoshop Express, TADAA HD Pro Camera, VSCO, Camera +, TouchRetouch, Afterlight 2, Enlight, Mextures*

**Anti-Theft Apps:** *Not My Phone, The Truth Spy, Prey Anti-Theft, Find My Phone, Find My Device, Cerberus, Lookout, mSpy, Flexispy, Hidden Anti Theft, Where's My Droid*

## Cruising

**Cruise Ship Calendar:** *cruisecal.com, cruisetimetables.com, cruisetoports.com, cruisesouthampton.com/cruises, destinationsouthampton.com/cruise/cruise-list, cruisemapper.com, whatsinport.com, southamptonvts.co.uk, cruisetoports.com, crew-center.com*

**Cruise Comparison Sites:** *comparethatcruise.com, dealchecker.co.uk/cruise.html, travelsupermarket.com/en-gb/cruises, cruisecompete.com, icelolly.com/cruise, https://cruises.cheapcaribbean.com, expedia.com/cruises, cruisewatch.com, costcotravel.com, tripadvisor.com/cruises, kayak.com/cruises, cruisecompare.co.uk*

**Cruise Deals:** *cruisedirect.com, vivavoyage.co.uk, cruise.co.uk, cruise118.com, planetcruise.com, cruise deals.co.uk, iglucruise.com, cruise1st.co.uk, vacationstogo.com, onlinevacationcenter.com, crucon.com, icruise.com, cruise.com, cruisecompete.com, cruise-addicts.com, orbitz.com, small-cruise-ships.com, cruisesonly.com, cruisesheet.com, avoyatravel.com, tourradar.com/f/ocean-cruise*

**Cruise Info:** *lifewellcruised.com, fodors.com/cruises, cruisecritic.com/ports, cruisecrocodile.com, cruisemapper.com/ports, avidcruiser.com/port-profiles*

**Cruise Reviews:** *avidcruiser.com, cruisecritic.com, cruisemates.com, tripadvisor.co.uk, cruisereviews.com, cruisediva.com, iqcruising.com, thetravelmagazine.net/reviews/cruise-reviews, iglucruise.com/cruise-reviews, cruiseline.com/reviews, cruise.co.uk/cruise-reviews*

**Cruise Shopping:** *cruisefashion.com, travelsmith.com, global.llbean.com, alpinetrek.co.uk, jack-wolfskin.co.uk, glovii.com, practicaltravelgear.com, nomadtravel.co.uk, astonbourne.co.uk, completeoutdoors.co.uk, encompassrl.com, foreverunique.co.uk/dresses/cruise-dresses.html*

**Duty-free:** *dutyfreeinformation.com/jet2-com-duty-free-shopping, gov.uk/duty-free-goods/arrivals-from-eu-countries, dfreeshop.com/cigarettes, worlddutyfree.com*

## Travel Money

**ATM Locator:** *mastercard.us/en-us/consumers/get-support/find-nearest-atm.html, network.americanexpress.com/globalnetwork/atm_locator, visa.com/atmlocator/#(page:home), https://branchlocator.santander.com/?defaultlanguage=en, link.co.uk/consumers/locator, mastercard.com/interactivelocator/atm.html*

**Wire/Send/Receive Money:** *transferwise.com, westernunion.com, moneygram.com, xoom.com, riamoneytransfer.co.uk, worldremit.com, worldfirst.com, xe.com, currencytransfer.com, oanda.com, hifx.co.uk, postoffice.co.uk/travel-money*

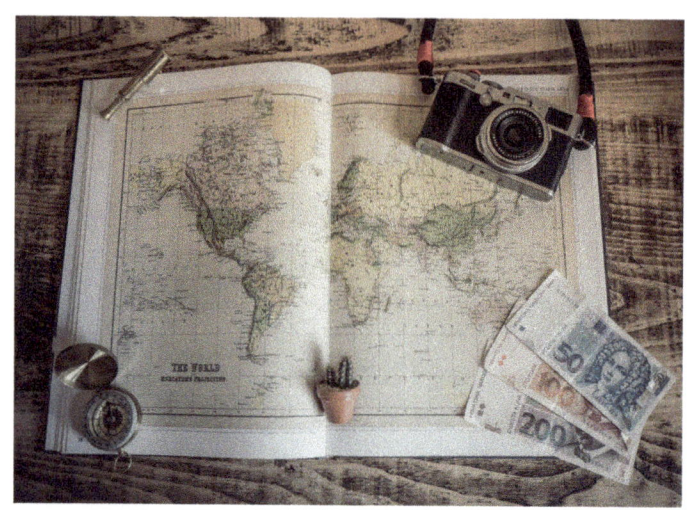

*Credit: Chris Lawton, Unsplash*

# Directory

**Currency Converters:** xrates.org, currency-convertor.org.uk, oanda.com, convertmymoney.com, cuex.com/en, travelex.com/currency-converter, xe.com

**Money Exchange:** leftovercurrency.com, travelexae.com, travelex.co.uk, currencies.co.uk, comparetransfer.com, worldfirst.com, fairfx.com, bestforeignexchange.com, money.co.uk, bestexchangerates.com

**Credit Card Comparison Sites:** cardhub.com, comparethemarket.com/credit-cards, moneysavingexpert.com/borrowing, experian.co.uk/consumer/credit-cards, money.co.uk, gocompare.com/credit-cards, bankrate.com, creditcards.com

**Top Travel Credit Cards:** Tandem Bank Cashback, Tandem Bank Journey, Santander Zero, Barclaycard Platinum Cashback Plus, Halifax Clarity, Creation Everyday, MBNA Horizon Cashback, Post Office Platinum, Starling Bank, Aqua Reward, 118 118 Money, Virgin Money Travel

**Best Prepaid Cards:** EasyFx One Card Personal, FairFx Euro/Dollar Card, Virgin Money Prepaid, WeSwap Global Prepaid Mastercard, Caxton FxCurrency Card, Revolut Standard Pre-Paid Card, Revolut Premium Prepaid Card, Post Office Travel Money Card

**VAT & Tax Refunds:** global-blue.com, premiertaxfree.com

## Communication

**Stay Connected:** mobal.com, telestial.com, skype.com, callingcards.com, speedypin.com, skype.com, mobal.com

**Wi-Fi Connections:** hotspot-locations.com, jaunted.com, wififreespot.com, cybercaptive.com, openwifispots.com, Wi-Fihotspotlist.com, wefi-com/wefi-app, appsapk.com/avast-Wi-Fi-finder, Wi-Fimapper

**SIM Cards:** T-Mobile One Plus, Orange International, Orange Holiday Europe SIM, Three Advanced Plan, O2 international SIM Card, Vodafone Data SIM for Europe, Lebara, Lyca Mobile, WorldSIM International SIM Card, SimOptions International SIM Card

# The Autonomous Cruiser

**Free Call Apps:** *Skype, Facebook Messenger, Facetime, WhatsApp Messenger, LINE, Viber, Snapchat, Hangouts, KakaoTalk, Maaii, imo*

*Please Note: Certain phone apps are banned in Azerbaijan, Belize, China, Iran, Kuwait, Morocco, Oman, Pakistan, Paraguay and UAE. Check the restrictions of your destination.*

## Foreign Language

**Phrase books/ Language Learning:** *barnesandnoble.com, pimsleur.com, bbc.co.uk/languages, omniglot.com, linguee.com, linguanaut.com, duolingo.com, hellotalk.com, hinative.com, triplingo.com, elanlanguages.com/en*

> **Don't Ask:**
> France was okay, but why did everyone speak French?

**Online translators:** *translate.google.com, babelfish.com, collinsdictionary.com/translator, online-translator.com, worldlingo.co.uk, tradukka.com, en.pons.com*

**Translator apps:** *iTranslate, Google Translate, Trip Lingo, Say Hi, iHandy Translator, Text Grabber, Odyssey Translator, Bing, Way Go, Speak & Translate, Naver Papago, Textgrabber*

## Government Services

**Travel Advice:** *gov.uk/foreign-travel-advice, gov.uk/visit-europe-brexit, fco.gov.uk*

**Embassy Finder:** *embassyworld.com, usembassy.gov, embassy-finder.com, ivisa.com/embassies, embassy.goabroad.com*

**Passport Service:** *gov.uk/browse/abroad/passports, postoffice.co.uk/passport-check-send, itseasy.com, passportsandvisas.com/passport, gov.uk/passport-services-disabled*

**Expedited Passports:** *britishpassportsuk.co.uk/same-day-urgent-passport-application.html, gov.uk/get-a-passport-urgently*

# Directory

**Travel Health Advice & Vaccinations:** *cdc.gov, iamat.org, gov.uk/global-health-insurance-card, nhs.uk/conditions/travel-vaccinations, travelhealthpro.org.uk, cdc.gov/travel, masta-travel-health.com, istm.org, tripprep.com, who.int, https://www.fitfortravel.nhs.uk*

**Visa Service:** *travelvisapro.com, statravel.co.uk/tourist-visa.htm, trailfinders.com/visas, cic.gc.ca, passportsandvisas.com/visas, border.gov.au, esta.co.uk, cbp.dhs.gov, indianvisaonline.gov.in, evisa.gov.tr/en, evisas.online, thetravelvisacompany.co.uk, cibtvisas.co.uk, visahq.co.uk, itseasy.com*

# Cruise Line Directory

## Ocean Cruise Lines

### AIDA Cruises
Owned by Carnival Corporation
Website: aida.de (cruise.co.uk/lines/aida-cruises)
Email: *Contact form via website*
Tel: 0381 20 27 08 08

### American Cruise Lines
Privately owned
Website: americancruiselines.com
Email: *Inquiry@americancruiselines.com*
Tel: +1 203 458 5700

### Azamara Club Cruises
Owned by Royal Caribbean Cruises Ltd
Website: azamaraclubcruises.com
Email: *AzamaraGuestRelations@AzamaraClubCruises.com*
Tel: 0344 493 4016

### Bahamas Paradise Cruise Line
Owned by former executives from the defunct Celebration Cruise Line
Website: bahamasparadisecruise.com
Email: *information@cruiseBP.com*
Tel: +1 800 374 4363

# The Autonomous Cruiser

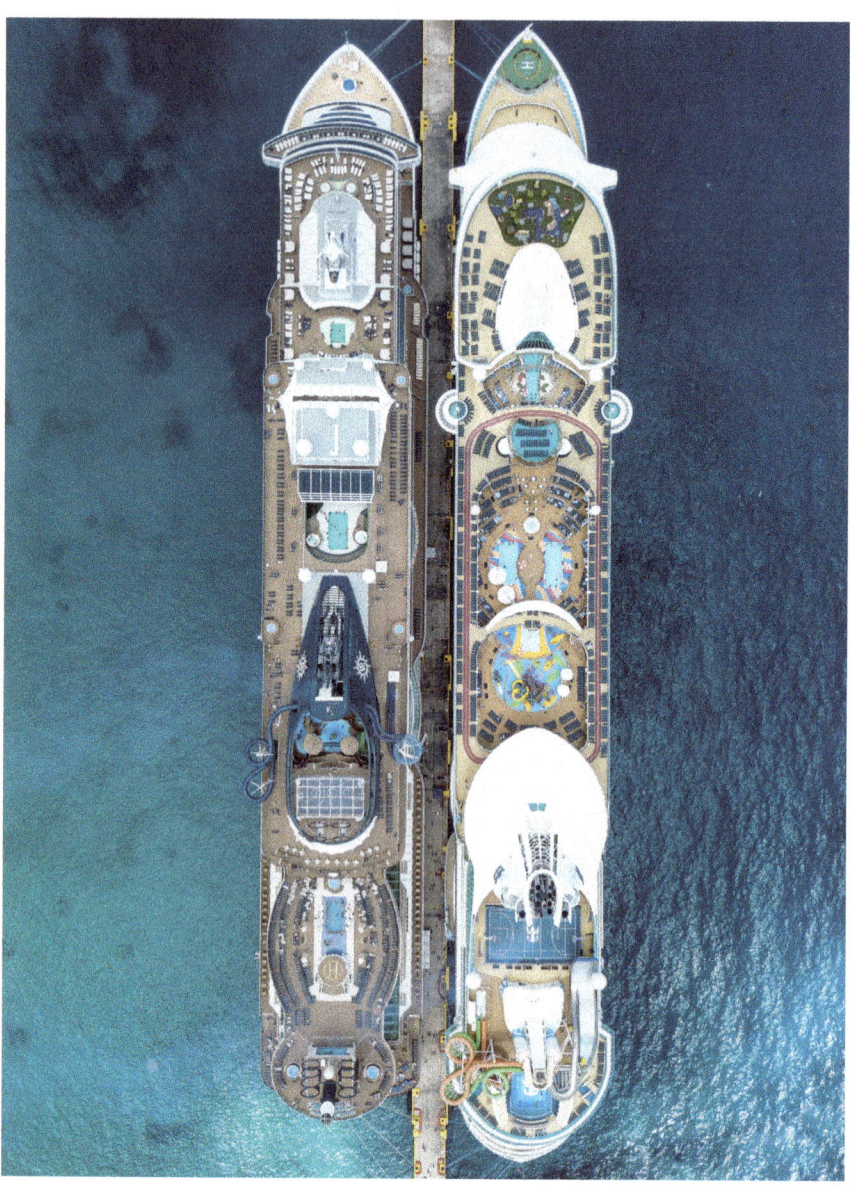

Credit: Costa Maya, Mexico RC Liberty of the seas (right), MSC Seaside (left), Costa Maya, Mexico - Brandon Nelson, Unsplash

# Directory

**Birka Cruises**
Owned by Rederiaktiebolaget Eckerö
Website: birkavikingastaden.se/en
Email: *kundsupport@birka.se*
Tel: +46 812 004 000

**Blue Lagoon Cruises**
Owned by South Sea Cruises under Fijian Holdings
Website: bluelagooncruises.com
Email: *reservations@bluelagooncruises.com*
Tel: +679 675 0500

**Captain Cook Cruises**
Owned by SeaLink Travel Group
Website: captaincook.com.au
Email: *Sydney@captaincook.com.au*
Tel : +61 893 253 341

**Carnival Cruise Line**
Owned by Carnival Corporation
Website: carnival.com
Email: *Contact form via website*
Tel: +1 800 764 7419

**Celebrity Cruises**
Owned by Royal Caribbean Cruises Ltd
Website: celebritycruises.com
Email: *customerrelationsuk@celebritycruises.com*
Tel: 01932 834 127

**Celestyal Cruises**
Owned by Louis plc
Website: celestyalcruises.uk
Email: *info@celestyalcruises.gr*
Tel: +1 877 337 4665

**Club Med Cruises**
Privately owned Chinese company
Website: clubmed.co.uk
Email: *uk@clubmed.com*
Tel: 0845 367 6767

**Costa Cruises**
Owned by Carnival Corporation
Website: costacruises.co.uk
Email: *bookings@uk.costa.it*
Tel: 0800 389 0622

# The Autonomous Cruiser

**Crystal Cruises**
Owned by Genting Hong Kong
Website: crystalcruises.com
Email: *CruiseQuestions@crystalcruises.com*
Tel: 0207 399 7601

**Cunard Line**
Owned by Carnival Corporation
Website: cunard.com
Email: *customerservices@cunard.co.uk*
Tel: 0344 338 8641

**Discover Egypt**
Owned by Platinum Holidays Ltd
Website: discoveregypt.co.uk
Email: *sales@discoveregypt.co.uk*
Tel: 0207 407 2111

**Disney Cruise Line**
Owned by Walt Disney Corporation
Website: disneycruise.disney.go.com
Email: *disneytraveluk@disneyonline.com*
Tel: +1 407 566 3500

**Dream Cruises**
Owned by Genting Hong Kong
Website: dreamcruiseline.com/en
Email: *reservations.en@gentingcruises.com*
Tel: +1 607 520 7119

**Fred. Olsen Cruise Lines**
Owned by the Fred. Olsen Group
Website: fredolsencruises.com
Email: *internet@fredolsen.co.uk*
Tel: 01473 292 200

**FTI Cruises**
Owned by FTI Group
Website: fti-cruises.com/en.html
Email: *service@fti-cruises.de*
Tel: +49 897 1045 7207

**Grand Circle Cruise Line**
Owned by Grand Circle Corporation
Website: gct.com
Email: *support@oattravel.com*
Tel: +1 800 221 2610

# Directory

**Holland America Line**
Owned by Carnival Corporation
Website: hollandamerica.com
Email: *guestrelations@hollandamerica.com*
Tel: 877 932 4259

**Majestic Cruises (aka Majestic International Cruises)**
Owned by Kollakis Group
Website: majesticcruises.gr
Email: *info@majesticcruises.gr*
Tel: +30 210 891 2600

**Mano Cruise**
Owned by Moshe Mano
Website: cruise.mano.co.il
Email: *Contact form via website*
Tel: +972 3 8288

**Marella Cruises**
Owned by TUI Group
Website: tui.co.uk/cruise
Email: *Contact form via website*
Tel: 0203 451 2682

**MSC Cruises**
Privately owned by the Aponte family
Website: msccruises.com
Email: *Contact form via website*
Tel: 0203 426 3010

**Norwegian Cruise Line**
Owned by Genting Hong Kong
Website: ncl.com
Email: *Contact form via website*
Tel: 0333 241 2319

**Oceania Cruises**
Owned by Norwegian Cruise Line Holdings Ltd
Website: oceaniacruises.com
Email: *guestrelations@oceaniacruises.com*
Tel: 0345 505 1920

**P&O Cruises**
Owned by Carnival Corporation
Website: pocruises.com
Email: *reservations@pocruises.com*
Tel: 0345 355 5111

# The Autonomous Cruiser

**P&O Cruises Australia**
Owned by Carnival Corporation
Website: pocruises.com.au
Email: *information@pocruises.com.au*
Tel: +612 9432 8500

**Paul Gauguin Cruise Line**
Owned by Norwegian Cruise Line
Website: paulgauguincruiseline.com
Email: *Contact form via website*
Tel: +1 425 440 6171

**Peace Boat Cruises**
Owned by Yoshioka Tatsuya
Website: peaceboat.org/english
Email: *pbglobal@peaceboat.gr.jp*
Tel: +81 333 638 047

**Pearl Seas Cruises**
Owned by American Cruise Lines
Website: pearlseacruises.com
Email: *Inquiry@PearlSeasCruises.com*
Tel: 0808 101 2713

**Phoenix Reisen**
Privately owned by Zurnieden family
Website: phoenixreisen.com
Email: *Contact form via website*
Tel: +49 228 92600

**Princess Cruises**
Owned by Carnival Corporation
Website: princess.com
Email: *enquiry@princesscruises.com*
Tel: 0843 374 4444

**Regent Seven Seas Cruises**
Owned by Norwegian Cruise Line Holdings Ltd
Website: rssc.com
Email: *Contact form via website*
Tel: 023 8068 2280

**Royal Caribbean International**
Owned by Royal Caribbean Cruises Ltd
Website: royalcaribbean.co.uk
Email: *Contact form via website*
Tel: 0844 493 4005

# Directory

**Saga Cruises**
Owned by Saga Group
Website: travel.saga.co.uk
Email: *reservations@saga.co.uk*
Tel: 01303 771 111

**Scenic Luxury Cruises & Tours**
Privately owned by Glen Moroney
Website: scenic.co.uk
Email: *Contact form via website*
Tel: 0161 236 2444

**Seabourn Cruise Line**
Owned by Carnival Corporation
Website: seabourn.com
Email: *Contact form via website*
Tel: 0845 070 0500

**SeaDream Yacht Club**
Privately owned by Atle Brynestad
Website: seadream.com
Email: *info@seadream.com*
Tel: +1 305 631 6100

**Silversea Cruises**
Royal Caribbean Cruises Ltd
Website: silversea.com
Email: *Contact form via website*
Tel: 0844 251 0837

**Star Cruises**
Owned by Genting Hong Kong
Website: starcruises.com
Email: *reservations.en@gentingcruises.com*
Tel: +1 852 2317 7711

**TUI Cruises**
Owned by TUI AG & Royal Caribbean Cruises Ltd
Website: tuicruises.com
Email: *info@tuicruises.com*
Tel: 0845 682 0190

**Virgin Voyages**
Owned by the Virgin Group and Bain Capital
Website: virginvoyages.com
Email: *Contact form via website*
Tel: 0203 003 4919

# The Autonomous Cruiser

**Voyages to Antiquity**
Privately owned by Gerry Herrod
Website: voyagestoantiquity.com
Email: *reservations@voyagestoantiquity.com*
Tel: 01865 302 550

**Windstar Cruises**
Owned by Xanterra Parks & Resorts Inc.
Website: windstarcruises.com
Email: *info@windstarcruises.com*
Tel: 0207 940 4488

## Expedition & Adventure Cruise Lines

For those that want something different to that of a typical cruise, expedition and adventure voyages offer journeys to the more remote areas of the world. You will be swapping the theatre productions and comedy clubs for lectures presented by geologists, naturalists, scientists and photography specialists.

**Aurora Expeditions**
Privately owned by Greg & Margaret Mortimer
Website: auroraexpeditions.com.au
Email: *Contact form via website*
Tel: +61 2 9252 1033

**Australis**
Owned by Chileans
Website: australis.com/site/en
Email: *sales@australis.com*
Tel: +1 800 743 0119

**Celebrity Xperience**
Owned by: Royal Caribbean Cruises Ltd
Website: celebritycruises.com
Email: *customerrelationsuk@celebritycruises.com*
Tel: 0844 493 2043

**Exclusive Expeditions**
Privately owned
Website: exclusiveexpeditions.co.uk
Email: *Contact form via website*
Tel: 0808 164 4210

# Directory

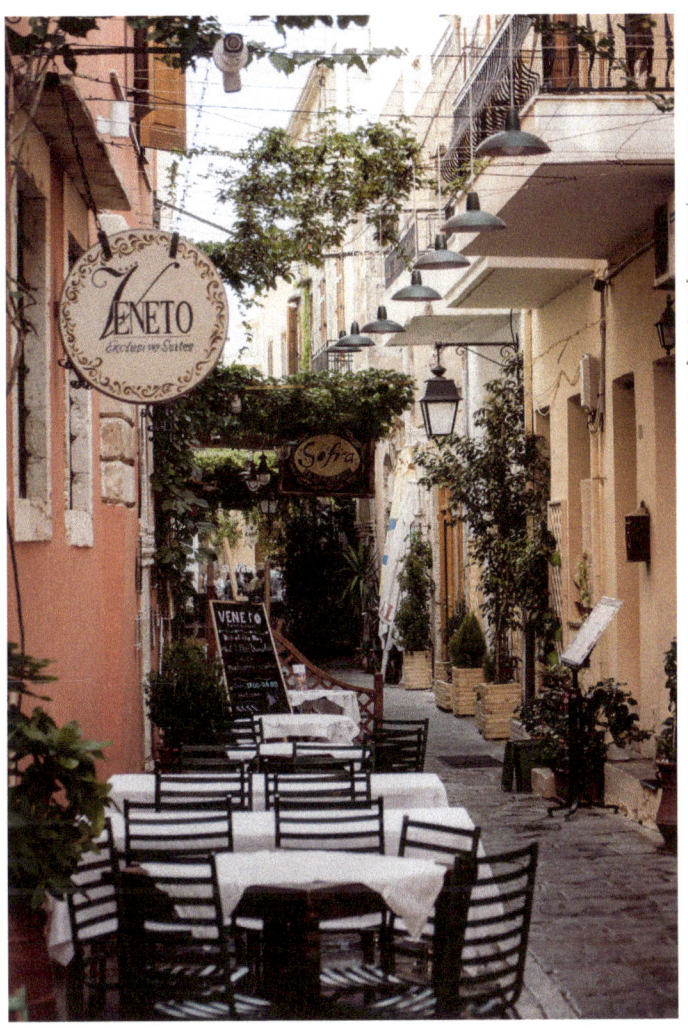

*Credit: Greece - Yuliya Kosolapova, Unsplash*

**Hansa Touristik**
Privately owned by Kilian family
Website: hansatouristik.de
Email: *info@hansatouristik.de*
Tel: +49 421 2232 5940

**Hapag-Lloyd Cruises**
Owned by TUI Group
Website: hl-cruises.com
Email: *Contact form via website*
Tel: +49 403 001 4600

# The Autonomous Cruiser

**Hebridean Cruises**
Owned by All Leisure Holidays Ltd
Website: hebridean.co.uk
Email: *enquiries@hebridean.co.uk*
Tel: 01756 704 704

**Hurtigruten**
Owned by TDR Capital
Website: hurtigruten.co.uk
Email: *uk.sales@hurtigruten.com*
Tel: 0203 603 8702

**Lindblad Expeditions**
Owned by Lindblad Expeditions
Website: expeditions.com
Email: *explore@expeditions.com*
Tel: +1 877 872 8154

**The Majestic Line**
Privately owned by Andy Thomas & Ken Grant
Website: themajesticline.co.uk
Email: *info@themajesticline.co.uk*
Tel: 01369 707 951

**National Geographic Expeditions**
Owned by Lindblad Expeditions
Website: nationalgeographicexpeditions.co.uk
Email: *Contact form via website*
Tel: 0203 105 0644

**Noble Caledonia**
Privately owned by Katarina Salén & Per Magnus Sander
Website: noble-caledonia.co.uk
Email: *info@noble-caledonia.co.uk*
Tel: 0207 752 0000

**North Pacific Expeditions**
Privately owned by Teevin family
Website: northpacificexpeditions.com
Email: *info@NorthPacificExpeditions.com*
Tel: +1 206 886 8107

**Oceanwide Expeditions**
Privately owned by Michael van Gessel
Website: oceanwide-expeditions.com
Email: *info@oceanwide-expeditions.com*
Tel: +31 118 410 410

# Directory

**Poseidon Expeditions**
Owned by Denis Vasilev Poseidon Arctic Voyages
Website: poseidonexpeditions.com
Email: *sales@poseidonexpeditions.com*
Tel: 0203 369 0020

**Ponant**
Owned by ARTEMIS Group
Website: enponant.com
Email: *Contact form via website*
Tel: +1 888 400 1082

**Quark Expeditions**
Owned by Travelopia
Website: quarkexpeditions.com
Email: *Contact form via website*
Tel: 01494 464 080

**ROL Cruise**
Privately owned by Jeremy Dickinson
Website: rolcruise.co.uk
Email: *customerservices@rolcruise.co.uk*
Tel: 0800 204 4635

**ROW Adventure (aka Unbound Travel)**
Privately owned by Peter Grubb & Betsy Bound
Website: rowadventures.com
Email: *info@rowadventures.com*
Tel: 0208 770 2517

**Sea Cloud Cruises**
Owned by Royal Caribbean Cruises Ltd
Website: seacloud.com
Email: *info@seacloud.com*
Tel: +49 403 095 9250

**Scenic Luxury Cruises & Tours**
Privately owned by Glen Moroney
Website: scenic.co.uk
Email: *Contact form via website*
Tel: 0161 236 2444

**Seabourn Cruise Line**
Owned by Carnival Corporation
Website: seabourn.com
Email: *Contact form via website*
Tel: +1 206 626 9179

**Silversea Cruises**
Royal Caribbean Cruises Ltd
Website: silversea.com
Email: *Contact form via website*
Tel: +44 844 251 0837

**St Hilda Sea Adventures**
Privately owned
Website: sthildaseaadventures.co.uk
Email: *info@sthildaseaadventures.co.uk*
Tel: 07745 550 988

**Star Clippers**
Owned by Star Clippers Ltd
Website: starclippers.com
Email: *info@starclippers.com*
Tel: 0845 200 6145

**Swoop Arctic**
Owned by Luke Errington
Website: swoop-arctic.com
Email: *polaradvice@swooptravel.co.uk*
Tel: 0117 369 0296

**True North**
Owned by Mark Stothard & Craig Howson
Website: truenorth.com.au
Email: *Contact form via website*
Tel: +61 891 921 829

**UnCruise Adventures**
Owned by Inner Sea Discoveries Alaska Inc
Website: uncruise.com
Email: *sales@uncruise.com*
Tel: 800 100 08 003

**Viking Ocean Cruises**
Privately owned by investors
Website: vikingcruises.co.uk
Email: *Contact form via website*
Tel: 0800 458 6900

# Directory

## River Cruises

River cruises travel along inland waterways and since a lot of places grew up around the major rivers in the world, you are able to dock in the heart of the city. With no tidal movement, seasickness or long days at sea a lot of travellers opt for this sort of tranquil cruise.

**A-Rosa (Germany)**
Privately owned
Website: arosa-cruises.com
Email: *Contact form via website*
Tel: +49 381 440 400

**1AVista (Germany)**
Privately owned
Website: 1avista.de
Email: *info@1avista.de*
Tel: 0221 99 800 800

**AmaWaterways (USA)**
Owned by Rudi Schreiner & Kristen Karst
Website: amawaterways.co.uk
Email: *info@amawaterways.com*
Tel: 0333 305 3909

**American Cruise Lines (USA)**
Owned by Charles A Robertson
Website: americancruiselines.com
Email: *inquiry@americancruiselines.com*
Tel: +1 800 460 4518

**American Queen Steamboat Company (USA)**
Owned by Hornblower Marine Services
Website: aqsc.com
Email: *info@aqsc.com*
Tel: +1 888 749 5280

**Aqua Expeditions (Peru)**
Owned by Francesco Galli Zugaro
Website: aquaexpeditions.com
Email: *Contact form via website*
Tel: +65 6270 4002

# The Autonomous Cruiser

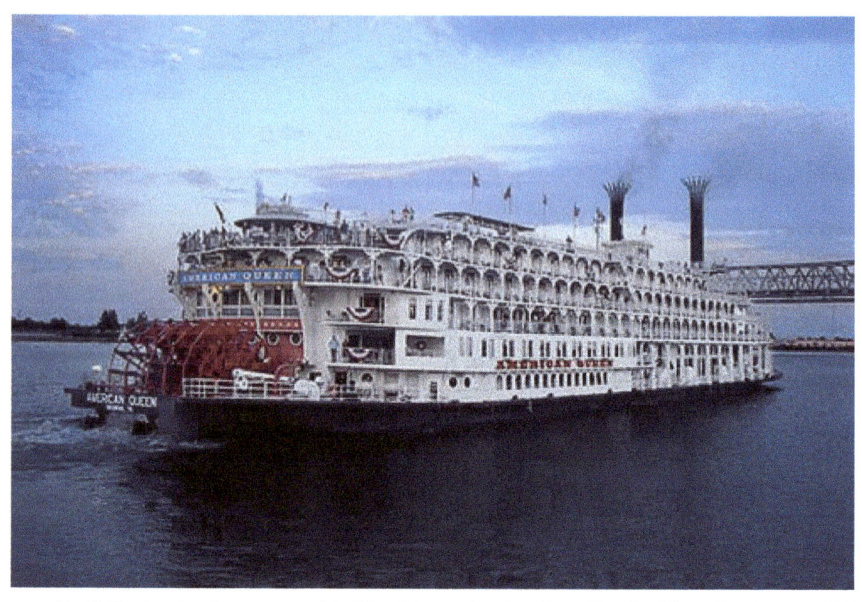

*Credit: The American Queen approaching New Orleans - American Queen Steamboat Operating Company, LLC*

**Australian Pacific Touring (Australia)**
Owned by Geoff McGeary
Website: aptouring.co.uk
Email: *info@aptouring.co.uk*
Tel: 0800 012 6683

**Avalon Waterways (USA)**
Owned by Group Voyagers, Inc (aka 'Globus family of brands')
Website: avalonwaterways.com
Email: *enquiries@globusfamily.com.au*
Tel: 0330 058 8243

**CroisiEurope (French)**
Owned by the Croisières family
Website: croisieurope.co.uk
Email: *Contact form via website*
Tel: +32 2 514 1154

**CrystalCruises (Japan)**
Owned by Genting Hong Kong
Website: crystalcruises.co.uk
Email: *askcrystal@crystalcruises.com*
Tel: 0207 399 7601

# Directory

**DouroAzul (Portugal)**
Owned by Mário Ferreira
Website: douroazul.com
Email: *reservas@douroazul.pt*
Tel: +351 223 402 500

**Emerald Waterways (USA)**
Owned by Glen Moroney
Website: emeraldwaterways.co.uk
Email: *Contact form via website*
Tel: 0808 159 4193

**European Waterways (UK)**
Privately owned
Website: europeanwaterways.com
Email: *sales@europeanwaterways.com*
Tel: 01753 598 555

**Fred. Olsen (UK)**
Owned by Bonheur and Ganger Rolf
Website: fredolsencruises.com
Email: *guest.services@fredolsen.co.uk*
Tel: 01473 292 200

**Grand Circle Cruise Line (USA)**
Owned by Alan & Harriet Lewis
Website: gct.com
Email: *support@oattravel.com*
Tel: +1 800 221 2610

**Great Lakes Cruise Company (USA)**
Privately owned by the Conlin family
Website: greatlakescruising.com
Email: *info@greatlakescruising.com*
Tel: +1 888 891 0203

**Hansa Touristik (Germany)**
Privately owned by the Kilian family
Website: hansatouristik.de
Email: *info@hansatouristik.de*
Tel: 0711 22 931 690

**Lüftner Cruises (Austria)**
Privately owned by Lüftner family
Website: lueftner-cruises.com
Email: *lueftner@lueftner-cruises.com*
Tel: +43 512 365 781

# The Autonomous Cruiser

**Mosturflot Cruise Company (Russia)**
Owned by the Moscow River Shipping Company
Website: mosturflot.com
Email: *info@mosturflot.com*
Tel: +7 495 221 8070

**Nicko Cruises (Germany)**
Owned by Mystic Invest
Website: nicko-cruises.co.uk
Email: *info@nicko-cruises.de*
Tel: 01223 568 904

**Pandaw River Expeditions**
Privately owned
Website: pandaw.com
Email: *information@pandaw.com*
Tel: 0208 396 7320

**Phoenix Reisen (Germany)**
Privately owned the Zurnieden family
Website: phoenixreisen.com
Email: *contact form via website*
Tel: +49 228 92 600

**Reisebüro Mittelthurgau (Switzerland)**
Owned by the Twerenbold Group
Website: mittelthurgau.ch
Email: *info@mittelthurgau.ch*
Tel: +41 71 626 8585

**Riviera River Cruises (UK)**
Owned by Phoenix Equity Partners & Silverfleet Capital
Website: rivierarivercruises.com
Email: *info@rivieratravel.co.uk*
Tel: 01283 742 317

**Saga (UK)**
Owned by the Saga Group
Website: saga.co.uk
Email: *reservations@saga.co.uk*
Tel: 0800 096 0082

**Scenic (Australia)**
Owned by Transit Scenic Tours
Website: scenic.co.uk
Email: *Contact form via website*
Tel: 0161 236 2444

# Directory

**Tauck River Cruises (USA)**
Privately owned by the Tauck family
Website: tauck.co.uk
Email: *tauckreservations@tauck.co.uk*
Tel: 0800 810 8020

**TUI River Cruises**
Owned by TUI AG & Royal Caribbean Cruises Ltd
Website: *tui.co.uk/river-cruises*
Email: *Contact form via website*
Tel: 0800 975 4477

**Uniworld River Cruises (USA)**
Owned by The Travel Corporation Group
Website: uniworld.com
Email: *enquiries@uniworld.com*
Tel: 0808 168 9110

**Viking River Cruises (USA)**
Privately owned
Website: vikingrivercruises.co.uk
Email: *Contact form via website*
Tel: 0800 319 6660

**Vodohod Russian River Cruises (Russia)**
Owned by UCL Holding
Website: russiancruisecompany.com
Email: *office@russiancruisecompany.com*
Tel: +1 888 960 0365

## Cargo, Container & Freighter Ship Voyages

While container ship travel might not be for everyone, it does offer up a new type of adventure which is a little off the beaten track. Listed is a comprehensive list of companies to help you decide whether this type of cruising is for you.

**Aranui**
Owned by Compagnie Polynésienne de Transport Maritime (aka C.P.T.M)
Website: aranui.com
Email: *reservations@aranui.com*
Tel: +1 800 972 7268

**CMA CGM Freighter Cruises**
Owned by Jacques Saadé
Website: cma-cgm.com
Email: *contact@partirencargo.com*

## The Autonomous Cruiser

Tel: +33 488 919 000

**Cargo Ship Voyages**
Owned by Seabreaks Ltd
Website: cargoshipvoyages.com
Email: *info@cargoshipvoyages.com*
Tel: 01983 303 314

**The Cruise People**
Owned by Kevin Griffin
Website: cruisepeople.co.uk
Email: *passageenquiry@aol.com*
Tel: 0207 723 2450

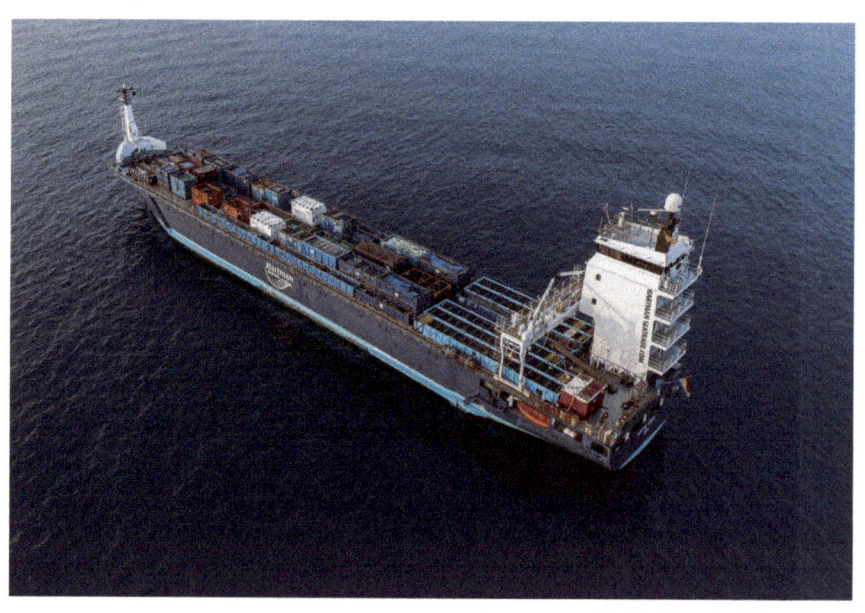

*Credit: Alexander Bobrov, Pexels*

**Freighter Expeditions**
Owned by the Concierge Travel Group
Website: freighterexpeditions.com.au
Email: *enquiries@conciergetraveller.com.au*
Tel: +61 2 8270 4899

**Freighter Travel, New Zealand**
Owned by Hawkes Bay Travel Centre
Website: freightertravel.co.nz
Email: *hamish@freightertravel.co.nz*
Tel: +64 6 843 7702

# Directory

**Grimaldi Lines Freighter Travel**
Owned by the Grimaldi Group
Website: grimaldi-freightercruises.com/en
Email: *gfc@grimaldi.napoli.it*
Tel: +39 081 496 444

**Maris Freighter Cruises.com**
Owned by Maris USA Ltd
Website: freightercruises.com
Email: *Contact form via website*
Tel: +1 800 99 62747

**Mundy Adventures**
Owned by Edwina Barbara Lonsdale & Matthew Philip Lonsdale
Website: mundyadventures.co.uk/cruises
Email: *Contact form via website*
Tel: 0207 399 7630

**NSB Freighter Cruises**
Owned by REEDEREI NSB
Bookings through partners Hamburg Sued Travel
Website: hamburgsued-frachtschiffreisen.de
Email: *frachtschiff@hamburgsued-reiseagentur.de*
Tel: +49 403 705 157

**Patricia UK Voyages (incorporating Strand Voyages)**
Owned by General Lighthouse Authority (GLA)
Website: wildwings.co.uk
Email: *thvpatricia@wildwings.co.uk*
Tel: 0117 9658 333

**PZM Polish Steamship Company, Szczecin**
Owned by Polsteam
Website: cruisepeople.co.uk/pzm.htm
Email: *passageenquiry@aol.com*
Tel: 0207 723 2450

**Rickmers – Line Freighter Travel**
Owned by Rickmers Group
Website: cruisepeople.co.uk/rickmers.htm
Email: *passageenquiry@aol.com*
Tel: 0207 723 2450

### Sea Travel Ltd
Owned by Sea Travel Ltd
Website: seatravelltd.com
Email: *mail@seatravelltd.co.uk*
Tel: 0203 371 9484

### Slow Travel Experience
Privately owned by Arne Gudde
Website: langsamreisen.de/en
Email: *mail@slowtravel-experience.com*
Tel: +49 30 609 863 930

## Cruise Lingo Glossary

Cruise virgins can get confused by the ship's lingo, most of which is never heard on land, so to get you started here are some of the most common nautical terms you might come across whilst onboard.

### A
**adrift:** floating at random
**aft:** rear of ship
**aground:** lying on or touching the ground under shallow water
**amidship:** in the middle of a ship
**anchor:** a device used to moor a ship to the bottom of a sea
**astern:** at the back or behind the stern
**atrium:** central passenger area, usually referring to the lobby or foyer
**atoll:** ring-shaped reef or island
**autopilot:** mechanical, electrical or hydraulic self-steering device
**aweigh:** anchor hanging clear of the bottom of the ocean bed

### B
**bail:** to remove water from a boat
**ballast:** weight in the keel to provide stability to the ship
**batten down:** to close or make watertight and prepare for heavy weather
**beam:** width of a ship at its widest point
**bearing:** direction a ship is heading relative to North, measured clockwise
**berth:** cabin bed or space where a ship is docked
**bow:** forward part of a ship
**bridge:** command centre where the ship is steered from
**bulkhead:** a vertical partition dividing the hull into compartments
**bunkers:** fuel storage area
**buoy:** a navigational floating aid to mark a location

## C

**calm:** absence of storms, high winds or rough activity of water
**capsize:** to overturn in the water
**cast off:** to let go of a cable/rope securing ship to a quay
**cay:** (pronounced key) small sandy island on the surface of a coral reef
**cenote:** natural groundwater swimming holes
**centrum:** another name for atrium used on some American ships
**channel:** a navigable waterway often marked with navigational aids
**chart:** a nautical map
**circumnavigate:** to travel around something
**course:** the direction the ship is heading
**crow's nest:** viewing platform or lookout post
**cruise card:** plastic, credit card sized ID issued on embarkation
**cruise director:** a member of the ship's personnel responsible for onboard entertainment and guest activities
**current:** horizontal movement of water caused by tides or wind

## D

**debarkation:** the process of disembarking guests from the ship
**deck plan:** map of the ship
**disembark:** to get off the ship
**distress signal:** a sign that a ship is in danger and a request for help
**dock:** a float or pier to which the ship can be tied
**downwind:** in the same direction as the wind is blowing
**draft:** depth below the waterline to the bottom of a ship's hull
**dry dock:** when a ship is taken out of water to be serviced or upgraded

## E

**ebb:** receding movement of the tide
**embark:** to board a ship
**embarkation:** the process for checking in passengers prior to sailing from the homeport
**enrichment program:** onboard activities, events, talks and seminars designed to enhance a passenger's cruise experience
**even keel:** the ship is floating in a level and smooth manner

## F

**fathom:** a unit of nautical depth equal to six feet
**forward:** towards the front of the ship
**funnel:** ship's smoke flue

## G

**galley:** the cook room or kitchen of a ship
**gangway:** a ramp between a ship and the land
**gross registered tonnage:** how big and heavy a ship is

## H

**hatch:** an operable opening in a ship's deck
**heading:** direction is which ship's bow is pointing
**helm:** steering mechanism of a ship, typically a tiller or a wheel
**helmsman:** crew member responsible for steering
**hold:** storage area below deck
**hull:** body or frame of a ship

## I

**Inaugural cruise:** (also maiden) a cruise ship's first journey with paying passengers
**inboard:** within a ship
**international dateline:** an imaginary line running down the Pacific Ocean that separates one day from another

## K

**keel:** an extension of the hull that extends below the water
**knot:** unit of speed equal to one nautical mile per hour

## L

**landmark:** a recognizable feature used for navigation
**latitude:** angular distance north or south of the earth's equator
**league:** distance measurement of three nautical miles
**leave:** permission to be absent or time away from work
**lee:** (also leeward) the side of the ship away from the wind
**lido:** deck with outdoor swimming pool
**list:** tilt or careen to one side
**longitude:** angular distance east or west of the Greenwich meridian
**loyalty programme:** reward scheme for repeat passengers

## M

**manifest:** a list of the passenger, crew, and cargo being carried by a ship
**man overboard:** a cry of help announcing a person has fallen over the side of a ship
**mast:** a tall, slim pole or post used to support the sails or flags on a ship
**meridian:** a line of constant longitude
**midship:** pertaining to the halfway point of a ship
**mooring:** holding a ship in place with lines at a berth
**muster station:** the place for passengers to assemble in the event of an emergency

## N

**nautical mile:** one minute of latitude, about 1.15 statute miles or 6000 feet
**neap tide:** tides that occur during the first and third quarter phases of the moon
**norovirus:** a common form of gastroenteritis causing vomiting and diarrhoea

## O

**offshore:** located in the sea away from the coast
**onboard credit:** added spending money applied to your onboard bill
**open seating:** dinner service with no fixed time where tables are not assigned

# Directory

## P
**parallel:** a line of constant latitude
**passenger-crew ratio:** the number of crew available to serve each guest
**pier:** a raised platform suspended by posts built from the shore out over water
**pilot:** local navigational expert for the port of call
**pitch:** (also pitching) to dip the bow and stern alternately
**plot:** to draw a ship's course on a nautical chart
**pontoon:** a floating structure that serves as a dock used when tendering
**port**: (also portside) left side of a ship when facing the bow
**porthole:** small circular window set into the hull of a ship
**prow:** the forward part of a ship's hull
**pullman bed:** a foldaway bed that pulls down from the bulkhead (wall) or the deckhead (ceiling) during the daytime
**purser:** (also bursar) finance officer of a ship

## Q
**quay:** (pronounced key) stone or metal structure alongside or projecting into water used for loading and unloading ships

## R
**radar:** a system for detecting objects in the distance by sending out radio waves that are reflected off the object and back to the source
**repositioning cruise:** a one-way itinerary that brings a ship from one region to another when a cruise season ends and another begins
**rig:** (also rigging) a series of cables, chains, and lines
**roll:** (also rolling) side-to-side movement of the ship
**rudder:** an underwater appendage that controls the direction of a ship

## S
**satellite navigator:** the global positioning system (GPS)§
**seaworthy:** in fit condition to sail on the sea
**secure:** to fasten to a dock or cleat
**ship's log:** an official book that records the daily events
**shoulder season:** period of travel between high and low season
**skiff:** (also Zodiac) a small, flat-bottomed open boat used for shore or shoreline excursions
**slip:** a berth or space for a ship to moor
**stabilisers:** wing like retractable fins that extend from the side of a ship to reduce excess rolling in rough seas
**starboard:** right side of a ship when facing the bow
**steer:** to guide the course of a ship by means of a rudder, or steering wheel
**stern:** the rear or back of a ship
**stowaway:** a person who conceals themselves on a ship to avoid paying the fare
**swell:** wind-generated rolling waves

**T**
**tender:** a small boat used to ferry people from the ship to the shore, often used when the harbour isn't deep enough for the ship to dock
**tendered:** ship anchored in open water
**tide:** cyclic rise and fall of sea level caused by the gravitational pull of the sun and the moon
**transfer:** typically refers to transportation from an airport or hotel to and from the ship
**turnaround day:** the day the ship returns to home port, disembarks passengers from the previous cruise and then embarks a new set for the next cruise

**U**
**underway:** a journey in progress
**upper berth:** fixed bunk on a ship above another bed
**upwind:** against the direction of the wind

**V**
**veer:** a sudden change of direction
**virtual balcony:** floor to ceiling display screen that transforms an inside cabin to one that looks like it has a vista of the outside

**W**
**wake:** path left behind a ship on the surface of the water
**watch:** period of time on duty when the crew guard the safe operation of a ship
**waterline:** where the water's surface meets the hull
**weigh anchor:** to raise the anchor when ready to start sailing
**winch:** a mechanical device to increase the tension in a line or cable
**windward:** towards the wind

**Z**
**Zodiac:** (also skiff) inflatable boats used by expedition ships for shore or shoreline excursion

# Ship's Codes

Although each cruise line uses its own set of codes, the majority of vessels, especially passenger ships, use universal emergency signals to alert the crew on board of certain situations. Signals can be in the form of blasts on alarm bells, sounds on the ship's whistle or code names paged over the PA system.

**Alpha Team, Alpha Team, Alpha Team:** fire emergency
**Alpha, Alpha, Alpha:** medical emergency
**Bravo, Bravo, Bravo**: a fire or other serious incident onboard

# Directory

**Charlie, Charlie, Charlie:** security threat or upcoming helicopter winch operation
**Code Blue:** usually means a medical emergency
**Code Red:** an outbreak of an infectious illness usually resulting in passenger(s) being confined to their cabin
**Code Green:** early stages of an outbreak of illness and alerts crew that standard cleaning operating procedures should follow. This means cleaning cabins twice a day, wiping down handrails, etc
**Code Yellow:** requires more enhanced cleaning of high-touch areas such as elevator buttons, handles, railings, restrooms, phones, computer keyboards, etc
**Delta, Delta, Delta:** indicates the ship has sustained damage or a possible biohazard
**Echo, Echo, Echo:** possible collision with another ship or the shore. On some ships it means danger of high winds while in port. It alerts the crew responsible for the gangway, thrusters etc to get into position and be ready for new manoeuvres
**Kilo, Kilo, Kilo:** a general signal for the crew to report to emergency stations
**Mr Skylight:** minor emergency
**Mayday:** distress signal over marine radio indicating there is imminent danger to life or to the vessel itself
**Oscar, Oscar, Oscar/Mr Mob:** 'man overboard'. Can also be signalled with three prolonged blasts on the ship's whistle and general alarm bell (Morse code for Oscar)
**Papa, Papa, Papa**: pollution problem or oil spill
**Pan-Pan:** distress signal over marine radio indicating there is an urgent situation but there is no imminent danger to anyone's life or the vessel
**Priority 1:** the possibility of fire
**Priority 2:** there is a leak on the ship
**Purell, Purell, Purell:** cleanup (vomit) followed by a location
**PVI:** public vomiting incident
**Red Parties, Red Parties, Red Parties**: fire or possible fire on board the ship. The message is immediately followed by information about where the fire is
**Operation Brightstar**: serious injury or medical emergency that needs immediate attention
**Operation Rising Star:** someone has died onboard
**Sierra:** stretcher is needed
**Star Code, Star Code, Star Code:** medical emergency
**Zulu, Zulu, Zulu:** fight onboard

Seven or more short blasts on the ship's whistle followed by one long blast is the signal to gather at your muster stations.

Continuous ringing of the general alarm bell for ten seconds and a continuous sounding of the ship's whistle for ten seconds signals fire and emergency.

# The Autonomous Cruiser

## Tender Ports

The list below is correct at the time of writing and is meant only as a guide as the need for a tender depends on the size of ship, docking priority allocated to a specific cruise line, port traffic, and certain weather, sea, swell, current and tidal conditions.

Newer piers and docking facilities are being built on a daily basis, so what was once a tender port might now offer a quayside berth. Newer, unexplored destinations are also being added to itineraries in an attempt to entice new bookings, so as always it is best to check with the cruise company before booking.

\* tender might be operational if there is an overload of ships docking on the same day or a cruise ship is too large to dock.

**Antarctica and South Atlantic**
Grytviken, South Georgia and the South Sandwich Islands
Inaccessible Island, St Helena
Nightingale Island, St Helena
Port Stanley, Falkland Islands

**Asia**
Benoa (Denpasar), Bali, Indonesia
Boracay, Philippines
Celukan Bawang, Bali, Indonesia
Galle, Sri Lanka
George Town, Penang, Malaysia *
Halong Bay, Hanoi, Vietnam
Hundred Islands, Philippines
Ishigaki, Japan
Jayapura, Indonesia
Jeju, South Korea
Ko Kood, Thailand
Komodo Island, Indonesia
Ko Samui, Thailand
Lembar, Lombok, Indonesia
Malacca, Malaysia
Male, Maldives
Miyakojima (Hirara), Japan
Nha Trang, Vietnam
Padang Bay, Bali, Indonesia
Phuket, Thailand *
Porto Malai, Langkawi, Malaysia

> **Don't Ask:**
> What a lovely beach, why didn't you tell me we would be so near the sea!

# Directory

Probolinggo, Java, Indonesia
Sabang, Pulau Weh, Indonesia
Senggigi, Indonesia
Sihanoukville, Cambodia *
Similan Islands, Thailand
Surabaya, Java, Indonesia
Trincomalee, Sri Lanka
Uligamu, Maldives

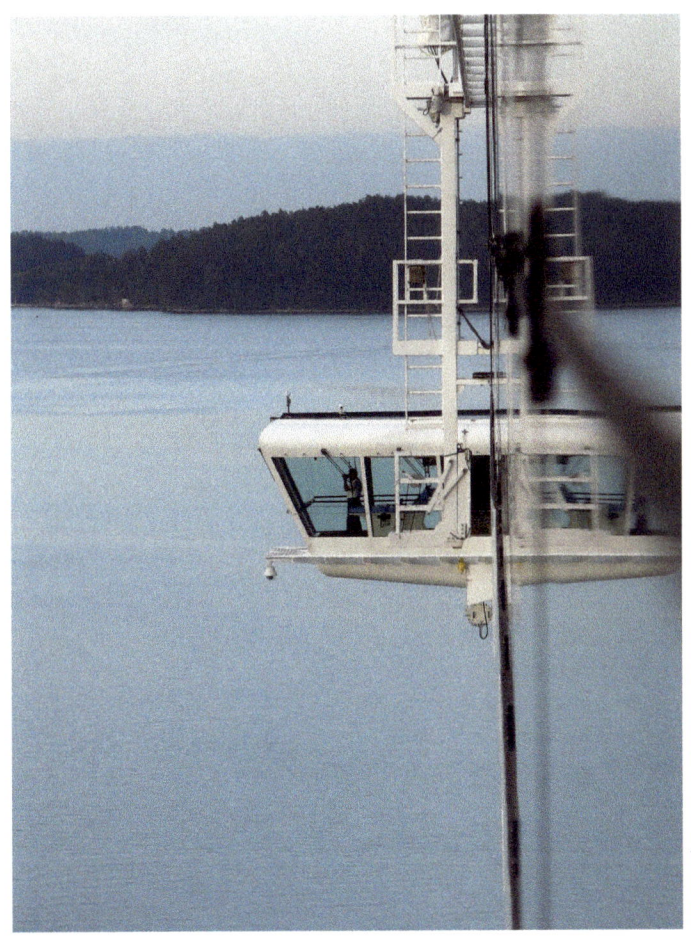

*Credit: View from the Bridge*

**Australasia, New Zealand, and South Pacific**
Airlie Beach, Queensland, Australia
Akaroa (Christchurch), New Zealand
Alofi, Niue Island
Alotau, Papua New Guinea

# The Autonomous Cruiser

Avatoru, Rangiroa, French Polynesia
Bahia de' Opunohu, Moorea, French, Polynesia
Bay of Islands, New Zealand
Bora Bora, French Polynesia
Cascade, Norfolk Island
Champagne Bay, Espiritu Santo, Vanuatu
Christmas Island (Kiritimati Island), Kiribati, Australia
Conflict Island, Papua New Guinea
Dravuni Island, Fiji
Eden, New South Wales, Australia
Esperance, Western Australia, Australia
Exmouth, Western Australia, Australia
Fakarava, Tuamotu, French Polynesia
Fanning Island (Tabuaeran Island), Kiribati, Australia
Geelong, Victoria, Australia
Ghizo Island, Solomon Islands
Gisborne, New Zealand
Gladstone, Queensland, Australia
Hamilton Island, Queensland, Australia
Hapatoni, Marquesas Islands, French Polynesia
Hiva Oa, Marquesa Islands, French Polynesia
Huahine, French Polynesia
Kaikoura, New Zealand
Kingston, Norfolk Island, Australia
Kiriwina, Trobriand Islands, Papua New Guinea
Kitava Island, Trobriand Islands, Papua New Guinea
Kuri Bay, Western Australia, Australia
Kuto Bay, Île des Pins (Isle of Pines), New Caledonia
Lifou, Loyalty Island, New Caledonia
Luganville, Espiritu Santo, Vanuatu
Mare, New Caledonia
Mooloolaba, Queensland, Australia
Moreton Island, Queensland, Australia
Mystery Island (Inyeug Islet), Vanuatu
Nuku'alofa, Tonga
Nuku Hiva, (Taiohae), French Polynesia
Oban (Halfmoon Bay), New Zealand
Ouvea (Wadrilla), Loyalty Island, New Caledonia
Penneshaw, Kangaroo Island, Australia
Phillip Island, Victoria, Australia
Port Arthur, Tasmania, Australia
Port Denarau, Denarau Island, Fiji
Port Douglas, Queensland, Australia

# Directory

Port Vila, Vanuatu
Rabaul, Papua New Guinea *
Rangiroa, Tuamotus, French Polynesia
Rarotonga, Cook Islands, New Zealand
Russell (Bay of Islands), New Zealand
Savusavu, Vanua Levi, Fiji
Tabuaeran (Fanning Island), Kiribati
Tadine, Mare, New Caledonia
Tahuata, Marquesa Islands, French Polynesia
Timaru, New Zealand
Townsville, Queensland, Australia
Vava'u, Tonga
Waitangi (Bay of Islands), New Zealand
Wala, Vanuatu
Whitsunday Islands, Queensland, Australia
Yorkeys Knob (Cairns), Queensland, Australia

**Canada**
Alert Bay, British Columbia
Baie-Comeau, Quebec
Cap-aux-Meules, îles de la Madeleine, Quebec
Charlottetown, Prince Edward Island *
Corner Brook, Newfoundland
Gaspésie, Quebec
Klemtu, British Columbia
Nanaimo, British Columbia
Red Bay, Newfoundland and Labrador
Saguenay, Quebec *
Saint Antony, Newfoundland and Labrador
Sydney, Nova Scotia *

**USA**
Astoria, Oregon *
Bar Harbor, Maine
Catalina Island, California
Gloucester, Massachusetts
Icy Strait Point, Alaska *
Juneau, Alaska *
Kailua Kona, Hawaii
Ketchikan, Alaska *
Key West, Florida *
Kona, Hawaii Island, Hawaii
Lahaina, Maui, Hawaii
Monterey, California

# The Autonomous Cruiser

Newport, Rhode Island
Nome, Alaska
Oak Bluffs, Massachusetts
Rockland, Maine
Salem, Massachusetts
Santa Barbara, California
Santa Catalina Island, California
Sitka, Alaska *

**North Atlantic**
Saint Pierre et Miquelon, France (French archipelago off the North American continent)

**Caribbean**
Basseterre, St Kitts *
Cap Cana (Punta Cana), Dominican Republic
Charlestown, Nevis *
Charlotteville, Tobago *
Cienfuegos, Cuba*
Cruz Bay, St. John, US Virgin Islands
Deshaies, Guadeloupe
George Town, Grand Cayman, Cayman Islands *
Great Harbour, Jost van Dyke, British Virgin Islands
Great Stirrup Cay, Bahamas
Gustavia, Saint Barthelemy (St Barts)
Half Moon Cay, Bahamas
Iles du Salut (Devil's Island), French Guiana
Isabel Segunda, Vieques, Puerto Rico
Isla Catalina, Dominican Republic
Ocho Rios, Jamaica *
Port Elizabeth, Bequia, Saint Vincent and the Grenadines
Princess Cays, Bahamas
Punta Cana, Dominican Republic
Road Bay, Anguilla
Road Town, Tortola, British Virgin Islands *
Rodney Bay, Saint Lucia
Roseau, Dominica *
Saint Georges, Grenada*
Saint John, US Virgin Islands
Saint Thomas, US Virgin Islands*
Saline Bay, Mayreau, Saint Vincent and the Grenadines
Samana, Dominican Republic
Santa Catalina, Dominican Republic
Spanish Town, Virgin Gorda, British Virgin Islands

Terre-de-Haut, Îles des Saintes, Guadeloupe
Tortola, British Virgin Islands *
Trois Ilets, Martinique

**Europe, Africa, and Middle East**
Ajaccio, Corsica, France *
Alghero, Sardinia
Amalfi, Campania, Italy
Antibes (Cannes), France
Bandol, France
Bantry, Republic of Ireland
Bonifacio, Corsica, France
Calvi, Corsica, France
Cannes, Monte Carlo, France
Cavalaire-Sur-Mer, France
Ciutadella de Menorca, Spain
Cork (Cobh), Ireland *
Dartmouth, United Kingdom
Dubrovnik, Croatia *
Dunmore East (Waterford), Ireland
Edinburgh, Scotland, United Kingdom *
Elba, Italy
Falmouth, United Kingdom*
Fishguard, Wales, United Kingdom
Fort William, Scotland, United Kingdom
Fréjus, France
Glengarriff, Ireland
Golfo Aranci (Costa Smeralda), Italy
Guernsey, Channel Islands, United Kingdom
Helsingborg, Sweden
Holy Loch, Scotland, United Kingdom
Horta, Azores, Portugal
Hvar, Croatia
Ile-Rousse, France
Ilfracombe, United Kingdom
Inverness (Invergordon), Scotland, United Kingdom
Korčula, Croatia
Korsakov, (Sakhalin Island), Russia
Kotor, Montenegro *
Le Lavandou, France
Le Palais, France
Lerwick, Shetland Islands *
L'Île-Rousse, Corsica, France
Mgarr, Gozo, Malta

# The Autonomous Cruiser

Monte Carlo, Monaco *
Mossel Bay, South Africa *
Naples, Italy *
Nice, France
Nosy Be, Madagascar
Nynäshamn, Sweden*
Oban, Scotland, United Kingdom
Peñíscola, Spain
Petropavlovsk, Russia
Plymouth, United Kingdom*
Ponza, Italy
Portimao, Portugal
Port Mahón, Menorca, Spain
Portoferraio, Elba, Italy
Portofino, Liguria, Italy
Porto Santo Island, Portugal
Portovenere (Cinque Terre), Italy
Portree, Isle of Skye, Scotland, United Kingdom
Primosten, Croatia
Propriano, Corsica *
Pula, Croatia *
Rapallo, Italy
Rejika, Croatia
Rosas (Roses), Spain
Saint Helier, Jersey*
Saint Malo, France
Saint Mary's (Tresco), Isles of Scilly, United Kingdom
Saint Peter Port, Guernsey, Channel Islands
Saint Tropez, France
San Antonio (Ibiza), Spain
Sanary-sur-Mer, France
San Remo, Liguria, Italy
San Sebastián de la Gomera, Canary Islands, Spain
Santa Margherita Ligure (Portofino), Italy
Saranda, Albania *
Sète (Montpellier), France
Sibenik, Croatia
Sir Bani Yas Island, United Arab Emirates
South Queensferry, Edinburgh, Scotland, United Kingdom
Split, Croatia *
Stockholm, Sweden *
Stornoway, Isle of Lewis, Outer Hebrides, Scotland, United Kingdom
Suez (Suez Canal), Egypt

Summer Isles, Scotland
Syracuse, Italy
Taormina, Italy
Tobermory, Isle of Mull, Scotland
Tôlanaro (Taolagnaro), Madagascar
Ullapool, Scotland
Villefranche (Nice), France
Visby, Sweden
Walvis Bay, Namibia
Xlendi (Victoria), Gozo, Malta
Yalta, Ukraine

**Greece/ Turkey**
Agios Nikólaos, Crete, Greece
Antalya, Turkey * (new cruise port due for completion 2023)
Argostoli, Kefalonia (Cephalonia), Greece *
Bozcaada, Bozcaada (Tenedos), Turkey
Delos, Greece
Gythion (Sparta & Mystras), Greece
Hydra, Nisos Hydra, Greece
Istanbul, Turkey *
Katakolon (Olympia), Greece
Kérkira, Nisos Kérkira (Corfu), Greece
Kos, Nisos Kos, Greece
Marmaris, Turkey
Megisti (Kastellorizo), Greece
Milos, Greece
Monemvasia, Greece
Mykonos, Greece
Myrina, Nisos Limnos, Greece
Náfplion, Greece
Naxos, Greece
Nydri, Greece
Pátmos, Greece
Santorini (Thira), Greece
Spétsai, Nisos Spétsai (Spetses), Greece
Syvota, Greece
Zakynthos, Greece

**Greenland, Iceland, Norway**
Åndalsnes, Norway
Bergen, Norway *
Djúpivogur, Iceland
Flam, Norway *

# The Autonomous Cruiser

Geiranger, Norway *
Grundarfjördur, Iceland *
Heimaey, West Men Islands, Iceland*
Hellesylt, Norway
Honningsvåg, Norway*
Ísafjördur, Iceland
Kangerlussuaq, Greenland
Leknes, Lofoten Islands, Norway
Nanortalik, Greenland
Narsarsuaq, Greenland
Ny Ålesund, Norway
Olden, Nordfjord, Norway *
Paamiut (formerly Frederikshåb), Greenland
Pyramiden, Spitsbergen, Svalbard
Qaqortoq (Julianehåb), Greenland
Storstappen Island, Norway
Tasiilaq, Greenland
Vigur, Iceland

**South and Central America**
Abraao, Ilha Grande, Brazil
Alta Do Chau, Brazil
Armação dos Búzios, Brazil
Banana Coast (Trujillo), Honduras
Belize City, Belize
Boca da Valeria, Brazil
Boca dos Botos, Brazil
Buzios, Brazil
Cabo Frio, Brazil
Cabo San Lucas, Baja California Sur, Mexico
Castro, Isla Chiloé, Chile
Cozumel, Mexico *
Fuerte Amador, Panama
Gatun Lake, (Colon), Panama
Golfito, Costa Rica
Guajara, Brazil
Hanga, Easter Island, Chile
Harvest Caye, Belize *
Icoaraci, (Belem), Brazil
Ilhabela, São Sebastião Island, Brazil
Ilheus, Brazil
Isla de Providencia, Colombia
Isla Robinson Crusoe, Chile
Loreto, Baja California Sur, Mexico

**Directory**

Los Cabos, Mexico
Manzanillo, Mexico
Margarita Island, Venezuela *
Parati, Brazil
Parintins, Brazil
Playa del Carmen, Mexico
Porto Belo, Brazil
Puerto Chacabuco, Chile *
Puerto Chiapas, Mexico
Puerto Montt, Chile *
Puerto Vallarta, Mexico *
Punta Arenas, Chile
Punta del Este, Uruguay
Quepos, Costa Rica
Recife, Brazil
Roatan, Bay Islands, Honduras *
San Andres, Colombia
San Blas Islands, Panama
San Juan Del Sur, Nicaragua *
Ushuaia, Argentina
Vila do Abraão, Brazil
Zihuatanejo, Mexico

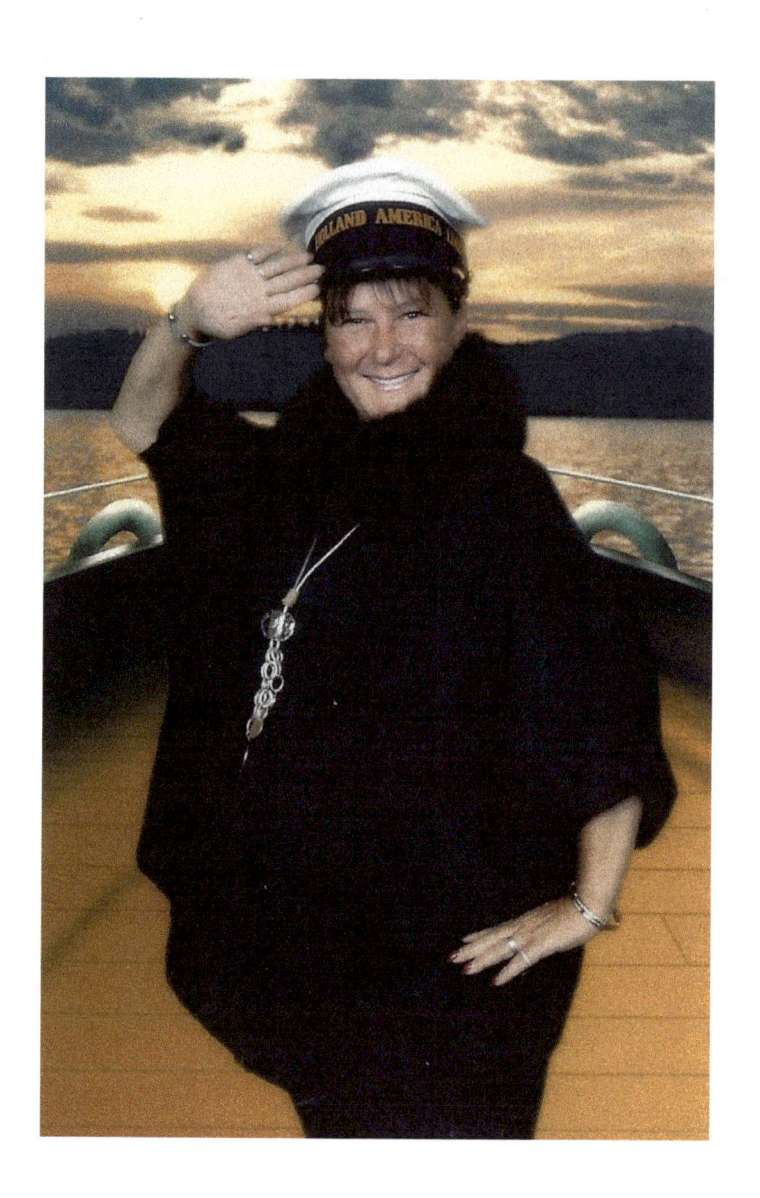

# About the Author

Daughter of the late British singer Matt Monro, Michele has been a seasoned cruiser for 42 years and has worked at sea for the last 11, bringing her unique brand of talks on her late father to Celebrity Cruises, P&O, Princess Cruises, Cunard, Cruise and Maritime, Fred. Olsen and Royal Caribbean.

A member of the Society of Authors, Michele's book *The Singer's Singer: The Life and Music of Matt Monro*, a touching biography of the man and much-loved performer who sang 'Born Free', 'From Russia With Love', 'Walk Away' and 'Portrait of My Love', has already been reprinted five times since its release and has been a hit across Europe, Australia, S.E. Asia and the United States. The author was presented with an Irwin Award for Best International Campaign from the book publicists of Southern California, and Titan Publishing presented the author with another award for Outstanding Sales.

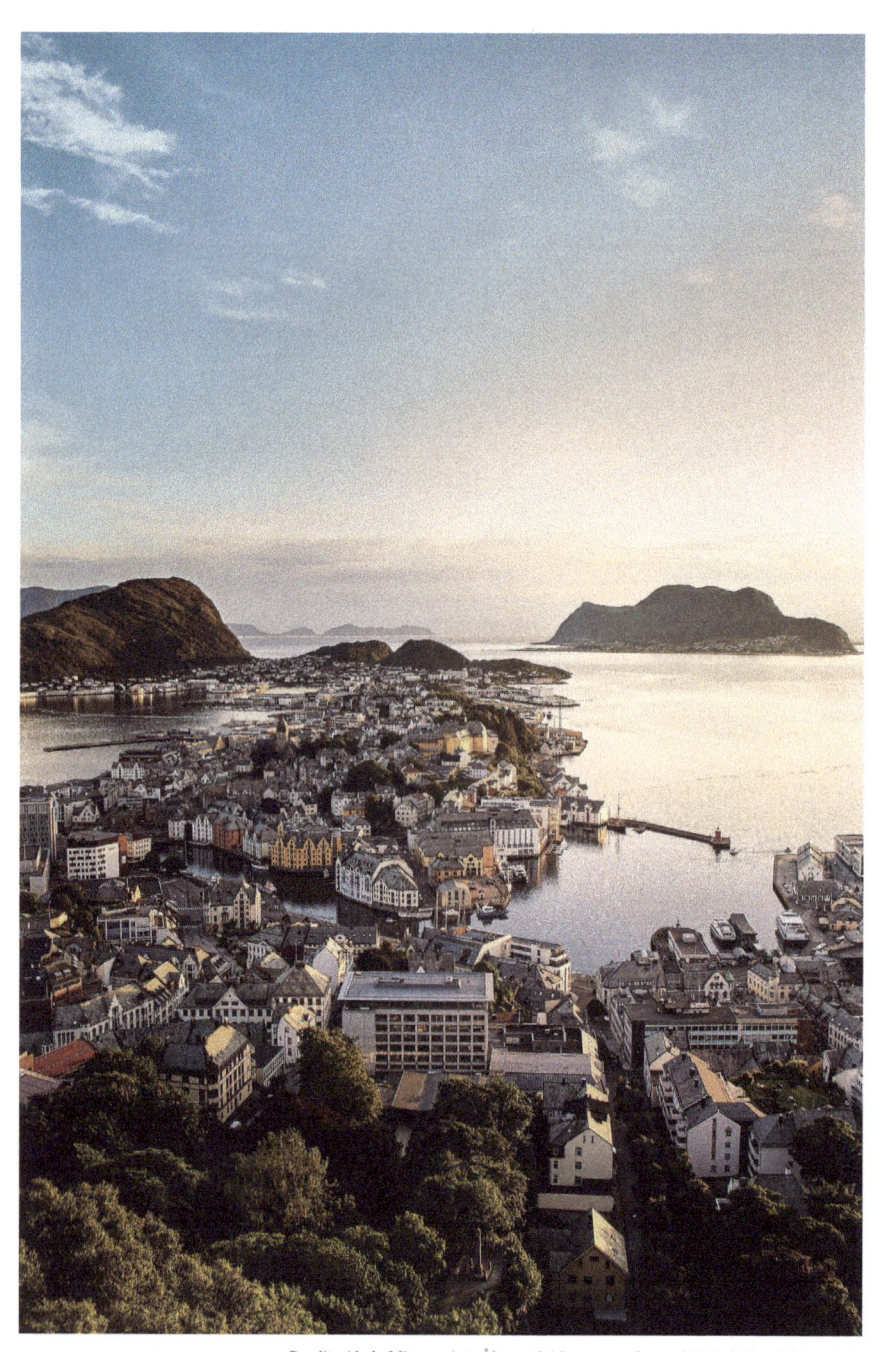

Credit: Aksla Viewpoint, Ålesund, Norway - Jarand K. Løkeland, Unsplash

# Contributions

This project has been over three years in the making and could not have been written without the vast amount of help I've received from all corners of the globe. Some offered reams of material while others contributed one fact, a single photograph or one piece of the jigsaw, but they all were equally important.

I would like to thank all the UK ports, tourist information sectors, cruise companies, mobility and disability services, institutions, archive departments, small firms, website owners, photographers, YouTube contributors, newspapers, passenger interviews and individuals whose contributions, assistance, and permissions have made the preparation of this book possible.

Finally, I need to thank my son, the most important person in my life, who spent months editing, shaping and improving this book, and gave me the confidence to fulfil another dream.

CPSIA information can be obtained
at www.ICGtesting.com
Printed in the USA
LVHW010229170222
711209LV00003B/5

9 781913 340964